THE MINDER BRAIN

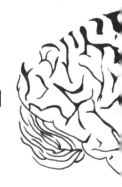

T0338623

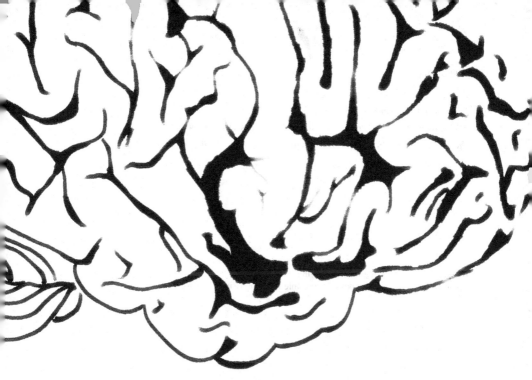

THE MINDER BRAIN

JOE HERBERT

Cambridge University, UK

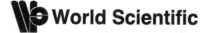

NEW JERSEY • LONDON • SINGAPORE • BEIJING • SHANGHAI • HONG KONG • TAIPEI • CHENNAI

Published by

World Scientific Publishing Co. Pte. Ltd.
5 Toh Tuck Link, Singapore 596224
USA office: 27 Warren Street, Suite 401-402, Hackensack, NJ 07601
UK office: 57 Shelton Street, Covent Garden, London WC2H 9HE

British Library Cataloguing-in-Publication Data
A catalogue record for this book is available from the British Library.

THE MINDER BRAIN
How Your Brain Keeps You Alive, Protects You from Danger, and
Ensures that You Reproduce

ISBN-13 978-981-270-394-1
ISBN-10 981-270-394-2
ISBN-13 978-981-270-395-8 (pbk)
ISBN-10 981-270-395-0 (pbk)

Typeset by Stallion Press
Email: enquiries@stallionpress.com

Printed in Singapore.

For Rachel, Daniel and Oliver, and in memory of Elisabeth.

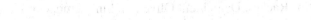

Foreword

Like most scientists, I am incurably excited by what I do. Not by the drudgery of getting grants, sitting on committees, writing reports, or dealing with increasingly convoluted administration; but that's all part of the deal. What really matters in knowing that each Monday you go into the laboratory and think, talk or even do something that just might lift a tiny corner of the vast curtain of ignorance that surrounds our knowledge of that incredible 1500 grams of tissue we call the brain. For amongst those cells and tangled fibres lie you and me. Ambition, genius, thought, imagination, love, hate, greed and, above all, consciousness of ourselves as alive and as part of our world — all this is somehow enabled by the brain. The brain is the person, and if it goes wrong, a person is ruined. This book is about part of what the brain does — a role of which many of us are hardly aware of but one that has ensured, over the millennia, that there are still humans on the earth. Despite famine, drought, wars, cold, infections and hostile environments of all sorts, we survive as a species though not always as individuals. All this time, our brains have been coping with most of what fate throws at us, a process that some call adaptation. How does the brain do it? How does it know what's needed? How does it enable us to provide that need? How much do we depend on our own brains, or on those of others? That's what this book is about; thinking about it is not only immensely challenging, it's also immense fun.

Nothing is more telling than the criticism or applause of friends and colleagues; I sent them chapters nervously. Barry Keverne was my first post-doc when I went to Cambridge all those years ago, and is now a distinguished behavioural scientist; Michael Hastings also worked with me many years ago and is now prominent in the field of circadian neurobiology;

Tirril Harris and George Brown are close collaborators and eminent sociologists, Richard le Page is a colleague and a parasitologist from my College and a skilled writer to boot, and Jeremy Prynne, another College colleague, is not only a stylist of repute but also a poet of distinction; Richard Green, an eminent psychiatrist and a notable author, has been a friend for 40 years, Anna Wirz is well-known for her work on rhythms, Jenny Barna, a biochemist, has been a most friendly and informed critic, Catherine Snow is an eminent linguist, Debbie Ganz is a skilled science and technical writer. Some read a chapter or two, others most of the book. Distinguished and busy, but immeasurably generous, people; I am deeply grateful to them all, and to Ching Ting Ang, my indefatigable editor and Surah Boobis, who prepared the index.

My University has provided — and goes on providing — a marvellously encouraging environment for research. Cambridge is rightly world-famous, because the people there are not only very good and creative, but also very companionable and generous with their time, their expertise and amenities. Every day is a tutorial, every week opens new doors, every year sees influxes of more bright people to stimulate, educate and sometimes infuriate the rest of us. In Cambridge, if you don't know something, pick up a phone or send an email and you'll find someone who does, and who is prepared to tell you about it. Beware of thinking how good you are, for within so short a time you'll meet someone better! My College, Gonville and Caius, is one of the glories of Cambridge. Our students treasure their all-too-short three years there; teaching them is a pleasure which the years don't diminish. My fellow Fellows provide not only persistent entertainment and friendship, but the sort of intellectual work-outs many would pay for. I have been blessed with a succession of delightful colleagues, collaborators, post-docs, graduate students and technicians; some have worked with me for lengthy years (and still do). Many of the ideas in this book, I am sure, depend on them. You can't do modern science without funds. Over the years the Wellcome Trust, that most imaginative institution, has been a constant provider. And. . . like all scientists, I am deeply aware that my family not only support me, but also tolerate me (in a slightly puzzled way): the absences (both physical and mental), the long hours, the not-so-good pay. My book is therefore dedicated to them with deepest gratitude.

You will find, alongside the text, quotations from two sources: scientific papers, to give those who are unfamiliar with professional science a feel for how scientists write about their subject, that they often disagree, and to provide support and illumination for what I say in the text; and brief extracts from a variety of 'literary' sources that I've enjoyed over the years. The latter idea derives from an excellent book called 'The Sickening Mind' by my former colleague Paul Martin, who makes the point that novelists and poets are much better than scientists at depicting life in all its variety; since this book is concerned about how the brain represents and deals with the vicissitudes of those lives, I have used their skill to show what it is I am trying to explain. Re-reading these books has added to the pleasure of writing mine.

Contents

Chapter 1

The Brain as a Survival Machine

This is Charles Darwin writing in 1859: "It is most necessary...
never to forget that every single organic being around us may be said to
be striving to the utmost to increase its numbers; that each lives by a
struggle at some period of its life; that heavy destruction inevitably falls
either on the young or old.... Lighten any check, mitigate the
destruction ever so little, and the number of the species will almost
instantaneously increase to any amount. The face of Nature may be
compared to a yielding surface, with ten thousand sharp wedges packed
close together and driven inwards by incessant blows....". This book is
about how we use our brain in this struggle for existence. It is about
how parts of our brain, inherited from our mammalian ancestors, are
dedicated to make sure we survive, although we are hardly aware
of them; and about how these work together with more recently
acquired brain structures to guide us through life, keeping us safe and
sound for the most part, so that we pass our qualities on to succeeding
generations.

You, like everyone else, have a warm, soft, rather moist, body, needing
regular intakes of usable energy. You are here because your parents had
the will and opportunity to reproduce. But you live in a tough world.
Food, water and essential minerals like salt are not easily available in the
environment from which you originally evolved. You have to want them
and to know where to look to find them. You have to keep warm in the
cold, or keep cool if the weather gets too hot. You have to find a mate, if
you are to pass on something of yourself to succeeding generations. Your
ancestors will have had to avoid being eaten by another species, whilst
making sure that they themselves were effective predators. You are in

competitions for many of the things you need, including a mate, with others of your own kind. To survive, you have to adapt. That is, you need the means to mould your behaviour to take account of how your world is, and to change your behaviour when it changes. Some of these changes may be sudden, others slow. Some arrive without warning, others are more predictable. Adaptation means not only changing your behaviour. Your body needs to adapt as well, making sure that it tells you what it needs to keep you going, and that it is resilient at moments of difficulty or shortage. So you survive into better times. No matter that you now live in a world we think of as technologically advanced. No matter that there are some who think that the modern world has removed some of the selection pressures on humans to which other animals are customarily exposed — true, if true at all, for only a small segment of humanity. You still carry with you many of the features that made your ancestors such a success. Otherwise, you would not be around today. The very fact that these qualities are now used in circumstances hardly imaginable, even a few centuries ago, is a tribute to your adaptive capacity.

Your brain not only keeps you alive, well and — as far as it can — out of danger, it also enables you to deal with life's emergencies. This may be a period of food shortage, or dehydration, or intense cold, or a confrontation with a larger, stronger rival, or the demands of giving birth or rearing young or preserving a territory, escaping from danger or keeping down a difficult job or coping with a bereavement. Such a demand may be short-lived and sharp; it may be long and unremitting; or intermittent and unpredictable. A general name for such an event, or set of events is 'stress'. Actually, a better word is 'stressor', meaning some external or internal event that induces 'stress' — the state of demand. Stressors can arise from the physiological world — too little food, too much heat and so on — or from the social and psychological one — a fight, arguments with friends, an unsatisfactory relationship, a demanding job. These are all examples of the need to adapt, and adaptation needs a brain. We will discuss stress more in Chapter 4.

This book is about the role of the brain in everyday life — adapting to intermittent emergencies such as stress. Modern ideas on adaptation began in the 19th century. Claude Bernard, like many other great scientists, is known for only a little of what he actually did. He was particularly

Social and Physical Evolution

Owing to the struggle for life, variations, if they be in any degree profitable to the individuals of a species, in their infinitely complex relations to other organic beings and to their physical conditions of life, will tend to the preservation of such individuals, and will generally be inherited by the offspring. The offspring, also, will thus have a better chance of surviving, for, of the many individuals of any species which are born, but a small number can survive. I have called this principle, by which a slight variation, if useful, is preserved, by the term 'natural selection', in order to mark its relation to man's power of selection. But the expression often used by Mr Herbert Spencer of the survival of the fittest is more accurate, and is sometimes equally convenient.

> Charles Darwin. (1872) *The origin of species.* Sixth ed.
> Ed. R E Leakey (Hill and Wang, NewYork.)

In recent years, historians have come to see that the most far-reaching change which grew out of the Renaissance was the evolution of the scientific method of inquiry. They have, therefore, given to the period of growth in science between 1500 and 1700 a new name, the Scientific Revolution . . . . Butterfield . . . says . . . that it 'outshines everything since the rise of Christianity and reduces the Renaissance and reformation to the rank of mere episodes'. . . . It was in the first place an intellectual revolution: it taught men to think differently. Only later was this put to a new practical use, in the Industrial Revolution about 1800, which gave our civilisation its outward character.

> J Bronowski, B Mazlish. (1960) *The western intellectual tradition.*
> (Hutchinson, London.)

. . . A sense of genetic unity, kinship, and deep history are among the values that bond us to the living environment. They are survival mechanisms for ourselves and our species. . . . biological diversity is an investment in immortality.

> Edmund O Wilson. (2002) *The future of life.*
> (Little, Brown and Co., London.)

To transform a weed into a cultivated plant, a wild beast into a domestic animal . . . to make stout, water-tight pottery out of clay which is friable and unstable . . . to work out techniques, often long and complex, which permit cultivation without soil or alternatively without water; to change toxic roots or interested in digestion, and worked on the way that the liver converts fats and sugars such as glucose in the food to glycogen, a form in which energy is stored. He recognised that the body needed to maintain levels in the blood of important molecules like glucose despite the fact that they were not always available. Hence, his dictum which resonates down the centuries: a constant internal environment is the condition for free life (*La fixité du milieu intérieur est la condition de la vie libre*). You walk around an inconstant, unpredictable and often unsatisfactory world carrying your own private, much more consistent, world with you — the inside of your body. But you have to keep it that way, despite the buffeting it gets from the outside world, a process now called 'homeostasis'. Some great scientists, like Bernard, tend to be resistant to the ideas of others — in his case, those of Darwin. Bernard was a 'generalist': he was interested in general properties of the body, not with individual differences. This does not detract from the stature of Darwin, who was fascinated by the importance of individuality, and showed how small variations in an individual's characters (a longer leg, a sharper claw, a less obvious colour etc.) might make it more or less 'fit;' that is, change the odds ever so little for or against its favour when conditions became tough. Not only were physical features important: slight advantages in the ability to communicate, to be a more effective parent, to learn a new skill, or to recognise a dangerous situation were all part of the Darwinian theory of selection. These abilities depend upon a brain. So, too, does the ability to know when to use your sharper claw to attack, or run away on your longer legs, or to summon help from those whom you know may offer it.

On their journey through time, everyone brings their individual qualities, which may give them an advantage over others, or at least an increased chance of dealing with the exigencies of their uncertain world. In the terrible siege of Leningrad (St Petersburg) in 1942, between 600,000 and 1 million people died of cold and starvation. But some survived. This was not a random event. Though no doubt chance played a part, other factors tipped the balance between who would live and who would die. Much would have depended on the brain, whose ability to adapt to demands varies from individual to individual, and from time to time, within the same person. This, as we shall, see, is as critical a factor as any other in success or failure, and in determining the cost that even success seeds into foodstuffs. . . there is no doubt that all these achievements required a genuinely scientific attitude, sustained and watchful interest and desire for knowledge for its own sake. For only a small proportion of observations and experiments . . . could have yielded practical and immediately useful results.

C Levi-Strauss. (1962) *The savage mind.*
(Weidenfeld and Nicolson, London.)

Some 10,000 years ago, certain human populations in the near east changed their way of life from that of hunting community to one based on the domestication of plants and animals . . . . The surplus food produced by the farmers could support large numbers of people, who could become labourers, artisans, soldiers, artists, politicians and scientists . . . . It should be emphasised however, that the change was wholly cultural; it took place far too quickly and too recently to be associated with biological changes in individuals.

D Pilbeam. (1970) *The evolution of man.*
(Thames and Hudson, London.)

Darwin's contemporaries saw at once what a heavy blow he was striking against piety. His theory entailed the inference that we are here today not because God reciprocates our love, forgives our sins, and attends to our entreaties but because each of our oceanic and terrestrial foremothers was lucky enough to elude her predators long enough to reproduce.

F C Crews. (2001) *New York Review of Books.*

may entail. Darwin showed us that studying physiological or behavioural control systems, important though this is, is not enough: we also need to know about how they vary between individuals, and how individuals thus vary in their effectiveness to deal with demand.

The brain is not a simple or uniform structure, so we have to ask whether there are parts of it that are more concerned than others with the story I want to tell. To answer this is not as easy as you might think. Suppose that you wake in the middle of the night, and feel hungry. You reach out a hand to turn on the bedside lamp. You get out of bed and put on a sweater. You walk downstairs quietly, so as not to wake others, go into the kitchen, open the door of the fridge and look for something to eat. You select a piece of cheese. Then, you scan the tins of food on the shelf above the fridge, reading the labels. You see one that you fancy and open it with a can-opener. You put it all on the plate, sit down and eat, though you find you have eaten enough before all the food has gone. So you store the remainder in the fridge for tomorrow.

You have just performed an adaptive response: you have defended your body against a too-low blood glucose — though you had no idea that this was the underlying cause of your behaviour. During the series of actions that make up your response, a large part of your brain has been used. It has detected the fall in your blood glucose levels. It has woken up. It has generated the sensation of hunger. It has motivated you to get food. It has decided to go and find some, and has remembered where food is to be found. It has allowed you to feel the light switch. It is also responsible for your knowing what a light switch is. It has recognised that as you get out of bed you are getting cold, and remembered that putting on a sweater can counteract cold. It has enabled you to perform the rather complicated actions of actually putting the sweater on. It has enabled you to walk downstairs without falling over. It has remembered that there are others asleep, and that is it anti-social to wake them — that is, there will be social repercussions (cost) if you do. It has recognised a fridge. It has also recognised a food object. Your brain enables you to read, and to translate what you read into food. That is, you know from the symbols on the tin — also recognised as such by your brain — that inside is a certain sort of food. The skill of opening a tin is only possible because your brain enables you to do so. You eat, using motor patterns generated

Open thy mind, the truth is coming; know,
When the articulations of the brain
Has been perfected in the embryo,

Then the First Mover turns to it, full fain
Of nature's triumph, and inbreathes a rare
New spirit, filled with virtue to constrain

To its own substance whatso active there
It finds, and make one single soul complete,
Alive, and sensitive, and self-aware.

Dante. *The divine comedy. II. Purgatory.*
Canto XXV. Translated by D L Sayers.
(Penguin Books, Harmondsworth.)

All that is noble and excellent and all that is worst in human commerce
has been thought to derive from the brain, a sort of gland that secretes
lofty ideas and superior morals when healthy and oozes destructive plans
when diseased.

F Gonzalez-Crussi. (1986) *Notes of an anatomist.*
(Picador, London.)

Killer instinct. General use, to describe the quality of extreme seriousness
thought to be required to win in sport and life.

Nigel Rees. (1996) *Dictionary of cliches.*
(Cassell, London.)

Nature, that fram'd us of four elements
Warring within our breasts for regiment,
Doth teach us all to have aspiring minds:
Our souls, whose faculties can comprehend
The wondrous architecture of the world,
And measure every wandering plant's course,
Still climbing after knowledge infinite,
And always moving as the restless spheres,
Wills us to ware ourselves and never rest,
Until we reach the ripest fruit of all,

by your brain. Signals from your body go to your brain, telling you when you have eaten enough. Your brain recalls that food is costly, and that there are means of preserving it for later, and that you will be hungry again quite soon. A great mixture of what psychologists would call motivation, emotion, memory and cognition, and what neuroscientists would call sensory and motor function. Does this mean that to understand the role of the brain in adaptation, we have to discuss everything we know about it?

Fortunately not. This is because we know that parts of the brain are specialised for particular functions. For example, there is a complex pathway in the brain, starting at the eyes and responsible for vision. This is the visual 'system,' and it enables what we call 'seeing'. Another set of nerve cells and pathways enable us to move. The arrangement of the motor system, as it is called, is rather distinct from the visual one, so that damage to it (for example, following a stroke) can cause paralysis — loss of movement — without blindness. Yet another part of the brain takes the information received by the sensory pathways and uses it to form an imprint, which we call memory. Next time we see, or hear, or feel the same sensation, we may be able to recall having experienced it before. Even more complex functions, like recognising a particular friend (or a fridge), or being able to read, are the responsibility of other parts of the brain. Damage to any one of them will interfere with that function, leaving others intact. These parts of the brain may be used for adaptive purposes (as in our night-time scenario) but they also have other uses. 'Seeing' is what the visual system does: you 'see' for many reasons, one of which is to be able to adapt. But the visual system is not a dedicated adaptation system: it does not tell you that you need to adapt, or how to do it: it provides the means (or part of them). You 'move' all the time; sometimes as part of adaptation, but for many other reasons. During the episode of your nocturnal feast, you used many of these parts of the brain. But many of them can be used in other, and quite different contexts. Later that day, you may play a game of tennis, or read your e-mail, watch television, or go to the office and write a memo. You will interact with colleagues and friends. You will use many of the same areas of the brain that were so useful during your midnight meal. None of these parts of the brain is dedicated to survival, though clearly essential for it.

That perfect bliss and sole felicity,
The sweet fruition of an earthly crown.
> Christopher Marlowe. (1564–1593) *From: Tamburlaine the great.*

. . . The intellectual, to my mind, is more in touch with humanity than is the confident scientist, who patronizes the past, over-simplifies the present, and envisages a future where his leadership will be accepted. . . . It is high time he came out of his ivory laboratory. We want him to plan for our bodies. We do not want him to plan for our minds, and we cannot accept, so far, his assurance that he will not.
> E M Forster. (1951) *Two cheers for democracy.*
> (Edward Arnold, London.)

But there is a brain system which has, as its main function, our preservation and that of our species. This part of the brain is particularly concerned with making sure that we do the things that maximise our health, keep us in good condition, and reproduce. As part of all these functions, it detects threats to our survival, recognises what they are, and devises the strategy by which we will overcome or compensate for these demands. It is clear that such an adaptation system cannot work on its own. No good being hungry or thirsty if you cannot move to where there is food or water, or recognise it when you see it. That means there must be co-operation between different parts of the brain, obvious enough. But none of these other systems has survival, adaptation and procreation as its major concern. We need a brain system that recognises our needs, and how to go about meeting them. A brain system that also keeps us out of trouble as well as continuously assessing threats to our wellbeing. A system that enables the right adaptive response, whether this means a particular sort of behaviour, or an appropriate pattern of hormone secretion, or alterations in the response of the 'emergency' nervous system — the process of coping, as some would call it. We have one: it is a part of the brain called the limbic system. It is a very special part of the brain, and it is the focus of this book.

Whoever it was that first cut across a human brain will never be known. Our inability to see things that are obvious until someone else points them out probably means that brains were cut up countless times before someone realised that the inside of this curious, wrinkled structure was not all the same. There are areas that appear almost white but others that are decidedly darker. Moreover, if our early observer had seen enough cut-up brains, he (she, perhaps) would have noticed that the arrangements of these lighter and darker areas are very similar from brain to brain. The inside of the brain appears to have a structure. The paler areas came to be called 'white matter', and the darker ones 'grey matter', suitably neutral and descriptive terms that give no clue to either their structure or function. This did not stop those with a passion for labelling from giving the different areas names. Names are important for at least two reasons: they define objects as distinct (that is, one area of grey matter from another), and they may also give a clue as to its supposed function or significance. The problem for the early anatomists of the brain is that

We all assume that the future will be like the past — it is the essential but unprovable premise of all our inductive inferences, as Hume noted. Mother nature (the designer-developer realized in the processes of natural selection) makes the same assumption. In many regards, things stay the same: gravity continues to exert its force, water continues to evaporate, organisms continue to need to replenish and protect their body water, looming things continue to subtend ever-larger portions of the retina and so on. Where generalities like these are at issue, mother nature provides long-term solutions to problems: hard-wired, gravity based which-way-is-up detectors, hard-wired thirst alarms, hard-wired duck-when-something-looms circuits. Other things change, but predictably, in cycles, and mother nature responds to them with other hard-wired devices, such as winter-coat-growing mechanisms triggered by temperature shifts, and built-in alarm clocks to govern the waking and sleeping cycles of nocturnal and diurnal animals. But sometimes the opportunities and vicissitudes in the environment are relatively unpredictable by mother nature or anyone — they are, or are influenced by, processes that are chaotic. In these cases, no one stereotyped design will accommodate itself to all eventualities, so better organisms will be those that can redesign themselves to some degree to meet the conditions they encounter.

Daniel C Dennett. (1991) *Consciousness explained.*
(Little, Brown and Co., New York.)

I hope I am not giving the impression that Davey's whole life was centred around his health. He was fully occupied with his work, writing and editing a literary review, but his health was his hobby, and, as such, more in evidence during his spare time, the time when I saw most of him. How he enjoyed it! He seemed to regard his body with the affectionate preoccupation of a farmer towards a pig — not a good doer, the small one of the litter, which must somehow be made to be a credit to the farm. He weighed it, sunned it, aired it, exercised it, and gave it special diets, new kinds of patent food and medicine, but all in vain. It never put on so much as a single ounce of weight, it never became a credit to the farm, but, somehow, it lived, enjoying good things, enjoying its life, though falling victim to the ills that flesh is heir to, and other, imaginary ills as they had very little real knowledge of what the different parts of the brain did. That, of course, did not stop the name-calling, or even speculative ideas — based on rather little evidence — on what they might do. Many of the names given to parts of the brain are based on appearance, or a fancied resemblance to other objects in the (medieval) world. Note, however, that the idea that the different regions of the brain might have different functions is itself important. Parcelling the brain into definable areas is what we would now call the modular approach to brain function. We think of a complex structure like the brain as made up of a number of sub-components, just as, for example, the engine of a car is constructed from a number of different components (carburettor, cylinder block, distributor etc.).

But is the brain an assembly of distinct components, each with a defined and separate function? One of the many difficulties in studying how the brain works is precisely because it is not arranged in this way. That does not mean that one cannot assign specific functions to anatomically recognisable parts of the brain. Indeed one can: for example, the great cortical mantle (the cerebral cortex) that forms most of the outside of the brain and gives it its typically wrinkled or folded appearance has areas that we know are concerned with identifiable actions. One is responsible for generating movement, another for analysing incoming visual information, yet another for receiving sensation from the skin (which we interpret as 'touch') and so on. Similar functional boundaries have been recognised in other parts of the brain, the so-called sub-cortical areas. That is not an issue. What is, however, is whether there are clearly defined boundaries between these areas, either anatomically — where does one begin, or the other end or functionally — is there a circumscribed areas of the brain that has an equally precise function? The answer to both questions is a resounding 'no.' Take vision, one of the better-understood parts of the cerebral cortex.

We know that nearly all information from the eyes ends up in a rather small area of cerebral cortex at the back of the brain. This is the visual cortex. That is why a bang on the back of your head makes you 'see stars'. But from this region, visual information is passed forwards to other parts of the cortex, each part doing different things — extracting particular bits of information out of the mass of data arriving from your eyes at the *well, through which it was nursed with unfailing care, with concentrated attention, by the good farmer and his wife.*

Nancy Mitford. (1945) *The pursuit of love.*
(Hamish Hamilton, London.)

What's this flesh? A little crudded milk, fantastical puff-paste. Our bodies are weaker than those paper-prisons boys use to keep flies in; more contemptible, since ours is to preserve earthworms.

John Webster. (1623) *The duchess of Malfi.*

These memories are the memorials and pledges of the vital hours of a lifetime. These hours of afflatus in the human spirit, the springs of art, are, in their mystery, akin to the epochs of history, when a race which for centuries has lived content, unknown, behind its own frontiers, digging, eating, sleeping, begetting, doing what was requisite for survival and nothing else, will, for a generation or two, stupefy the world, bring to birth and nurture a teeming brood of genius, droop soon with the weight of its grandeur, fall, but leave behind a record of new rewards won for all mankind; the vision fades, the soul sickens, and the routine of survival starts again.

Evelyn Waugh. (1945) *Brideshead revisited.*
(Penguin Books, Harmondsworth.)

visual cortex. The processing itself gets ever more complex as it passes forward, but there is no clear boundary at which we may say that visual information has ceased to be processed. It mingles with other sorts of information — for example, from the 'language' part of the brain, so you can read when you see a collection of words, or with the part that stores memories so you can recognise a familiar face and so on. You cannot cut out a chunk of brain and say 'this is the seeing brain' because the brain uses many parts to decode visual information, and 'seeing' by itself is not a very useful brain activity: you need to do something with the information. The same arguments go for the movement ('motor') parts of the brain and for any other brain area. If you were to lose a limb, or your sight, then the areas of the cortex responsive to sensation or vision will alter their boundaries. This is a long-winded way of saying that the brain works as a whole, there are parts that specialise in particular aspect of the things it has to do, but these parts interconnect and interact with one another, and that the brain itself is malleable.

So how do we reconcile this notion of a functionally and anatomically blended brain with the apparently opposite idea of brain 'systems'? By taking a much more flexible (and intellectually less comfortable) position: we are looking at a impressionist gouache, rather than a geometric design. The analogy with parts of the car has broken down: the brain is not the kind of machine we are familiar with in our mechanical world, but it is a machine nevertheless. Certain parts of the brain can, indeed, be confidently said to have a single (or a set of related) functions: but there are many areas where this is not so. This does not meant that they do not have a definable role, only that we need to describe this in a different way. The bottom line, however, is that if we are to recognise a 'system' in the brain, we have both to give it a physical reality (that is, say which parts of the brain are in our system) and a functional one (what it does that distinguishes it from other parts of the brain). Let's see whether this applies to the limbic system.

Limbic means 'edge' or 'border' and was originally applied to the brain by the great French neurologist Paul Broca. Broca is actually famous for his recognition that there was a special part of the brain responsible for spoken language, but, like many talented scientists, he was a versatile man. He gave the name 'the great limbic lobe' to a part of the

The Human Brain

More than one writer has asked, why have some animals had their mental powers more highly developed than others, as such development would be advantageous to all? Why have not apes acquired the intellectual powers of man? Various causes could be assigned; but they are conjectural, and their relative probability cannot be weighed.

> Charles Darwin. (1872) *The origin of species.* Sixth ed.
> Ed. R E Leakey (Hill and Wang, New York.)

The brain is waking and with it, the mind is returning. It is as if the milky way entered upon some cosmic dance. Swiftly, the head-mass becomes an enchanted loom where millions of flashing shuttles weave a dissolving pattern, always a meaningful pattern though never an abiding one; a shifting harmony of sub-patterns.

> C S Sherrington. (1940) *Man on his nature.*
> (Penguin Books, London.)

Each nerve cell receives connections from other nerve cells at sites called synapses. But here is an astonishing fact — there are about one million billion connections in the cortical sheet. If you were to count them, one connection (or synapse) per second, you would finish counting some thirty-two million years after you began.

Indeed, the chemical and electrical dynamics of the brain resemble the sound and light patterns and the movement and growth patterns of a jungle more than they do the activities of an electrical company.

> G Edelman. (1992) *Bright air, brilliant fire.*
> (Allen Lane, London.)

About two decades ago, a new science was launched, variously called neurobiology, brain research or neuroscience. This statement will offend many who would divine a much earlier origin for the subject. But I would say that the recognition that many individual research workers from a variety of university departments and other institutions, with backgrounds in very different disciplines, share a common objective — the explanation of the functions of the brain — dates from only about 20 years ago.

> C Blakemore. (1986) The nature of explanation in
> the study of the brain. In: *Functions of the brain.*
> Ed. C Coen, pp. 181–200. (Clarendon Press, Oxford.)

cortex which, he thought, formed the inside border (or boundary) of the cerebral cortex of the mammalian brain. In the human brain, this is a C-shaped region that is coiled round the inside of the cerebral hemispheres. So it was an anatomical definition, and one limited to the cortex. Judson Herrick, an American comparative neuroanatomist, found out that Broca's limbic lobe had a somewhat less elaborate structure than the rest of the cortex, and he suggested it might be concerned with more 'primitive' functions, such as feeding and sex, leaving the other parts of the cortex to deal with 'higher' mental activities. Others thought it was particularly concerned with the sense of smell. But it was James Papez who dropped the real bombshell. In 1937, he pointed out that the limbic cortex was actually connected to a variety of other structures, and that these formed a sort of cerebral loop (such interconnected circuits were much in vogue at the time as a way of understanding brain function). Finally, he proposed that this circuit was the neural basis of emotion.

The significance of this idea should not be underestimated. It proposed that there was a dedicated system in the brain that was responsible for an emotional state, without specifying in any way how the brain might actually generate an emotion. So there might be separate brain structures responsible for 'thoughts' and 'feelings'. This was a striking idea, though not a new one: it implies that the two sorts of mental activity are carried out in separate parts of the brain (Papez called them 'streams'). It also implies that somehow, they have to be amalgamated if one is to associate a particular sensation or event with its attendant emotion. It is important to note that Papez described emotion as the only function of the limbic system.

The term 'limbic system' was introduced by Paul MacLean, following a visit to James Papez, in 1952. MacLean had a panoramic view of the way the brain was built. He proposed what he called the 'triune brain'; that is, the brain actually consisted of three concentric structures which, he thought, were typical of the brains of reptiles, more primitive mammals and 'higher' mammals, respectively. The middle one corresponded, largely, to the limbic system. He originally called the limbic system the 'visceral' brain, because he thought it responsible for processing sensation from the viscera (including the gut), though he associated it also with smell. The phrase 'gut feeling' may occur to you, as you try to relate this idea to that of an emotional state.

Science progresses by way of metaphor and analogy. Electricity is likened to a fluid, valency bonds to hooks and eyes, atoms to billiard balls. The science of the brain is no exception to this rule. Descartes, in the seventeenth century, likened the brain to the intricate hydraulic mechanisms of his day; the nineteenth and early twentieth centuries saw a powerful analogy to the telegraph cable and the telephone exchange; nowadays, in the late twentieth century, the computer metaphor is all-pervasive. Metaphors and analogies both help and bias our understanding. The power of the computer analogy perhaps prevents us from seeing the brain from other equally significant viewpoints. In particular, it prevents us from seeing the brain as if it were an immense gland. Yet, this view has much to commend it. Neurons can be seen not so much as relays or on/off valves but as secretory cells. The electrical phenomena of electrotonic and action potentials can, on this analogy, be seen merely as triggers for the release of secretions — the neurotransmitters and modulators.

C U M Smith. (1989) *Elements of molecular neurobiology*. First ed. (Wiley and Sons, Chichester.)

There are some who say that 'emotion' is an insufficient criterion for defining a brain system, others that the function of the limbic system is too vague for it to be a valid concept. Both are incorrect arguments, though for different reasons. There is no doubt that one very important function of the limbic system is the generation, expression and recognition of emotion. There is also equally no doubt that this is not its only function. Emotion is an essential ingredient of survival. In its absence — for example, without the ability to experience fear — no animal, including any of us, would survive for very long. But you need more than an emotional response to survive. By slavishly following Papez's original idea (still good but a limited one), these critics have mistaken a component of what the limbic system does for its entire function. Emotion is part of what it does. A part of what? Promoting survival of course; and to survive, as Darwin taught us, we need to adapt. Since adaptation is a complex but coherent activity, it comes as no surprise that there are parts of the limbic system that are principally concerned with elements of the ability to adapt other than emotion. Emotional responses have to fit in with the rest of this process, but are an essential part of it. Just because there are parts of the limbic system that do not seem to be directly concerned with emotion does not refute the validity of the system as a whole. It only means we need to redefine what it does. It is our survival machine. No other part of the brain can do what the limbic system does. Those who have argued that the concept of the 'limbic system' depends on emotion alone or that it is so all-embracing and vague that it includes the whole brain have missed these essential points. This misapprehension has even found its way into august works of reference, such as Gray's Anatomy. Perhaps a future edition will take a more thoughtful approach.

Many distinguished neuroscientists have pondered the limits of the limbic system. Walle Nauta emphasised its role in bringing together internal ('visceral') and external stimuli, and included parts of the midbrain (those that receive information from the viscera) as well as the hypothalamus. Rudolf Nieuwenhuys (another example of the tradition of outstanding Dutch neuroanatomists) added other areas of the forebrain, and some bits of brainstem, particularly those that have nerve cells containing the monoamines, such as noradrenaline and serotonin into the

Those Rules of old discover'd, not deviz'd,
Are nature still, but nature methodiz'd;
Nature, like Liberty, is but restrained
By the same laws which first herself ordain'd.
Alexander Pope. (1688–1744) *From: An essay on criticism.*

Freud was in his fortieth year when Studies in Hysteria appeared —almost
at that crucial age after which, it is often speculated, no scientist ever
achieves much that is worthwhile. Yet, 1895 was to mark the beginning of
an extraordinary five years of activity. . . later in the year, he wrote, in a few
weeks, an elegant paper in which he tried to describe psychical processes
in terms of quantifiable forces, an attempt in which he only just failed to
outline the neurone theory put forward by Wilhelm von Waldeyer the
following year, and describing the nervous system in terms of neurones . . . .
Ronald W Clark. (1980) *Freud. The man and the cause.*
(Jonathan Cape, London.)

Nervous systems that are hard-wired are lightweight, energy-efficient, and
fine for organisms that cope with stereotyped environments on a
limited budget. Fancier brains, thanks to their plasticity, are capable not
just of stereotyped anticipation, but also of adjusting to trends . . . . For
truly highpowered control, what you want is an anticipation machine that
will adjust itself in major ways in a few milliseconds, and for that you need
a virtuoso future-producer, a system that can think ahead, avoid ruts in its
own activity, solve problems in advance of encountering them, and recognize
entirely novel harbingers of good and ill. For all our foolishness, we
human beings are vastly better equipped for that task than any other
self-controllers, and it is our enormous brains that make this possible.
Daniel C Dennett. (1991) *Consciousness explained.*
(Little, Brown and Co., NewYork.)

Also people think they're not computers because they have feelings and
computers don't have feelings. But feelings are just having a picture on
the screen in your head of what is going to happen tomorrow or next year,
or what might have happened instead of what did happen, and if it is a
happy picture they smile and if it is a sad picture they cry.
Mark Haddon. (2004) *The curious incident*
of the dog in the night-time. (Vintage, London.)

'greater limbic system'. We will have much more to say about these intriguing neurochemicals later in this book (Chapter 3). He also pointed out that the limbic system has many nerve cells that contain a wide variety of another type of chemical signal, the peptides. Some brainstem nerve cells also have similar peptides, so he included these as well. We will say much more about peptides as well (Chapter 2), for within these chemicals, I believe, lies a good part of the code for successful adaptation.

The limbic system is like other systems. It is made up of a number of neural components, represented by chunks of brain that have two properties: they are connected together, and they have a common function. In the case of the visual system, it is for seeing; for the motor system, it is for locomotion; as for the limbic system, it is for the preservation of self and species. The first proposition of this book is that this is the part of the brain that specialises in adaptation and survival. The second is that the limbic system has a number of ways of making sure we overcome physical, social or psychological challenges: note that preservation requires us to cope with them all. Effective adaptation to events such as lack of water, or a confrontation with a dangerous antagonist, is a complex business. You need to do the things that enhance adaptation (that is, behave appropriately), your nervous system needs to take the necessary actions to stabilise your physiology in the face of deficiency or demand, and the whole process is helped enormously by changes in the secretion of your hormones. The limbic system formulates this co-ordinated set of reactions by which such demands are met. The third proposition is that the limbic system has its own way of working. Though it shares many of the features of other parts of the brain, it has some peculiarities of its own. The most important one is that it uses a chemical code to formulate adaptation to challenges. If we understood this code, we would know a lot more about how this part of the brain is so good at what it does. Since our survival depends on our limbic system, we need to know how it works. Finally, we have to think about situations in which, despite its best efforts, the limbic system cannot cope, and adaptation is insufficient. What are the consequences, either personal or for the social group or even for the species, of failure? And what about success? As we shall see, even if we do succeed in overcoming the current challenge in some way, there may be a price to pay, such as an increased chance of

Arguments Against the Limbic System

The term, "limbic system," has come into vogue during the past decade or two, but it is difficult to find either anatomical or physiological justification for lumping a diverse, multi-functional collection of cortical areas and subcortical structures together as the *limbic system*, and this designation appears not to have sufficient descriptive value to justify its continued use.

> L Van Atta, J Sutin. (1972) Relationships among amygdaloid
> and other limbic structures in influencing activity of
> lateral hypothalamic neurons. In: *The neurobiology of*
> *the amygdala*. Ed. B E Eleftheriou, pp. 343–369.
> (Plenum Press, New York.)

We have seen that a large and increasing number of brain structures and functions has been implicated with the limbic system. This heterogeneous collection cannot be defined by a single criterion. . . . The limbic system is not a piece of nature given to us. It is just one out of many scientific concepts. From an empirical point of view this concept is not adequate and there is nothing to justify its continuing use in a general and indiscriminate sense. . . . It may turn out that the limbic system becomes more and more obsolete as our knowledge increases. But so far it has a very important role to play: it meets our need and desire for explanatory concepts in the neurosciences which is reflected in the influence that the limbic system has in many areas of the neurosciences. . . . The term, however, is simple and enjoys universal recognition: everyone thinks he knows what is meant when he hears it.

> R Kotter, N Meyer. (1992) The limbic system:
> A review of its empirical foundation.
> *Behavioural Brain Research* **52**, pp. 105–127.

If the limbic system is the emotion system, then studies showing which brain areas are involved in emotion should tell us where the limbic system is. But this is backward reasoning. The goal of the limbic system theory was to tell us where emotion is in the brain on the basis of knowing something about the evolution of brain structure. To use research on emotion to find the limbic system turns this criterion around. Research on emotion can tell us where the emotion system is in the brain, but not where the limbic system is. Either the limbic system exists or it does not. Since there are no independent criteria for telling us where it is, I have to say that it does not exist.

> J LeDoux. (1998) *The emotional brain*.
> (Weidenfeld and Nicolson, London.)

illness. Whether the triumph is worth the price is something else the brain may be able to tell us. That is our fourth proposition.

But our brains are more than a limbic system. Surrounding this ancient and highly successful limbic survival machine is another, even more complex, but typically human structure: the cerebral cortex. All mammals have a cortex, but the human brain is distinguished from others by the size and complexity of its cortex, not its limbic system. So the human brain brings to the problem of survival not only an efficient limbic system, but also the analytical, decision-making, concept-forming abilities of the huge human cortex. This is going to have a dramatic impact on how the human brain solves the survival problem, and the number of people on earth shows how well it has done. I am going to suggest that the two parts of the brain use rather different ways of working. Your cortex is a very large, unique, biological computer (nothing like the computer on your desk), and it encodes and decodes information by using a huge number of — perhaps quite simple — neural 'circuits' or assemblies of nerve cells. The 'code' it uses is thus based on way these assemblies function together. Your limbic system, as we have already suggested, has a different method: it uses a complex chemical code to signal its operation. It is a sort of huge gland. Now, it is important not to over-stress these differences: the cortex also uses chemical signals (though a bit differently to the limbic system) and the arrangement of nerve cells in the limbic system matters as it does in the cortex (though for different reasons). But your limbic system looks rather similar to that of other mammals, even a rat; it is your cortex that distinguishes you as a human being. And they have to work together, if you are to survive the rough and tumble of the real world. An important objective of this book is to discuss how the cortex and limbic system interact and depend on each other, as they surely do, so that humans solve their ancient survival problems in distinctively human ways.

It is not easy for a scientist to think about ignorance as opposed to knowledge, but we should acknowledge the limits of our understanding of the brain. We should never forget that, at the start of the twenty-first century, the brain remains a profound mystery, despite all the cohorts of neuroscientists, the masses of papers, the erudite books, in a way that is not true for other parts of the body. No mystery about the heart, or liver, or lungs or gut: we know the principles of how they work. Not so for the brain.

What is undeniable is that the hypotheses of Papez and Maclean have served the essential function of stimulating enormous amounts of research on the neural basis of emotion, so much so that the belief in a limbic system is entrenched in the literature and attempts to reappraise it may seem eccentric . . . But it is now equally clear that the areas included within the limbic system do not function as a system specialized for emotional processing, as opposed to other forms of information processing. Indeed, the hippocampus, while clearly the centrepiece of the limbic system concept, is not at all the centrepiece of the brain's emotional system. This structure and some of those connected with it, including those of the Papez circuit, are now widely accepted to be involved more with cognitive processes including mnemonic functions, perhaps especially spatial short-term memory. . . . It would appear to be of doubtful utility to continue to explore the function, or functions, of the limbic system since the anatomical criteria for defining it are at best imprecise and its purported unitary function in emotion is untenable.

Gray's anatomy. (1995) 38th ed.
(Churchill Livingstone, New York.)

I cannot tell you precisely how your brain makes you feel hungry, or feel fear, or recognise a friend, though I can tell you something about which parts of the brain might be involved in each of these functions, and some general ideas about how those areas work. This is not despair, but reality. We need to recognise the limits of our knowledge, even in the optimistic world of the neuroscientist. However, there are some things we do know.

We know that your limbic system ensures that you eat when you need to, or that your body tides you over bad times when your have to fast. It makes you feel thirsty when your body runs short of water, or defends you against involuntary dehydration; to seek out extra salt when you run low on this essential molecule, or restrict salt loss from the body if supplies are scarce. It drives you to put on a sweater when the weather is cold, or makes you shiver if you cannot find one; it wakes you up in time for the day, and puts you to sleep at night; it makes you like those things that are good for you, and avoid situations that may harm you; if you are harmed, it takes the necessary steps to help you mend; it makes sure that enough of us breed, and that we take care of our young, and each other, so that there will be members of our species to follow us in future generations. It makes us fight for survival; live in social groups; respond to the demands of others; and seek help when we need it.

It brings joy and sadness, success and failure, love and hate, sometimes illness, as part of the deal. What do we know about how it does all this? What happens if it fails? This is what this book is all about.

But before we go any further, I want to say something about 'you' and 'your brain.' You will see I have used both terms rather interchangeably. In fact, 'you' — the individual you — is largely (some would say exclusively) your brain. Other parts of your body may be unique — your fingerprints, for example, but your brain is what defines you as a person and as an individual. As someone said, a brain transplant is the only situation where it is much better to be the donor. There are various ways to talk about the brain. Sometimes, it makes sense to say the brain (or parts of it) does this or that, or performs functions through the agency of the rest of the body. Sometimes, it makes sense to say we use our brain to gather information about our environment, or to make best-choice decisions about actions or conduct. There can seem to be deep differences between the various ways of talking about the brain, particularly when one

... Arthur of England was a champion of civilization which is misrepresented in the history books.... In those despised Middle Ages of theirs, you could become the greatest man in the world, by simply having learning. And it is a mistake to believe that Arthur's civilization was weak in this famous science of ours. The scientists, although they happened to call them magicians at the time, invented almost as terrible things as we have invented — except that we have become accustomed to theirs by use. The greatest magicians, like Albertus Magnus, Friar Bacon, and Raymond Lully, knew several secrets which we have lost today, and discovered as a side issue what still appears to be the chief commodity of civilization, namely gunpowder. They were honoured for their learning, and Albert the Great was made a bishop. One of them who was called Baptista Porta seems to have invented the cinema — although he sensibly decided not to develop it.

T H White. (1958) *The once and future king.*
(Fontana/Collins, London.)

Scientists in modern times tend to specialise; few have the interdisciplinary base which would give them a view of the whole scene.
John Peyton. (2001) *Solly Zuckerman. A scientist out of the ordinary.*
(John Murray, London.)

Do you remember the bust of Socrates, the man who died rather than profess his belief in the gods of the time...? Take this bust in your mind's eye, colour the beard black, dashing it here and there with puffs of grey; clap the head thus made on a portly body of middle height, and the doctor is before you. Throw a veil over the upper part of the face and you might be in the company of a born vestreyman. Reveal the essential feature, the immense brows, and you know at once that you have to deal with that most formidable of all composite forces — a dreamer who thinks, a thinker who dreams.

Contemporary description of Karl Marx.
Francis Wheen. (1999) *Karl Marx.* (Fourth Estate, London.)

Enter the experts ... Enter the Science of Psychology. Officially installed in a cellar, it abolishes the art of knowing what people are like, and ensures that they are incomprehensible to themselves as well as to others.
E M Forster. (1951) *Two cheers for democracy.*
(Edward Arnold, London.)

considers issues like — what is a person, what is a conscious self, what is 'knowing' or what is an individual. Such issues have been much written about, mostly by philosophers, in books not at all like this one. These matters — important and intractable as they are — are not, in my view, central to the theme of this book. So when I write that either the 'brain' or 'you' 'knows' something or other and 'does' or 'decides' something else, and forget the apostrophes, you will understand.

Evolution of Man

So, there he stands, our vertical, hunting, weapon-toting, territorial, neotenous, brainy, naked ape, a primate by ancestry and a carnivore by adoption, ready to conquer the world. But he is a very new and experimental departure, and new models frequently have imperfections. For him, the main troubles will stem from the fact that his culturally operated advances will race ahead of any further genetic ones. His genes will lag behind, and he will be constantly reminded that, for all his environmentally-moulding achievements, he is still at heart a very naked ape.

Desmond Morris. (1967) *The naked ape.*

(Jonathan Cape, London.)

Our lives. . .are a constant dance between. . .surges of ancient emotions and their impulsive behaviours on the one hand, and the slower cognitions and admonishments of the evolutionarily later cerebral cortex on the other.

Ian Robertson. (1999) *Mind sculpture.*

(Bantam Books, London.)

E M Forster's novel *Where Angels Fear to Tread* gives a good example of teleology making the difference between description and explanation. Philip is trying to find out why his friend Caroline helped to bring about a marriage between Philip's sister and a young Italian man of whom Philip's family disapproves. After Caroline reports all the conversations she had with Philip's sister, Philip says, 'What you have given me is a description, not an explanation'. Everyone knows what Philip means by this — in asking for an explanation, he wants to learn Caroline's purposes. There is no purpose revealed in the laws of nature, and not knowing any other way of distinguishing description and explanation, Wittgenstein and my friend had concluded that these laws could not be explanations. Perhaps some of those who say that science describes but does not explain mean also to compare science unfavorably with theology, which they imagine to explain things by reference to some sort of divine purpose, a task declined by science.

Steven Weinberg. (2001) Can science explain everything? Anything?

New York Review of Books.

And Gandalf said: 'This is your realm, and the heart of the greater realm that shall be. The Third Age of the world is ended, and the new age is begun; and it is your task to order its beginning and to preserve what may be preserved. For though much has been saved, much must now pass away. . . . And all the lands that you see, and those that lie around them, shall be dwellings of men. For the time comes of the dominion of men, and the elder kindred shall fade or depart.'

J R R Tolkien. (1954) *The lord of the rings.*
(George Unwin and Allen, London.)

A sense of stupidity can easily descend on and darken the brain; and when I for one say I do not understand this or that, I do not necessarily imply the suspicion that there is nothing to be understood. In all sincerity, or stupidity, there are many of my own affairs that I do not understand.

G K Chesterton. (1958) Tagtug and the tree of knowledge.
In: *Essays and poems.* Ed. W Sheed.
(Penguin Books, Harmondsworth.)

So long as you write what you wish to write, that is all that matters; whether it matters for ages or only for hours, nobody can say. But to sacrifice a hair of the head of your vision, a shade of its colour, in deference to some headmaster with a silver pot on his head or to some professor with a measuring-rod up his sleeve, is the most abject treachery. . . .

Virginia Woolf. (1928) *A room of one's own.*
(Penguin Books, London.)

Doctor Jeddler was. . .a great philosopher, and the heart and mystery of his philosophy was to look upon the world as a gigantic practical joke.

Charles Dickens. *The battle for life.*

Never have I listened to such an extraordinary speech. At any other time, it would have been ludicrous, for here was a boy, with no sense of beauty and a puerile command of words, attempting to tackle themes which the greatest poets have found almost beyond their power. Eustace Robinson, aged fourteen, was standing in his nightshirt saluting, praising and blessing the great forces and manifestations of Nature.

He spoke first of night and stars and planets above his head, of the swarms of fireflies below, of the great rocks covered with anemones and shells that were slumbering in the invisible sea. He spoke of rivers and waterfalls, of the ripening bunches of grapes, of the smoking cone of Vesuvius and the hidden fire-channels that made up the smoke, of the myriads of lizards who were lying curled up in the crannies of the sultry earth, of the showers of white rose-leaves that were tangled in his hair. And then he spoke of the rain and the wind, by which all things are changed, of the air through which all things live, and of the woods in which all things can be hidden.

E M Forster. (1947) *Collected short stories.*
The story of a panic. (Penguin Books, London.)

When I was at school, I studied biology. I learned that in making their experiments scientists will take some group — bacteria, mice, people — and subject them to certain conditions. They compare the results with a second group which has not been disturbed. This second group is called the control group. It is the control group which enables the scientists to gauge the effect of his experiment. To judge the significance of what has occurred. In history, there are no control groups. There is no one to tell us what might have been. We weep over the might have been, but there is no might have been. There never was. It is supposed to be true that those who do not know history are condemned to repeat it. I don't believe knowing can save us. What is constant in history is greed and foolishness and a love of blood and this is a thing that even God — who knows all this can be known — seems powerless to change.

Cormac McCarthy. (1993) *All the pretty horses.*
(Vintage International.)

Zaphod lounged under a small palmtree on the bridge trying to bang his brain into shape with massive Pan Galactic Gargle Blasters. . .and Arthur took to his bed to flip through Ford's copy of The Hitch Hiker's Guide to the Galaxy. . .he came across this entry.

It said: 'The history of every major Galactic civilization tends to pass through three distinct and recognizable phases, those of survival, inquiry and sophistication, otherwise known as the how, why and where phases.

'For instance, the first phase is characterized by the question: How do we eat? And the second by the question Why do we eat? And the third by the question Where shall we have lunch?'

D Adams. (1979) *The hitch hikers guide to the galaxy.*

(Pan Books, London.)

Great scientists can kill their subject. Newton killed physics in Cambridge. What, it was asked, was there left to do? As a result the advances in science and technology on the Continent were ignored. So were Faraday in London and William Thomson (Lord Kelvin) in Glasgow. Obsessed by the belief that an undergraduate must learn what was true, Whewell opposed the study of modern science: he argued that not until a century had passed could we be certain that scientific theories were true. . . . After more than twenty years of. . .arid discussion it was at last decided to set up a committee on the teaching of experimental physics (in Cambridge). . . .

Noel Annan. (1999) *The dons. Mentors, eccentrics and geniuses.*

(Harper Collins, London.)

'Tis most true that many are possessed by an incurable itch to write. . . desirous of fame and honour, he will write no matter what. . .toiling for a frothy name among the vulgar masses. 'Tis pride and vanity eggs them on. They turn authors. . .to prove they have existed.

And if thou vouchsafe to read this treatise, it shall seem not otherwise to thee than the way to an ordinary traveller, sometimes fair, sometimes foul; here champaign, there enclosed; barren in one place, better soil in another. . . . I shall lead thee over steep mountains, though treacherous valleys, dew-clad meadows and rough plowed fields, through a variety of objects, that which thou shalt like and surely dislike.

Robert Burton. (1621) *The anatomy of melancholy.*

Chapter 2

A Chemical Code for Survival

A heap of cells is not an organism. A mass of people living side by side is not a society. The transition from a random collection of people who just happen to be near each other to a society requires communication: without it, each person is an individual, but only that. Nothing happens together, there is no co-operation, no sharing, no division of labour, no specialisation. People are able to communicate by telephone, email, letters and by speech. Underlying each of these physical methods of passing information is a common factor: language. Language is an arbitrary code for the symbolic representation of events. We can say more or less the same thing in Zulu, Arabic, English or French. The symbols are completely different in each case; however the information is the same. To act as an effective conduit of information, a language needs an agreed vocabulary (the code) a consistent and meaningful syntax (the order of words matters), a means for delivering this code (writing, speech etc), and a means for decoding it (understanding and interpreting the language: the receptor). If someone shouts 'look out' in Swahili, I, for one, will not duck. If I say 'good morning' to a native of Bengal, he may not respond. If someone learning English says to you 'this eat yes Friday' you may be puzzled for a moment.

Cells also communicate. They do not, of course, speak to each other. But they do have to send signals to other cells, and these signals are crucial if a mass of cells is to become an organ or a set of organs a body. Cells need to be influenced by other cells; the activity of other cells may be critical for them. They, in turn, need to signal other cells themselves, for similar reasons. Cells need to do things together, in the right sequence, or at the right time, or in the right circumstances. The body is buzzing

31

with messages. But the brain is the organ specialised for information decoding, storage and retrieval.

Peptides are remarkably suitable molecules for communication, which is why the body uses them so much for this purpose. The analogy between a spoken or written language and a chemical code can be over-stretched, but there are some obvious similarities. The English alphabet is made up of 26 letters. From these letters, an almost infinite number of words is composed. The number is so large because a word is defined by both the sequence of letters and their number. There can be words of extremely variable lengths, and some languages use much longer ones than others. But longer words do not necessarily contain more information than shorter ones. The set of words is the vocabulary and their agreed meaning is the semantics of a language. There are strings of letters that, in English, are non-words. Psychologists who study language use them all the time, not to each other (though sometimes one wonders) but as 'control' words. Languages also have a higher order organisation: the order of words, their syntax.

Peptides are chemicals in the body made up from an alphabet of 22 amino acids, and these are like coloured beads on a necklace or letters in a word. They can occur in any order (imagine each to be a differently coloured bead or a letter), and a peptide can have virtually any length, though most that are used for communication have between three and 100 amino acids. There is an indistinct boundary between 'peptides' and 'proteins'. Both are the same, really, though the word 'protein' is reserved for bigger peptides (those above about 200 amino acids). You can see immediately how the body can use peptides as chemical codes. After all, there are only 4 less amino acids than letters in the (English) alphabet, the language of Shakespeare, many great poets, our daily news, a mass of complex scientific information, and the major means of social communication and control. But any language has its limits. Philosophers debate the exact meaning of words, and whether there are ideas that cannot be encapsulated by language. Literary critics discuss the limits of language to express emotions and events. Scientists invent new words to represent new discoveries. Some languages do not have words that others have. There is the famous example of the many Inuit words for 'snow', though, sadly, the story seems not to be true.

Communication Between Brain Cells

We propose here to classify communicational phenomena between cells of the central nervous system under two general frames: 'wiring transmission' and 'volume transmission'. 'Wiring transmission' is defined as intercellular communication occurring through a well-defined connecting structure. . . . It includes synaptic transmission but also other types of intercellular communication through a connecting structure (e.g., gap junctions). 'Volume' transmission is characterised by signal diffusion in a three dimensional fashion with the brain extracellular fluid. . . . . Volume transmission includes short- and long-distance diffusion of signals. . . .

> L F Agnati, M Zoli, I Stromberg, K Fuxe. (1995) Intercellular communication in the brain: Wiring versus volume transmission. *Neuroscience* **69**, pp. 711–726.

It is an attractive notion to compare the complexity and variability of interneuronal communication with our language. Accordingly, a phone call and information transfer via a megaphone respectively would reflect wired and volume transmission to a certain extent (as would radio in the case of hormone action). A promising and necessarily reductive approach to understand the biological 'language' of. . . neuropeptides in the brain is to focus on single 'words'. . . to reduce the 'language' into its component parts without ignoring the fact that understanding single 'words' is just the beginning of understanding the 'language'.

> R Landgraf. (1995) Intracerebrally released vasopressin and oxytocin: Measurement, mechanisms and behavioural consequences. *Journal of Neuroendocrinology* **7**, pp. 243–253.

Despite the complexities of individual systems, neurocrine, endocrine, and growth factor-mediated signaling systems show striking similarities in the molecules they use for communication and in their signal-transduction mechanisms. . . . According to theorems for efficient and error-free encoding, the differences in rate and distance of information transfer and in noise interference between neurocrine, endocrine, and growth factor-mediated messages require different encoding strategies. These differences are reflected in the use of plurichemical transmission (to increase information content) or in the number and sequence of amino acids within peptide molecules (to protect against noise interference). . . . The data discussed are consistent with the role

If a cell can make a given peptide at the appropriate time, send it so that it is detected by another cell, and the second cell responds, we have the basis of a biological code. The existence of a set of peptides each with a defined 'meaning' (i.e., cellular response) is the semantics. The delivery system corresponds to speech or email or whatever in the world of 'real' coded language. Detection by the receptive cell is the decoding process (reading the message). Peptides are the words of a biological code, and amino acids are its letters. As it happens, biochemists have assigned a letter to each of the amino acids. Because 22 amino acids can be arranged in so many ways, and in strings of different lengths, we have an almost infinite chemical vocabulary. Is there also a syntax? Indeed there is. In many cases, the receipt of several peptides, either together or in sequence, will initiate a set of responses that depend on that sequence as well as on the constituent peptides making up the signal. Even scientists often refer to cells 'talking' to each other.

We think of the brain as the communication system, but all the cells in the body have to send messages to each other. The immune system is one of the better examples of a dispersed collection of cells that have to communicate. There isn't a tissue in the body that does not use peptides as codes. So far all the peptides we have considered are released by one set of cells and act either back on themselves, as a sort of feedback signal (autocrine communication), or on another set, separated only by a few microns (1 micron is 1 millionth of a metre, or 1 thousandth of a millimetre) (paracrine communication). They act as local hormones: that is, a chemical released by one cell that regulates another. That is fine if the cells belong to the same organ, and lie close to one another. But suppose cells need to send chemical signals to the cells of different organs; they may lie centimetres or even metres away. We need a delivery system. Luckily, we have one: the circulatory system. Because blood permeates almost all the body, signals released into it will eventually arrive at their target. These signals are the classical hormones, and form part of the hormonal (endocrine) system. Peptides make up quite a few of these hormones, though there are other sorts (codes) as well. There are peptides that control growth, and reproduction and many other activities. But the most famous of all is insulin. Insulin is a classical peptide hormone. It is released from the pancreas, and its chief action is to regulate glucose of regulatory peptides as signals in a universal structured code for biological communication.

E A Mayer, J P Baldi. (1991) Can regulatory peptides be regarded as words of a biological language? *American Journal of Physiology* **261**, pp. 171–84.

Our genes have to build a brain (to take day-to-day decisions for them). . . . The reason why they cannot manipulate our puppet strings directly is. . . time lag. Genes work by controlling protein synthesis, but it is slow. The whole point about behaviour, on the other hand, is that it is fast. It works on a time-scale not of months but of seconds and fractions of seconds. Something happens in the world, an owl flashes overhead, a rustle in the grass betrays prey, and in milliseconds nervous systems crackle into action, muscles leap, and someone's life is saved — or lost. Genes don't have reaction times like that. . . they can only do their best *in advance* by building a fast executive computer for themselves, and programming it in advance with rules and 'advice' to cope with as many eventualities as they can 'anticipate'. But life. . . offers too many different possibilities for all of them to be anticipated. . . . The genes have to 'instruct' their survival machines not in specifics but in the general strategies and tricks of the living trade.

R Dawkins. (1976) *The selfish gene.* (Oxford University Press, Oxford.)

levels in the blood and help glucose to enter the tissues that need it for energy. Let's look more closely at insulin.

Insulin in the blood is actually made up of two peptide chains joined together. But when it is first made in the pancreatic cell it is a much bigger molecule, and bits are chopped off by enzymes in the pancreas to make the blood-borne form. One of the pieces (called C-peptide) may itself have significant actions.

In effect, the pancreas is making two hormones from one parent molecule. This is very common. Sometimes many peptides are made from one parent. There can be alterations in the enzymes responsible for the chopping procedure, so a parent peptide may make different sets of daughters if circumstances alter.

There are not that many hormones that are essential for life (though most make it a lot better) but insulin is one. It is hard to realise that up until the 1930s, diabetes mellitus (diabetes for short) was a dreaded and invariably fatal disease. Because insulin-deficient diabetes (there is another form) usually affects young people, this was doubly tragic. No amount of desperate dieting saved them. Most were dead within 18 months of diagnosis. What was sadder is that the cause was known: insulin deficiency, but nothing could be done. It was even known that the pancreas had lots of insulin in it, but all efforts to extract it failed. This was because the pancreas has enzymes in it that are used to digest your food, but they also digested insulin during the attempted extraction process. Until, that is, a pair of Canadian scientists — one was a medical student at the time — hit upon a successful method. Almost overnight, diabetes, though still a serious disease, was treatable and nowadays diabetics live a relatively normal life span even though the current treatment is not perfect. Everyone will know at least one diabetic. In the 1920s hardly anyone did: they had all died. A transforming event had occurred in medicine which was utterly dependent on animal experiments. This may interest those who find such experimental work uncomfortable to think about, or who wonder whether work on animals is ever applicable to man.

The pancreas lies close to the gut, and is concerned closely with what goes on in the gastrointestinal system. The gut itself uses quite a few hormones to make sure it secretes the right enzymes as your lunch passes

Chemical Signals in the Brain

Evidently the physics and chemistry of the cell can do much with the help of final causes. Chemistry and physics account for much which the cell does, and for so much to which years ago physical science could at that time offer no clue, that it is justifiable to suppose that the still unexplained residue of the cell's behaviour will prove resoluble by chemistry and physics.

C S Sherrington. (1940) *Man on his nature.*
(Penguin Books, Harmondsworth, UK.)

The concepts of information theory, involving such factors as channel width, signal, noise and redundancy in a message are well known in the information technology industry and the optimal solution for a communications system depends on whether, for example, a message is being transmitted along a private wire from my word processor to its printer or greetings to a friend are being sent by satellite to the other side of the world. In terms of encoding the message for transmission, a number of factors affect the accuracy of information transfer. For example, error can be decreased by increasing redundancy within the message by using sequences of symbols rather than individual symbols.

M Peaker. (1992) Chemical signalling systems: The rules of the game.
Journal of Endocrinology **135**, pp. 1–4.

The distinction between transmitters, modulators and hormones has its heuristic value. It explains high speed and spatial precision on the one hand up to a theoretically unlimited variability in signalling on the other. Nevertheless, it is illusory to believe that the brain works in this way. Probably even simple information transfers use a combination of these modes of communication, e.g. a neuropeptide molecule released as a transmitter could subsequently act as a modulator suggesting that complex responses to a neuropeptide are likely to reflect a gradation from synaptic through non-synaptic to conventional hormonal actions.

R Landgraf. (1995) Intracerebrally released vasopressin and oxytocin:
Measurement, mechanisms and behavioural consequences.
Journal of Neuroendocrinology **7**, pp. 243–253.

It has been suggested that peptide molecules evolved very early and that the endocrine and nervous systems may express similar peptides. . . because they evolved from primitive cells that had already evolved these substances down it and digestion proceeds as it should. Secretin (the first hormone to be discovered), gastrin, motilin, vasoactive intestinal peptide (called VIP), substance P (the 'P' stands for 'peptide'), somatostatin, and the delightfully-named cholecystokinin (Greek for 'activates the bile', which is exactly what it does) are some. Some of the other names also give you a clue about what they do. We will meet them again, in a surprising place.

Suppose that you, a minor deity, have just invented hormones — that is, an endocrine system. You have worked long and hard, but your new system has some problems. Local (paracrine) communication is relatively easy: release some peptide, and it diffuses to the cell next door and does its stuff. But launching your precious peptide into the bloodstream is another matter. How does it know where to go? How will the cells you want to target actually recognise your peptide even if it arrives safe and sound? Your delivery system, the blood, is none too predictable. After all, blood goes practically everywhere. Imagine putting a letter in a postbox without knowing which town it would arrive in. Your only consolation is that, unlike some real mail systems I know about, the letter (hormone molecule) is collected straight away and disappears from view. You cannot rely on targeted delivery, so you have to opt for another way. This is to ensure that only the cells you want to respond to the peptide message have the necessary receptors (decoders). These molecules, themselves complex proteins, usually lie on the cell wall and a passing peptide molecule recognises its own receptor and locks onto it. As soon as it does so, the cell reacts to the hormone (endocrinologists tend to talk about 'locks and keys' to illustrate this point). But there may be more than one type of receptor for a hormone, and different receptors may do different things. A silly example illustrates this: the shout "duck" may cause one person to crouch, another to look for a particular type of bird. Same message, different receptor (decoder).

Only cells that are equipped with the right receptor(s) will respond to the hormone. Receptors are detection devices, and so the amount of hormone is important. If there is too little, the receptor will not detect it. This is not too much of a problem in paracrine, local, communication. Though the cells here also use receptors, the peptide is not diluted very much because it has not far to go. This is not the case for blood-borne for use in intracellular communication. . . . This notion does not explain why common messenger molecules were retained during the period that the unicellular organisms evolved into specialized cells that apparently no longer needed the molecules for intracellular communication.

I Kupfermann. (1991) Functional studies of cotransmission.
Physiological Reviews **71**, pp. 683–732.

Although transmitters provide a useful way to organize studies of the nervous system, they do not define functional units of information processing. In fact, the roles of different transmitter systems in transferring or integrating information are poorly understood. This problem is particularly evident when neurotransmission is defined broadly to include events lasting more than a few hundred milliseconds and spreading spatially beyond the receptor site. . . The functional distinctions between traditional 'fast-acting' transmitters, such as glutamate, and slow modulators, such as peptides, become blurred when the range of their effects is considered over behaviorally relevant time-scales of seconds and minutes.

B A Trimmer. (1999) The messenger is not the message; or is it?
In: *Beyond neurotransmission.* Ed. P S Katz, pp. 29–82.
(Oxford University Press, Oxford.)

hormones. So you have to design your endocrine system to deliver quite large amounts of peptide to make sure enough reaches the receptors on those distant cells. This can be expensive metabolically. More problems. The blood may contain substances that tend to chew up your peptide, so you may have to protect it in some way during its travel. Since a very effective peptide hormone system exists, we can be sure that these problems have been solved.

There is one part of the body that has developed a special blood delivery system to avoid some of these difficulties. It is quite a while now since we thought about the brain, but it has a major part to play in controlling hormones. One of the ways it does so is by producing peptides that themselves pass to the pituitary gland, which lies just under the brain. The pituitary is a major hormone control centre, and produces a whole range of (rather bigger) peptide hormones that go directly into the general blood stream, just like other endocrine glands. The clever bit is that the brain uses a special blood system to send its peptides to the pituitary. Perhaps it cannot make enough of these peptides, but whatever the reason, there is a very private system of blood vessels that run between the base of the brain (the hypothalamus) and only to the pituitary. This means that even a small injection of peptide from the brain cells (neurons) in the hypothalamus into this special blood delivery system will all go straight to the pituitary, with hardly any dilution. So the brain does not need to make much peptide. It is anatomically addressed. And small changes in the amount of peptide released into this blood system (called the pituitary portal system) will be faithfully reflected in changed action in the pituitary; so the control is better. There are some other neurons in the hypothalamus that behave like more conventional hormone-producing glands and secrete directly into the general blood stream. They are huge compared to other neurons, because they have to make such large amounts of peptide. That is probably why the special system exists — to avoid having lots of enormous nerve cells that are expensive in terms of space and energy.

About 40 years ago, there was a bout of intellectual fisticuffs on this very topic, waged by two academic heavyweights of the time. One claimed that the (anterior) pituitary had a nerve supply from the brain, and this was how it was controlled. The other, just as vehemently, asserted that there was a novel communication link between the two: the brain

It was during this term that I began to realize that Sebastian was a drunkard in quite a different sense to myself. I got drunk often, but through an excess of high spirits, in the love of the moment, and the wish to prolong and enhance it; Sebastian drank to escape. . . .
Julia used to say, "Poor Sebastian. It is something chemical in him".
That was the cant phrase of the time, derived from heavens knows what misconception of popular science. "There's something chemical between them" was used to explain the over-mastering hate or love of any two people. It was the old concept of determinism in a new form. I do not believe there was anything chemical in my friend.

Evelyn Waugh. (1945) *Brideshead revisited.*

Open thy mind, the truth is coming; know,
When the articulations of the brain
Has been perfected in the embryo,

Then the First Mover turns to it, full fain
Of nature's triumph, and inbreathes a rare
New spirit, filled with virtue to constrain

To its own substance whatso active there
It finds, and make one single soul complete,
Alive, and sensitive, and self-aware.

Dante. *The divine comedy. II. Purgatory. Canto XXV Trans D L Sayers.* (Penguin Books, Hammondsworth.)

I do not believe that gifts, whether of mind or character, can be weighed like sugar or butter, not even in Cambridge, where they are so adept at putting people into classes and fixing caps on their heads and letters after their names.

Virginia Woolf. (1928) *A room of one's own.*
(Penguin Books, London.)

Why was there jealousy — not just for him, but for lots of people? Why did it start up? It was related to love in some way, but that way wasn't quantifiable or comprehensible. Why did it suddenly start wailing in his head, like a ground-warning system in an aircraft: six and a half seconds, secreted a 'factor' into a special blood system, which started from the brain and ended in the pituitary. That is, there was a chemically coded message from the brain to the pituitary. This was a revolutionary idea at the time. It was also right.

As it happens, I was at this time a young student of the first protagonist, the brilliant and charismatic Solly Zuckerman. He was most famous as a major influence on governmental science policy in the UK for several decades (he eventually became Lord Zuckerman). Sadly, he was wrong about the pituitary. His adversary was Geoffrey Harris (GW Harris), not so charismatic, but a better bench scientist (and never ennobled). Harris-Zuckerman debates (a polite label) enlivened scientific meetings of the time, and taught me that human nature sometimes gets in the way of good science. Harris is rightly revered as a founder of the science of neuroendocrinology (the interaction between the nervous and hormonal systems). Zuckerman, who had been at the centre of defence policy, by the end of his life had become a nuclear disarmer.

And so on to the brain, which is where we were heading all along. Other tissues use peptides to communicate so they can function properly. Guts squirm, muscles contract, glands secrete, but communication is what the brain does. Since it is so good at it, and, indeed, is there to help communication between other organs, we would hardly expect it to need peptides. These, we might think, are only for those organs that cannot use the computational and communication powers of the brain. The brain, after all, has nerve fibres to communicate and send specific messages. As with more rational scientific predictions than this, we are in a for a very big surprise. The brain is packed with peptides. If we examine the brain carefully, we find three important facts: the peptides are located in the nerve terminals — the part of the nerve cell that communicates with the next nerve cell. So they seem to be in a good position to act as transmitters or signalling molecules. Many of them have very familiar names; we have come across them in other parts of the body. The limbic system, the focus of our attention, is peculiarly rich both in the number and amount of peptides we find in it. Could it be that the brain is also taking advantage of the chemical coding capacity of peptides, and, if so, why does it need to do so? Are they doing something special there? What is their role in coping, adaptation and survival?

evasive action now. That was what it felt like sometimes, inside Graham's skull. And why did it pick on him? Was it some kind of fluky chemistry? Was it all dished out at birth? Did you get given jealousy the way you got given a big bottom or poor eyesight, both of which Graham suffered from? If so, maybe it wore off after a while; maybe there was only enough jealousy chemical in that soft box up there for a certain number of years. Perhaps, but Graham rather doubted it: he'd had a big bottom for years, and that showed no signs of easing up.

Julian Barnes. (1983) *Before she met me.*

(Picador, London.)

Now is the moment to think about how most nerve cells are connected and how they work. The cerebral cortex is thought by most neuroscientists to be primarily responsible for our ability to recognise things in the environment, whether by sight, sound or touch; for thinking, for making decisions about what to do or not to do, for certain forms of memory, and for being able to make complicated and skilled movements. Naturally enough, to be able to do all these things (and more) requires much computational power. This means huge numbers of nerve cells (neurons). Each neuron in the cortex (as elsewhere in the brain) is little electrochemical processor. It collects information from the chemicals released from other neurons onto its information-gathering system: mostly finger-like projections from its cell body (dendrites) on which end the terminals of other neurons. These chemicals, the transmitters of other neurons, can make the cell 'fire'; that is, send one or more (usually a series) of electrical impulses down the long process (the axon) that passes close to another neuron's dendrites, and releases a chemical of its own. Axons can be anything from a few millimeters to metres long. Where the axon goes determines which neuron next in the chain is affected. In the cortex, many neurons have a very precise arrangement: each one sends its axon to a limited set of other neurons. The precise pattern varies, but most people agree that the basis of the cortex's remarkable abilities is the complexity and variety of these connections. So the whole cerebral cortex is made up of billions of smaller components: each component is itself made up of many neurons connected together in a particular way. This wiring arrangement is clearly very important, though that does not mean it cannot change. The wiring, however, is not like that in a computer; the end of each nerve does not directly connect with another (as in a computer) but releases a chemical transmitter when the electrical impulse that is travelling down the axon reaches the chemical-filled terminal lying next to another nerve cell (this is called a synapse).

If the cortex is heavily dependent on the precise way the neurons are connected together, the chemicals used as transmitters must not disturb this arrangement. Many of the cortical neurons use as their transmitters rather simple molecules, such as single amino acids. A common one is glutamate (one amino acid), which activates the next neuron. Another is GABA (also a single amino acid: γ-amino-butyric acid), which has the opposite inhibitory effect. Furthermore, just to make sure that the network stays as it should, each nerve terminal is fixed close to the next nerve cell, so that the synaptic space between them is small, and any transmitter released will go directly onto the next neuron (and its receptors) and not wander off to stimulate (or inhibit) a neighbouring one. To be doubly sure, there are very efficient ways of sucking up the transmitter released, so that it stays where it should and its effects are time-limited. Glutamate and GABA are acting as faithful chemical 'on' or 'off' switches to the next neuron. Like saying either 'yes' or 'no'. The actions of both transmitters are certainly more complex than this because each has several different types of receptor, each doing different things, but this 'on/off' switching is a good part of what they do. Computational neuroscientists spend happy and productive hours modelling such neural networks on their powerful computers, trying to see if they can reproduce some of the known actions of the cortex, particularly its ability to learn. The bottom line is that the specific action of the standard cortical neuron depends mostly on its connections, which are very precise and rather limited and whether it inhibits or excites the other neurons with which it connects.

Down in the limbic system, something very different is happening. There are networks of peptide-containing neurons. Take a look at one or two. The first difference between cortical neurons and the limbic peptide neurons is the peptide. Not a simple, single-letter molecule at all, but a complex one with a string of letters and capable of conveying much more information than a simple amino acid. But what information? Now let us look at the connections the neuron makes. Unlike the cortex, with its reassuring strictness, the peptide neuron seems to meander, making a large number of connections. Intriguingly, there is no close association between the end of the peptide neuron (the synapse) and the receptors that respond to it. They can be quite a long way away, so the released peptide seems to have to percolate the brain. Since this may dilute it, we are intrigued to find that we need extraordinarily tiny amounts of peptide to affect the next neuron. Neurons are a 100 times more sensitive to peptides than the 'classical' single-letter amino acid transmitters like glutamate or GABA. And there is no sucking back up of peptides, no mechanisms to restrict them to a local neuron. The brain seems to be encouraging peptides to wander about and regulate any neurons in the neighbourhood which happen to have the right receptors. There are dozens of peptides, not just two or so, and some neurons seems to contain more than one. And each peptide may have several receptors, each decoding its message in a distinct way. Suddenly, we realise what all this could mean and that it is a familiar story. The brain seems to be using peptides like the local (paracrine) hormones that we know about in other organs. It's about time we did some experiments.

Let's go into the lab. There are a number of male rats ready. Some days previously, each has had a tiny tube inserted through its skull under anaesthesia into the brain ventricles. The brain ventricles are fluid-filled spaces inside the brain, and anything injected into them quickly reaches most of the brain substance. Now, the rats are walking around their cages completely unaware of this tube (people with certain brain conditions, for example high pressure in their ventricles, have similar tubes inserted, and feel nothing). On the shelf is a bottle labelled 'angiotensin II'. It has been diluted so that 10 microlitres (10 thousandths of a millilitre) contain just 25 picograms (a picogram is 10^{-12} or 0.000000000001 gram). Angiotensin II (ang-II for short) is a small peptide (8 amino acids). Like many other peptides, it is made from a much bigger precursor, and chopped down to its final size by a number of enzymes. There is quite a lot in the brain, nearly all of it in the limbic system.

We inject 10 microlitres (25 picograms) of angiotensin-II down the tube in one of the rats and into its ventricle. The rat's cage is empty, but now we put in a small amount of food. The rat, I should tell you, is neither food deprived nor thirsty. Absolutely nothing happens, though we wait for about 30 minutes. We repeat the experiment on another male rat. This time we put in a second (also male) rat. Apart from a few tentative sniffs, nothing much happens again. Undaunted, we try a third time. Now we put in the cage a tube equipped with a drinking spout and filled with water. After about 1 minute, the rat rushes over to the tube and drinks and drinks. About 10–15 millilitres, a large amount for a rat. Particularly one that was not thirsty. We discuss the actions of angiotensin II in adaptation more fully in Chapter 6.

Then, we try a different peptide called neuropeptide Y. This time the rat does not drink, it eats. And eats. No mating (in fact, it prefers eating food to mating with even an attractive female). It seems to want to eat, not do much else. We will discuss this in Chapter 5.

Finally, we try a third peptide. This time it is one called CRF (which stands for 'corticotropin-releasing factor'). Now the rat does not eat or drink, but looks very fearful, and if we put in that second male rat, is quite likely to attack it. More on this in Chapters 4 and 10.

It looks as if there might be a chemical 'code' in the limbic system for a range of important adaptive behaviours. Behaviours without which none of us would survive, but which are no good unless they happen under the right circumstances.

As you will read in the rest of this book, we are beginning to decode the actions of the peptides in the limbic system, and the story is starting to make sense. As we think about how the brain controls your appetite, your body temperature, your water intake, your sex-life, the way you treat your children, how you cope with stress, we will come across peptides, dozens of them. The limbic system responds to peptides to determine what you need. It uses its nerve fibres to deliver peptides to where they are needed, when need arises. These peptides carry the information both about what you need and what you need to do to survive.

But the limbic system uses other chemicals as well. If we analyse these chemicals, we find that there are large concentrations of a second sort — the amines.

Chapter 3

Serotonin, Steroids and Signalling

Though peptides are a major chemical code in the limbic system, they are not the only one. There are plenty of other communication molecules. One family is collectively called the 'amines', and one member of this family is serotonin. It has became rather famous in recent years.

Suppose you were to take small samples from all over the brain, and analyse them for their content of serotonin. You would find that all of them had quite a lot, though the amount varied from part to part. If you repeated this on several brains, making a note of which parts you sampled, you might well find that every time you did the experiment, you got approximately the same result. All of the brain seems to contain serotonin, but there are consistent differences in the amounts you find in different areas. You begin to recognise three features of serotonin: it is ubiquitous, it is found particularly in the grey matter of the brain, but its distribution is not uniform or random. There seems to be a pattern.

Now suppose you do something else. From those parts of the brain that contain particularly large amounts of serotonin, you take more samples, but this time, instead of putting them through a machine that measures levels of serotonin, you cut thin slices (about 20 microns thick), and treat them with a stain that shows up serotonin. You can see, by putting these thin slices under a good microscope, which of the cells in the brain actually contain serotonin. You are amazed to find that there are none. Instead, you see thin, irregular hair-like structures containing serotonin, which you recognise as nerve fibres. You are pleased to see that those areas that contained plenty of serotonin (as shown by the previous analysis) also have a rich higgledy-piggledy network of serotonin-containing fibres, whereas in others the network is much more sparse. So it looks as if all

No system is static; it is always in the process of becoming what it is not. Any putting together of changes is put together with the energy that will tear it apart. The winding down of one system is the winding up of another. The condition is circular: it doesn't matter where you apparently enter the cycle. Be Eurydice lost, and the energy of that system will put together the Orpheus who has lost you and the music with which he will gain entrance to the nether world. Be Orpheus, and the energy of that system will be scattered when the Thracian women tear you apart. Be the Thracian women, and your tearing-apart of Orpheus will release the energy that puts him together again with Eurydice unlost. Eurydice and Orpheus and the Thracian women are only the costumes: the actors are being lost, the losing and the finding, the gathering and the scattering. The actors are the action cycles continually moving in us and in all things.

Russell Hoban. (1973) *Introduction to household tales.* (Picador).

Ah Love! Could thou and I with Fate conspire
To grasp this sorry Scheme of Things entire,
Would not we shatter it to bits — and then
Re-mould it nearer to the Heart's Desire!

The Rubaiyat of Omar Khayyam.
Translated. (Edward Fitzgerald. Collins, London.)

Flittering and fretting
Among the philosophies created by its mind
Yet constrained to be an animal
Caught in the devastation of the
Pinnacle and abyss of self consciousness
Man

He must learn to laugh at himself
Remember what a mixture of self control
And unalterable nature
Those chemicals traversing his brain having
Taken aeons to evolve are not so easily thwarted
They contain his ideas
*   They may contain his God*

J C J Barna (1980). *Unpublished poem.*

the serotonin in the brain is contained in nerve fibres. But where are the serotonin-containing neurons? There must be some, because nerve fibres are processes from neurons. Luckily, you have been very painstaking, and have taken sections through most of the brain. You examine them systematically. You find more serotonin nerve fibres, though you go on seeing that the way they are distributed in the brain is not uniform. Some parts of brain have a dense network, in others the fibres are sparse and hard to see.

Suddenly, almost as you give up, you come across your first serotonin-containing nerve cell. Excitedly, you look through the rest of your sections of the brain. You see that there is a rather small collection of such cells. They are clustered in the part of the brain which you recognise as the midbrain: right at the back of the brain — in between the spinal cord and the main part of the brain (what Paul Maclean would call the 'reptilian' part mentioned in Chapter 1). A long way from the cortex, or even most of the limbic system. You notice that these serotonin neurons are clustered in several groups, though none of these groups is very large. Most neurons in the brain, you realise, do not contain serotonin. As you go further back into the brain stem you see the serotonin neurons disappear. All serotonin-containing neurons, it seems, are bunched together in a small part of the brain. But what about all those nerve fibres, that are found so far away in other parts of the brain? The whole brain seems permeated with serotonin nerve fibres.

Luckily, there is a way to find out, though it needs an experiment. You enlist the help of a colleague who has a special substance (called a neurotoxin) that selectively destroys serotonin neurons, and you get him to inject this into the area of the midbrain that contains these nerve cells. You wait a few days, then look at the midbrains of the rats that have received the neurotoxin. Since you are a well-trained scientist, you have also injected some saline (in which the neurotoxin is dissolved) into another set of rats, and you examine their midbrains as well. As you hoped, the midbrains of the rats treated with the neurotoxin now have no serotonin-containing neurons: the neurotoxin has killed there serotonin-containing neurons off. All the other neurons seem perfectly healthy. The rats given saline, have (to your relief) the normal number. But the really interesting part comes next. You now look at the rest of the brain. In the control animals, you

My impression is the Prozac, because it gives pleasure indirectly, by enhancing hedonic capacity and lowering barriers to ordinary social intercourse, generally increases person autonomy. . . .

Is Prozac a good thing? By now, asking about the virtue of Prozac — and I am referring here not to its use in severely depressed patients but, rather, to its availability to alter personality — may seem like asking whether it was a good thing for Freud to have discovered the unconscious. Once we are aware of the unconscious, once we have witnessed the effects of Prozac, it is impossible to imagine the modern world without them.

P D Kramer. (1994) *Listening to Prozac.*

(Penguin Books, New York.)

Thus, in brief, to our imagination cometh, by the outward sense or memory, some object to be known (residing in the foremost part of the brain) which he, misconceiving or amplifying, presently communicates to the heart, the seat of all affections. The pure spirits forthwith flock from the brain to the heart by certain secret channels, and signify what good or bad object was presented; which immediately bends itself to prosecute or avoid it, and, withal, draweth with it other humours to help it. So, in pleasure, concur great store of purer spirits; in sadness, much melancholy blood; in ire, choler. If the imagination be very apprehensive, intent and violent, it sends great stores of spirits to or from the heart, and makes a deeper impression, and greater tumult; as the humours in the body be likewise prepared, and the temperature itself ill or well disposed, the passions are longer and stronger: so that the first step and fountain of all our grievances in this kind is a distorted imagination, which, misinforming the heart, causeth all these distemperatures, alteration and confusion of sprits and humours . . . . The spirits so confounded . . . bad humours increased . . . and thick spirits engendered, with melancholy blood.

R Burton. (1641) *The anatomy of melancholy.*

see the usual networks of serotonin-containing nerve fibres. But no serotonin-fibres are to be seen in the neurotoxin-treated rats. The brain seems empty of serotonin. You do a few more experiments to make sure that the neurotoxin has not spread to other parts of the brain. No: its action is limited to the serotonin neurons in the midbrain.

There is only one interpretation, though it is a surprising one. All the extensive network of serotonin nerves that are found throughout the brain come from a few small groups of nerve cells lying deep in its base. Imagine a long wall covered in ivy; in some parts the ivy grows thickly, in others less so. But all this extensive network comes from a small cluster of roots at one end of the wall. So it is with serotonin in the brain. This means that serotonin has a widespread, pervasive effect in the brain, which will vary according to how rich the serotonin network is in that part, and which depends on the activity of a small collection of nerve cells lying deep in the midbrain. You predict that serotonin will have actions on all sorts of brain functions. Since you have already noticed that the limbic system has a noticeably rich serotonin-nerve supply, you suspect that the things that the limbic system does will be rather sensitive to serotonin. However, you also recall that other parts of the brain (for example, the cerebral cortex) also have serotonin-containing nerve fibres, and that these come from the same nerve cells that supply the limbic system. You suspect that the action of serotonin will be correspondingly pervasive, though not indiscriminate. You are absolutely right.

Serotonin occurs in many tissues, including the blood, where it was first discovered. Its name derives from the constricting effect it has on blood vessels. In the blood, it is found in high concentrations in the platelets, which are known to be essential for blood clotting, and serotonin helps limit bleeding after a cut. There is plenty of serotonin in the gut as well. As in the case of peptides, it is striking that the gut and the limbic system contain so much of the same neurochemical.

Serotonin is also known as 5HT, which stands for 5-hydroxy-tryptamine. This is actually a better name, since it represents the chemical structure of serotonin, whereas 'serotonin' reflects an action which has turned out not to be very interesting. Both names have survived and are used by neuroscientists. Some of the drugs that alter 5HT function are called 'SSRIs' (selective serotonin reuptake inhibitors), so even pharmacologists (who like

Serotonin Receptors

The explosive development of research in the serotoninergic system led to the discovery that different 5-HT receptors are involved in numerous physiopathological functions mediated by serotoninergic neurotransmission. Initially, the receptors were often suspected of being artifactual because the existence of multiple receptors was considered unrealistic. The results of recent studies. . . clearly confirm the reality of several types of serotonin receptors. . . . That multiple receptors exist. . . constitutes an important adaptive advantage. . . the multiplicity of 5-HT receptors allows differential interactions of 5-HT with biological tissues.

E Zifa, G Fillion. (1992) 5-hydroxytryptamine receptors.
Pharmacological Reviews **44**, pp. 401–449.

We demonstrate that mice without 5-HT1A receptors display decreased exploratory activity and increased fear of aversive environments. . . . These results demonstrate that 5-HT1A receptors are involved in the modulation of exploratory and fear-related behaviors and suggest that reductions in 5-HT1A receptor density due to genetic defects or environmental stressors might result in heightened anxiety.

S Ramboz *et al.* (1998) Serotonin receptor 1A knockout:
an animal model of anxiety-related disorder. *Proceedings of the
National Academy of Sciences, USA* **95**, pp. 14476–14481.

The current study shows that increased 5-HT2C receptor responsiveness accompanies isolation rearing in rats and may contribute to the enhanced response to stress and the increased neophobia (fear of new experience) seen in this animal model of trait anxiety.

K C F Fone, K Shalders, Z D Fox, R Arthur *et al.* (1996)
Increased 5-HT2C receptor responsiveness occurs on rearing
rats in social isolation. *Psychopharmacology* **123**, pp. 346–352.

. . . Removal of circulating corticosteroids by adrenalectomy causes up-regulation of 5-HT1A receptor expression and the addition of exogenous corticosteroids suppresses 5-HT1A receptor expression . . . . It seems clear that changes in hypothalamo-pituitary-adrenal axis function can result in dysregulation of the serotoninergic system.

S Wissink *et al.* (2000) Regulation of the rat serotonin-1A receptor gene by
corticosteroids. *Journal of Biological Chemistry* **275**, pp. 1321–1326.

to use chemical names) succumb to historical pressure. Drugs that act on serotonin are used to treat a variety of clinical conditions, including depression, excessive appetite, anxiety, unwanted aspects of sexuality, as well as in pain relief, as an anticonvulsant, in migraine and in the nausea that sometimes accompanies chemotherapy. They are also, of course, used 'recreationally'. An earlier generation took LSD (lysergic acid diethylamide), a drug that tended to induce hallucinations (sometimes they persisted). The present one prefers 'ecstasy' (MDMA: methylene-dioxy-methamphetamine), another drug which alters mood and social interaction. It can also increase your body temperature (occasionally fatally), or cause you to drink too much water. It is clear that our prediction that serotonin might have many important actions on the brain is being upheld. It is time we asked ourselves what exactly this chemical does in the brain. In particular, whether it plays any special role in adaptation or how we respond to stress. Does this explain its role in so many illnesses? And why do people who take drugs that increase serotonin say that they feel better?

How special is serotonin in the brain? The rather astonishing anatomical arrangement, whereby a small number of neurons deep in the brain supply serotonin-containing nerve fibres to the rest of the brain is not, as it happens, unique. There are at least three other chemical systems in the brain that bear a striking resemblance to the serotonin system. All of them start from clusters of nerve cells in the lower part of the brain, from which spread a network of nerve fibres to many other parts. This resemblance extends to the chemicals they use for neurotransmission. Instead of serotonin, the other three systems use either noradrenaline (called nor-epinephrine in the US), dopamine or acetylcholine. These are also quite simple molecules that have some chemical similarities to serotonin. However, there are two important differences. First, the cells that give rise to each system are quite distinct one from another — that is, there are separate clumps of neurons, each containing one or other of these transmitters. Second, the pattern of the distribution of their fibres to the rest of the brain is not the same for each. For example, the distribution of nerve fibres containing noradrenaline is quite different in the brain from that of dopamine. In fact, the two systems seem to try to avoid each other, even though (perhaps because) the two compounds are very closely

... Mice lacking serotonin 1A receptors throughout the brain showed pronounced anxiety-like behaviour... whereas selective restoration of the receptors in the forebrain restored normal behaviour.... Eliminating forebrains serotonin receptors during adult life... did not elicit anxiety-like behaviour. By contrast, the same procedure during gestation... did lead to pronounced anxiety-like behaviour. So forebrain serotonin receptors are needed during the development of newborns to modulate the predisposition to anxiety-like behaviour, but are no longer critical during adult life.

S H Snyder. (2002) Serotonin sustains serenity. *Nature* **416**, pp. 377–380.

related chemically. Serotonin and noradrenaline overlap somewhat more, but even in their case there are many areas that contain either a rich serotonin network or a noradrenaline one, but not both. Acetylcholine, a rather different molecule (but still chemically related), has its cells in the base of the forebrain, and its network largely limited to the cortex.

We will need to consider these other systems in their own right later. In each case, they are able to influence a wide area of the brain. Imagine the situation when one is active: there will be repercussions in a set of scattered parts of the brain. But this pattern will be a distinct one for each system since the pattern of nerve fibres of each family member is distinct. Secondly, if we focus too tightly on one system, forgetting about the others, we will lose sight of the fact that, at any one time, the brain is being affected by the combined action of the whole family. So what one is doing, to some degree, is dependent on the others. Now neuroscientists are only too human. They like to become expert in one field; indeed this is necessary if any one of them is to be able to cope with an enormous amount of information, learn some very difficult techniques, and contribute anything new.

The problem is that this tends to give rise to 'serotonin' or 'noradrenaline' or 'dopamine' experts, and so on. Each is busy with his/her own field. They hardly have time to glance at the others. Yet the brain is not built in this convenient way, nor does it function as a tightly-separated set of systems. If you alter the activity of noradrenaline, this may well have an effect on serotonin, but if you are a noradrenaline expert you may not notice (or even care). This has been a real problem. Some scientists have developed quite complex ideas of what, for example, serotonin might do in the brain: but not a mention of the other members of the family. In the next lab, all the talk is of noradrenaline and how, for example, it might influence 'arousal'. Not a thought about dopamine, or, indeed, functions other than that being studied.

Now back to serotonin. We can measure the electrical activity of serotonin neurons. Such an animal is totally unaware of the electrode in its brain, and behaves quite normally. At the moment, it is lying in the corner of the cage; but we notice that the electrodes in the serotonin nerve cells are sending out a signal about once every second (1 hertz, that is 1 pulse per second). So there seems to be 'baseline' activity: serotonin neurons

Otto Loewi, co-discoverer of neurotransmission, describes a dream revealing a way to prove their existence:

The night before Easter Sunday of that year 1920, I awoke, turned on the light, and jotted down a few notes on a tiny slip of thin paper. Then I fell asleep again. It occurred to me at six o'clock in the morning that during the night I had written down something most important, but I was unable to decipher the scrawl. The next night, at three o'clock, the idea returned. It was the design of an experiment to determine whether or not the hypothesis of chemical transmission that I had uttered seventeen years ago was correct. I got up immediately, went to the laboratory, and performed a simple experiment on a frog heart according to the nocturnal design.
(Loewi was awarded the Nobel Prize in 1936.)
E S Valenstein. (2002) The discovery of chemical transmitters.
Brain and Cognition **49**, pp. 73–95.

A commonly held hypothesis in neurobiology is that drugs and neurotransmitters bind to . . . receptors located at sites of termination of pathways containing the relevant transmitter. . . a logical expectation is that . . . the distribution of neurotransmitter receptors should closely resemble the locations of transmitter release. . . . One objective of the present commentary is to show that close transmitter/receptor matches are the exception rather than the rule. . . .
M Herkenham. (1987) Mismatches between neurotransmitters and
receptor localizations in brain: Observations and implication.
Neuroscience **23**, pp. 1–38.

tick over even at rest. That is not true for all the neurons in the brain. We leave the recording machine turned on, and watch what happens later on when the animal goes to sleep. We are intrigued to see that the serotonin cells go almost silent. If we were to continue our study, we would see a kind of daily rhythm in serotonin activity: active during the waking hours, much less so during sleep. Does this mean serotonin is concerned with sleep? There are some who thought so. Experiments on cats showed that reducing the levels of serotonin in the brain by using a drug also reduced sleep. But this did not occur in other species, and in cats the effect wore off, even though serotonin levels did not rise. Changes in serotonin may be an accompaniment of sleep (that is, an epiphenomenon), rather than a determinant. The difference is important: no good thinking of new sleeping pills based on changing serotonin if sleep is not regulated by it.

The really interesting result, however, occurs when we expose our animal to a mild psychological stress. We can put a rat into a cage belonging to another rat. Rats, like humans, find that being in someone else's territory is very stressful. Try walking uninvited into someone else's house. Despite the fact that the rat is not doing much in either situation, the activity of the serotonin system increases quite markedly. A stressed animal, it seems, activates its serotonin system. Why? And how does the serotonin system, buried deep in the midbrain, 'know' that the rat is stressed?

Let us pause for a moment, and remember that what we are measuring is electrical activity, though what we want to know about is the release of serotonin from the network of nerve fibres connected to the serotonin neurons. Neurons release their transmitters by firing off impulses down their fibres (axons). However, it is not that simple. One electrical impulse doesn't always mean one packet of transmitter; and doubling the impulse rate doesn't necessarily double transmitter release. However, if we also measure serotonin release in the parts of the brain containing the terminal network we get the same results: stress increases the release of serotonin. So we have to try to understand how serotonin fits in with our ideas on adaptation and the response to stress. Let's begin by considering what happens when we either increase or decrease serotonin levels in the brain, without stressing the animal.

You are standing at one end of a long corridor in a large building devoted to neuroscience research. Down one side is a number of doors, each a lab. Behind each door is a different, but equally intense, scientist. Hugely competitive, and deeply suspicious of each other, they do not talk much. The first lab works on the control of body temperature, the second on the release of hormones from the pituitary, the third on pain pathways in the brain, the fourth on eating behaviour, the fifth on sex behaviour, the sixth on learning. All of them, unknown to the others (communication is that bad) have been sent the same drug to test: it is one that they all know reduces the level of serotonin in the brain.

Behind each door there is equal excitement. All our scientists are getting positive results, and a positive result means a paper (an article in a scientific journal). Our first scientist finds that reducing serotonin also lowers body temperature: he concludes that serotonin controls this important physiological state. The second finds that the release of 'stress' hormones such as corticosterone from the adrenal gland is altered by lowering serotonin. She confidently concludes that serotonin regulates the pituitary. The third finds that pain responses are accentuated by the drug: serotonin is a pain-related neurochemical; a new door to pain relief? The fourth is pleased that her rats eat much more after being given the drug: serotonin reduces appetite. Obesity is a major problem; this might be a new treatment. The fifth dreams of gold after seeing that his rats mate much more vigorously: blocking serotonin might be an aphrodisiac. The sixth notices that his rats respond much more easily to a variety of stimuli, including distracting or alternative events: serotonin seems to make them more 'impulsive' or reactive. Since all our scientists are methodical people, they also try another drug that increases serotonin; and they get the (now expected) opposite result. All the doors open, and each scientist emerges, carrying a large brown envelope. You glance over their shoulders as they hurry past, ignoring each other. You see that each envelope is addressed to the editor of a different scientific journal: these, it seems, are the papers. The first is sending his to a physiological journal, the second to an endocrine one, the third to a clinical one, the fourth to a behavioural one and so on. All the papers will be published at about the same time, six months or so later. None will read the others', since the pain scientist is deeply uninterested in eating, and even the eating expert regards working on sex as slightly dubious. Perhaps this is the moment to emphasise that this is a slight caricature; most of the scientists that I know get on very well and do talk, though you might be surprised at their ignorance of each other's interests.

But serotonin is not altered only by acute stress or time of day. There is the remarkable finding that the brain's level of serotonin can be changed by what you eat. The brain makes serotonin from an amino acid called tryptophan, which enters the brain from the blood. You get your tryptophan from the proteins in your food. If you lower blood tryptophan, then brain serotonin drops, quite quickly, as well. Amongst other things, this can alter your mood, a fact which is used in clinical research on depression — as we see later. Serotonin may also reflect who you are or, more particularly, where you stand in your social group. There are some experiments suggesting that monkeys low in the social hierarchy have higher levels of serotonin. Serotonin may help protect stressed animals against some of the adverse effects of being bottom of the pile — no fun in the life of a monkey. More about this in Chapter 10. In fact, such a monkey looks distinctly depressed: we return to how depression and social life affect each other in another chapter (Chapter 12).

Leaving aside, for the moment, any Olympian attempt to synthesise a more general interpretation of all these results, we return to the subject of stress. It is clear that if serotonin is altered by stress (as it is) then this will affect a whole range of responses, and in rather a consistent way. In general, we might conclude, lowered serotonin results in reactions (whatever they may be) being intensified, whereas the opposite follows raised serotonin. Serotonin might act as a kind of neural volume control. This implies that altering serotonin may not affect the response itself, but the likelihood of it occurring in a given situation. In other words, the 'situation' (that is, the context in which the animal or person finds itself) determines what happens, but serotonin influences (or biases) the chance of it actually happening. Another way of putting it is that the impact of a stressor will be cushioned to a degree that depends upon the prevailing activity of the serotonin system.

This is rather a striking idea, though whether it can comfortably include all the experiments we have been watching is another matter. In humans, it might suggest that some people, facing a stress, become ill (e.g. depressed) if they do not have enough serotonin (discussed more fully in Chapter 12). However, further down the corridor, behind another door, is a pharmacology lab, and they have been getting results that complicate our rather simple view of serotonin and what it does in the brain.

When the midbrain serotonin neurons are activated, we can imagine a puff of serotonin being released from the nerve endings wherever in the brain there is a terminal serotonin network; the richer the network, the bigger the puff. But how does the rest of the brain know that anything has happened? Released serotonin enters the tiny space outside the nerve terminal (the synaptic cleft). At the opposite side of the cleft is part of the cell wall (membrane) of the next neuron. Only if this neuron can sense the release of serotonin, will the latter have any signalling or controlling function. Lying in the cell membrane is a very specialised, and rather complex protein structure, the receptor (similar, but not identical, to those for peptides discussed in Chapter 2). This is specially built to detect serotonin. Molecules of serotonin released into the cleft lock onto the receptor: pharmacologists call this 'binding'. Once serotonin has bound to the serotonin receptor, the next neuron can respond. That is, it 'knows' that serotonin has been released onto its cell surface. Dropping serotonin onto a cell without serotonin receptors does absolutely nothing at all. Neurons that receive a connection from the serotonin system usually have a plentiful supply of serotonin receptors, as you would expect. But there is a complication, and it is very important.

Not all the serotonin receptors are the same. They all bind serotonin, to some degree. But they have different protein structures, and what they do next (that is, what they do to the next neuron in the chain) differs. The brain has a whole family of serotonin receptors. Everyone agrees there are many, but exactly how many depends on opinion. Most scientists recognise at least seven different types, and there are subtypes within each type. The total is at least eleven, though pharmacologists have a habit of finding more and more. Thus, the response to serotonin will depend not only on how much serotonin, or where it is released, but on the mixture of receptor types on each responsive neuron. There is only one sort of serotonin; why are there so many different receptors for it?

The array of receptors has been a major boon to pharmaceutical companies. This is because different effects of serotonin can, to some degree, be related to different receptors. If a drug picked out one receptor rather than the others, it might be able to alter one function (say, eating), rather than another (say body temperature). This, of course, does not answer the 'why' question, unless you happen to believe in a deity that is particularly kind to pharmaceutical companies. Each receptor has a different sort of action. Some alter the entry of ions such as sodium or calcium into nerve cells. These will change the electrical properties of the cell membrane and either encourage or inhibit firing. Others change molecules inside the cells that have a number of actions (eg. activating enzymes, or altering the activity of genes) depending on which molecule is altered and the type of neuron in which this happens. So receptors increase the versatility of serotonin: it can do many more things in the brain than would be the case there only one serotonin receptor. Furthermore, each receptor type can be altered individually, for example by hormones. This allows a more refined control system on the action of serotonin in the brain. If only one (or two, or whatever) receptor types are increased (or decreased) then this will alter the balance of serotonin's action in a subtle way.

So many receptors vastly complicate the problem of understanding what serotonin does in the brain, and how this can change with time and circumstance. And there is more. As we have seen, serotonin is released into the synaptic cleft. Its action on the next cell (the post-synaptic neuron) depends, amongst other things, on its concentration in the cleft and how long its stays there. Serotonin neurons have a way of limiting the amount and duration of serotonin in the cleft by taking it back up again into the nerve terminal: a sort of neural vacuum cleaner. This is done by another receptor, called a re-uptake receptor, positioned on the membrane of the serotonin terminal itself, rather than the membrane of the next neuron. Anything blocking this receptor will increase the action of released serotonin. Now we can understand how SSRIs like Prozac work. They block the uptake receptor (hence their name) so effectively increasing serotonin's action. Other members of the amine family, such as noradrenaline and dopamine, also have multiple receptors (though serotonin seems to have the most), and a re-uptake mechanism. Remember that the serotonin system in the brain is only one member of a family, and that the family together probably represents less than 1 per cent of the total number of neurons in the brain. The immense complexity of serotonin is only a fraction of the total complexity of the brain. Is it any wonder that our understanding, not only of serotonin, but of the brain in general, is so incomplete? We begin to see that the statement that the human brain is the most complex object in the known world might be only too true. Your sympathy for neuroscientists deepens. But we cannot walk away; serotonin (and all the other neurochemicals) are simply too important in our lives not to be understood.

I have focussed on serotonin because it is a molecule that shows very well how a particular class of transmitter works in the brain. But, as we have already seen, it is only one member of a family. Dopamine is an equally interesting transmitter, though it is a rather less widespread in the brain. Thinking about what it might do is more easily done in another chapter (Chapter 5), but here we want to remind ourselves that it is part of the amine family, and has the peculiarities of that family. Noradrenaline is not only a member of the amine family in the brain, it is also a major hormone in the blood. It gets into the blood from the adrenal gland, not the brain. But, just like many other chemical signals that occur both in the body and the brain, the two can work together. For example, noradrenaline in the brain may increase 'arousal', it makes you more alert, and helps you focus your attention. Blood noradrenaline also goes up in states of arousal, for example when you are excited or frightened: it has major effects on raising blood pressure and heart rate, another bodily response to an arousing situation. Your survival in a tight spot may depend on your being alert. Drugs that block a particular noradrenaline receptor have been used to decrease anxiety (which is normally part of certain sorts of arousal, but can get out of hand). There is more on this in Chapter 4. But increasing serotonin also reduces anxiety.

The limbic system is full of these amines, which makes drug companies wonder whether they can produce 'limbic' drugs that pick out eating, or sex, or other limbic activities. I doubt it. Amines are not really a code in the limbic system in the same sense as peptides: there are too few of them, and not enough 'words'. But the important fact is that amines do things that are different from peptides. The major distinction is that amines seem to be able to alter a whole range of brain functions, whereas peptides are much more specific. That does not make them any less important or interesting. They may amplify or moderate the action of peptides. To understand more fully how the limbic system works, and how the brain copes with demand, we need to know much more about how these very different molecules co-operate with each other.

The third class of chemical signals I want to mention briefly here are the steroids. These are familiar molecules like testosterone, oestrogen, cortisol, progesterone. They are discussed much more fully in Chapters 4 and 8, but here we should note some important differences between steroids and the other chemicals we have been thinking about. The big difference between steroids and the other communication molecules (amino acids, peptides and amines) is that they enter the brain largely from the blood. They are made in the various hormone-producing (endocrine) glands in the body (e.g. the testis, ovary, adrenal). There is some evidence that the brain itself makes steroids, but most come from outside it. So there is no targeted 'delivery' system, no way of ensuring that steroids enter only parts of the brain. The whole brain is suffused with steroids. But there is a detection method making sure that the right parts of the brain respond to these chemical signals: only certain regions of the brain have the sort of receptor molecules that allow them to detect and respond to steroid hormones. No guesses where these are found in great profusion: the limbic system. Before we consider steroids in much more detail in other parts of this book, we need to note that they form the third great chemical code of the limbic system. Each of the three codes has, as you can see, its own peculiar features, but they work together. Together, they have kept you alive.

Chapter 4

The Brain and Stress

The idea of a state of stress is not at all new. Suppose we were to measure the heart rate and blood pressure of several people: one had just been told he had lost his job; the other had been attacked by a mugger in the street; a third had just lost a great deal of blood from a bleeding vein; and a fourth was exploring a rather dark, strange place that he found frightening. In all cases we are likely to find that the pulse quickens, the blood pressure rises, the face may grow pale and, were we to measure it, blood levels of adrenaline, the hormone secreted from the inner part of the adrenal gland, had gone up. These changes in the body, all the result of the increasing activity of the sympathetic nervous system, would not tell us which person was which. The sympathetic nervous system is a network of nerves that pass from the brain and spinal cord to activate heart, blood vessels, lungs and gut — it is our general emergency system. Note that the nature of the emergency is not specified; it could be anything that threatens us. Also note that how we react to this threat is not specified either: for example, we could either attempt to deal with it in a variety of ways or try to avoid it and run away.

This was what Walter Cannon meant, in a famous book published in 1932, when he described the sympathetic nervous system as being activated in readiness for either 'fight or flight,' the two very appropriate, but also very different, ways of tackling any (physical) threat. This system activates your heart, blood vessels and glands; it is not under your control. In an acute emergency, the body assumes that you will shortly need every muscle and every bit of attention to make sure you deal with the emergency as effectively as possible. You do not want to deflect unnecessary energy or resources onto parts of the body that are not essential for the immediate threat. This includes the gut: you can digest your lunch

65

later. So you divert blood from other areas to the muscles, and increase your heart rate and blood pressure to drive more blood every precious minute through them. You increase your blood glucose to fuel them with extra energy, and make sure your brain is extremely alert. The sympathetic nervous system does all this for you, very quickly. Since many threats will need this pattern of emergency reaction, it can usefully occur irrespective of what exactly the threat might be. It is what physiologists call an 'undifferentiated' response. You do something at once, and work out the details later. Your brain gambles on getting it right (or right enough). The odds must be in favour, since this undifferentiated way of dealing with acute stress has evidently proved effective. Mostly, we and our mammalian cousins, who have very similar sympathetic responses to an acute threat, live to fight or flee another day.

Cannon recognised that his 'fight or flight' response could be triggered by strong emotion, though he was less precise about whether any particular emotion was needed. And, of course, this leaves unanswered the vital question of how the brain generates the emotion in the first place. As you walk in the forest, you may come across a bear in the next clearing — a suitable moment for a flight response. But should it be an antelope, your reaction would be very different, and the sight of a weaker competitor might result in more fight than flight. A rustle in the undergrowth may also trigger a flight response, before you have time to know precisely what lies in wait. All this suggests that there must be room for some quite high level processing by the brain if the correct decision about how to respond behaviourally is to be made, even though the physical reaction of the sympathetic nervous system is undifferentiated. But is the emotion also undifferentiated? We might label the emotional response to an incipient (and perhaps unknown) threat as 'anxiety' or 'arousal' or even 'fear'. The exact nature of the emotion itself might not matter; it serves only to elicit the emergency response, leaving the slower, more deliberate, 'cognitive' parts of the brain to work out exactly what has happened later. We consider the difficult subject of the emotions again in Chapter 12.

If we accept this order of events, then the occurrence of stress (recognising the bear), triggers an emotional reaction, which in turn triggers the alterations in the body's physiological reaction through the agency of the sympathetic nervous system. The initial adaptation is coded

What is Stress?

Adaptability is probably the most distinctive characteristic of life. . . none of the great forces of inanimate matter are as successful as that alertness and adaptability to change which we designate as life — and the loss of which is death. Indeed there is perhaps even a certain parallelism between the degree of aliveness and the extent of adaptability in every animal — in every man.

The soldier who sustains wounds in battle, the mother who worries about her soldier son, the gambler who watches races — whether he wins or loses — the horse and the jockey he bet on: they are all under stress.

The beggar who suffers from hunger and the glutton who overeats, the little shopkeeper with his constant fears of bankruptcy and the rich merchant struggling for yet another million: they are all under stress.

The mother who tries to keep her children out of trouble, the child who scalds himself — they too, are under stress.

H H Selye. (1956) *The stress of life*. (McGraw-Hill, New York.)

In contemporary life, stress is more likely to depend on symbolic stimulus meanings than on physical features. It is our personal interpretation of real or imagined objects as actually or potentially harmful to our physical or psychological well-being that is most likely to cause us to be anxious and worried and ultimately depressed. In these cases, it is not so much the stimulus that causes stress so much as the interpretation we put upon it. We will not fully understand the psychology or biology of stress until we understand how environmental events come to acquire symbolic significance and thereby gain access to circuits that control the so-called stress responses. At the same time, from a clinical point of view, we will not fully understand how to control stress until we understand the mental events that initiate stress responses.

J E LeDoux. (1995) Setting 'stress' into motion. Brain mechanisms of stimulus evaluation. In: *Neurobiological and clinical consequences of stress: From normal adaptation to PTSD*. Eds. M J Friedman, D S Charney, A Y Deutch, pp. 124–134. (Lippincot-Raven, Philadelphia.)

. . . The modern working environment has become increasingly stressful. Changes in working patterns, combined with recession and unemployment, have meant two things for the majority of workers: greater demands and more uncertainty. Put together, these two ingredients make stress. It hardly needs by the way that the sympathetic nervous system alters the pattern of blood flow and glandular secretion in the body. This enables the initial behavioural response (fight or flight), leaving a more considered cognitive response for later — what is the bear doing there? How can I avoid it next time? Are there other bears around, and if so, where? So far, we have thought about all this without much consideration of the actual chemicals involved; but they are important.

Like all other nervous systems, the nerve cells making up the sympathetic nervous system are electrochemical machines. An electrical impulse passing down the nerve releases a chemical at the end of the nerve fibre (the synapse) which encodes what happens in the target tissue. The targets include glands (such as sweat glands), or muscle cells in the walls of blood vessels and in the heart. The chemical that is released by the sympathetic nerves is noradrenaline (called norepinephrine in the US). Here is our chemical code. Let's look at it.

Noradrenaline is so-called because it is adrenaline without a methyl (CH_3) group — that is what 'nor' means. It is rather a simple molecule, and is closely related to dopamine as well as adrenaline. It is released by the sympathetic nerves when they are activated. For many years, the whole of the sympathetic nervous system was thought to function together. Either you activated it or you did not. That view has been moderated somewhat recently, so that it is now thought that there are occasions when only part of the noradrenaline system can be active. The nerves themselves make fine, but quite wide, networks of endings in the target tissue (muscles, glands etc.). This means that although the release of noradrenaline can be limited to one or another target tissue, within the tissue itself there is a general response. Released noradrenaline is quickly sucked back up into the nerve endings, so it does not hang around for long after it has been released. Like other amines, once it is removed or metabolised, it is not used again.

One of the messages of this book is that there is a very blurred boundary between the way that chemical codes are used as neurotransmitters and as hormones, particularly in the limbic system. Noradrenaline is a marvellous example. Not only is it released by the nerve endings of the sympathetic nerves, it is also secreted from the adrenal gland (the hormone-producing gland above your kidney). The adrenal is two scientific proof, but research has confirmed that there is a close link between job security and psychological wellbeing. Many people now lack both.

Paul Martin. (1997) *The sickening mind.* (Harper Collins, London.)

Ours is not a perfect world. If it were, nations would beat their swords into plowshares, we would always find a parking spot, and the supermarket line we pick would always move the fastest. And our kidneys would filter our blood at just the right speed. But it is not a perfect world, and our bodies are forever buffeted by this imperfection. We can be seriously injured or become ill. The rains may fail, locusts may swarm, and we must spend a season hungry and walking miles to forage. We may be menaced by predators or by the aggressiveness of our own kind. Our hearts may be broken by loss. And we are smart enough to often anticipate these perturbations, or neurotic enough to decide irrationally that they are impending.

R M Sapolsky. (1992) *Stress, the aging brain, and the mechanisms of neuron death.* (MIT Press, Cambridge, Massachussetts.)

I have seen. . . a. . . rabbit dragging its hind-legs feebly and screaming while a stoat was still a dozen feet away and approaching its victim at a gentle gamble. . . It seemed to be quite healthy; I rescued it, but its eyes were already half-glazed, its heart violently palpitating, and its limbs trembling and unco-ordinated. It dies within half an hour, apparently of a heart attack on sighting or smelling the stoat. It is probable that rabbits have an innate fear of mustelids. . . .

R M Lockley. (1964) *The private life of the rabbit.*
(Andre Deutsch, London.)

concentric balls of cells: an outer layer (called the adrenal 'cortex') and an inner one (the adrenal 'medulla'). It is the latter that releases noradrenaline. The adrenal medulla is developed from the same cells as the sympathetic nervous system, but during development, the latter grow into nerve cells (with an attached nerve fibre etc.) whereas the adrenal medulla develops into gland-like cells. But both retain the same ability to release noradrenaline. The big difference is, whereas noradrenaline released from nerve terminals is limited to the region around the terminal (typical of a neurotransmitter), noradrenaline from the adrenal medulla whooshes into the bloodstream: that is, it is a typical hormone. An emergency situation releases noradrenaline from both the sympathetic nerves and the adrenal medulla. The two methods are good examples of 'anatomical' and 'chemical' addressing. The first means that there is a local and quite precise system (nerve fibres) for delivering a powerful chemical code (noradrenaline) within a particular tissue. The cells in that tissue will respond to the chemical signal provided they have the requisite receptors (receivers). Chemical addressing means that there is no limited delivery system, the chemical signal is distributed widely and generally (through the bloodstream in this case); it reaches most of the tissues, but cells only respond if they have the correct receptors. So anatomical addressing (channeled delivery) has two ways of directing the signal, chemical addressing has only one. The two addressing systems work together to help formulate the response to the emergency.

The adrenal medulla, unlike the sympathetic nervous system, also releases adrenaline. Noradrenaline and adrenaline are quite similar in their actions as well as their chemical structure (this is not always the case, sometimes a small change in a molecule profoundly alters its signalling properties), but there are some differences (e.g. on blood flow through muscles). There have been some attempts to show that the adrenal medulla releases different proportions of the two hormones under different conditions: for example, in 'anger' or 'fear'. If true, this would suggest that the adrenal had a differentiated response to particular emotional states, which would be fascinating. Unfortunately, it is not really convincing evidence. So why do we need both the adrenal medulla and the sympathetic nervous system? This seems to be an example of physiological redundancy: you can get on quite well without your adrenal medulla (but not your sympathetic nervous system). The adrenal medulla may be a kind of

The Body's Response to Stress

For more than 2000 years there has been a tradition in Western medicine that has equated health with harmony in physical and emotional life. In this tradition, disorders have been understood as disruptions of optimal relationships between different elements, and the restoration of health has been thought to require a restoration of balance. While we now know that this paradigm is oversimplified and for some disorders inaccurate, the concepts of harmony and balance nevertheless form the basis for an increasingly sophisticated model of how the body reacts with and adapts to a changing environment — a model of how what we call stress disturbs the body's normal homeostasis, and how in response the body mobilizes a group of highly specific mechanisms to defend and maintain this balance.

D Michelson, J Licinio, P W Gold. (1995) Mediation of the stress response by the hypothalamo-pituitary-adrenal axis. In: *Neurobiological And Clinical Consequences Of Stress: From Normal Adaptation To PTSD.* Eds. M J Friedman, D S Charney, A Y Deutch, pp. 225–238. (Lippincot-Raven, Philadelphia.)

The effects of stress on reproductive functions. . . depend on the type, duration and frequency of the stimulus. . . . There is. . . little doubt that though the early effect of stress may, at least under some circumstances, be stimulatory, prolonged or severe stimuli are accompanied by. . . a suppression of reproductive function. This phenomenon may have adaptive importance, that is, to 'conserve energy during hardship'.

C Rivier, S Rivest. (1991) Effect of stress on the activity of the hypothalamic-pituitary-gonadal axis: Peripheral and central mechanisms. *Biology of Reproduction* **45**, pp. 523–532.

(There are) two major components of the stress experience: effort and distress. The effort factor involves elements of interest, engagement, and determination. . . . an active way of coping, a striving to maintain control. The distress factor involves elements of dissatisfaction, boredom, uncertainty, and anxiety. It is associated with passive attitude and feelings of helplessness. . . . Effort with distress tends to be accompanied by increase of both catecholamine (noradrenaline) and cortisol secretion. . . . Effort without distress is a joyous state. . . . It is accompanied by increased catecholamine secretion. . . . Distress without effort implies feeling helpless, losing control, giving up. It is emergency backup or amplifying system that you only really need in extreme circumstances.

But does the release of noradrenaline (and adrenaline) do anything other than alter the heart and blood pressure and so on? In the late 19th century, two philosopher-psychologists (William James and Carl Lange) had an idea. Though they did not know about noradrenaline or the adrenal medulla, they did know that scary events resulted in increased heart rate, etc. and that this could be apparent to the individual concerned ('my heart is thumping'). They suggested, therefore, that the consequent emotional state (fear, anger etc.) might be the result of the brain becoming aware of these bodily states. In other words, the brain generated an emotion because the body told it something had happened, and, moreover (and this was the really interesting idea), the exact pattern of the changes in the body coded the emotional state — a certain pattern resulted in 'anger', another in 'fear' and so on. Do not underestimate the impact of this idea: it removes the control of emotion from brain to body. You will immediately see a problem with this: how does the body 'know' which pattern of response to generate without a preceding emotional state?

This idea has not really stood the test of time. The first difficulty with it is that the predicted differences in various emotional states in sympathetic and adrenal activation have not been found. Of course, this might be simply because we have not measured carefully enough, but the fact remains that an essential piece of evidence is lacking. Furthermore, if you give people the same dose of noradrenaline, you can get different emotional states. A classical experiment was to give volunteers noradrenaline (telling them it was a vitamin injection; this was done 40 years ago under rather different ethical conditions from today), and then see what emotions they reported. What they experienced was dependent on what was happening around them. If they saw something scary, they were more scared than they would otherwise be; if irritated, they became more angry and so on. Noradrenaline did not seem to generate emotion but to amplify it. I have to tell you that the experiment, classical though it may be, was not a very good one. The bottom line is that nobody believes that peripheral noradrenaline (or adrenaline) generates emotion by itself, though it may amplify emotions, particularly negative ones. Experiments in which both the adrenal medulla and the sympathetic nervous system have been generally accompanied by cortisol secretion, but catecholamines may be elevated too.

M Frankenhaeuser. (1980) A psychological framework for research on human stress and coping. In: *Achievement, stress and anxiety.* Ed. H W Krohne and L Laux, pp. 101–113. (Hemisphere Pub., Washington DC.)

Why is stress so important in chronic human disease? While transient stressors generally trigger adaptive responses, exaggerated or chronic activation of the stress system, particularly in vulnerable individuals, can have detrimental effects on a wide range of organ functions, including the brain, the immune system and the viscera.

E A Mayer and M S Fanselow. (2003) Dissecting the components of the central response to stress. *Nature Neuroscience* **6**, pp. 1011–1012.

removed have shown that rats can still learn to avoid unpleasant stimuli, and still show the behavioural signs of fear.

There are rare cases in humans of both these systems not developing since they both come from a common set of cells in the embryo, and these people, though they have many problems, are not fearless. But we are left with how to explain why peripheral noradrenaline may accentuate emotions such as fear. This is a problem because noradrenaline (and adrenaline) do not get into the brain from the blood. They are kept out by the so-called blood-brain barrier, which protects the brain from some chemicals in the blood. However, the brain can certainly detect changes in heart rate and blood pressure, and this may be the signal.

One reason that the brain keeps blood noradrenaline out may be that it has a noradrenaline system of its own. To let in peripheral noradrenaline would lead to confusion: how would the nerve cells of the brain know whether they were being 'addressed' by noradrenaline coming from the brain's private system or from the hormone liberated into the blood from the adrenals? The noradrenaline system in the brain is part of a family of systems, each with its own characteristic but related chemical transmitter (they are discussed more fully in Chapter 3). Like other members of this chemical family, which includes serotonin, as well as the closely-related dopamine and a compound called acetylcholine, the nerve cells using noradrenaline are clustered in small groups deep in the brainstem. From here, they send extensive networks of nerve fibres into many (but not all) parts of the upper brain (the forebrain) as well as down into the spinal cord. The limbic system is very richly supplied. So altered activity in the noradrenaline nerve cells of the brainstem will result in widespread changes in activity in many other parts of the brain, including the limbic system.

But what does noradrenaline do? Imagine you are on a seashore, and the waves are making a lot of noise. Someone shouts 'look-out' because of some incipient danger, but you cannot hear him against the background. Now suppose the waves are subdued, or your friend shouts louder, you hear him and take action. The waves are the 'noise' — they are not communicating specific information about an important change in your environment whereas the shout is the 'signal' — the information you need. Increasing the signal and/or decreasing the noise will improve your chances

Welcome O life! I go to encounter for the millionth time the reality of experience and to forge in the smithy of my soul the uncreated conscience of my race.

James Joyce. (1916) *A portrait of the artist as a young man.*

Of course they were frightened. They were frightened even before the creature began to crash up the stairs. The westerly was howling and threatening to drag the roof, screeching, up into the night. Clouds scudded across the top of the big skylight which always illuminated their dreams and nightmares. Through this frame they saw warty faces illuminated by thunderstorms. They watched for enemy bombers and, having freed themselves from the tight clamp of their mother's sleeping embrace, saw torn newspapers pass across the sky like migrating birds.

Peter Carey. (1985) *Illywhacker.* (Faber and Faber, London.)

Then a terrible silence fell upon us again. I was now standing up and watching a cat's-paw of wind that was running down one of the ridges opposite, turning the light green to dark as it travelled. A fanciful feeling of foreboding came over me; so I turned away, to find to my amazement, that all the others were also on their feet, watching it too.

It is not possible to describe coherently what happened next: but I, for one, am not ashamed to confess that, though the fair blue sky was above me, and the green spring woods beneath me, and the kindest of friends around me, yet I became terribly frightened, more frightened than I ever wish to become again, frightened in a way I have never known either before or after. And in the eyes of the others, too, I saw blank, expressionless fear, while their mouths strove in vain to speak and their hands to gesticulate. Yet all around us were prosperity, beauty, and peace, and all was motionless, save the cat's-paw of wind, now travelling up the ridge on which we stood.

E M Forster. (1947) *Collected short stories.*
The story of a panic. (Penguin Books, London.)

Nay, but the earth is kind to me,
Though I cry for a star, leaves and grasses, feather and flower,
Cover the foolish scar,

of detecting the warning. That is one thing noradrenaline does in the brain, and you can see how useful this could be in situations (e.g. danger) where you need your senses to be at their maximum sensitivity so your limbic system can take action.

One result of this is to increase brain states called either 'arousal' or 'attention'. Arousal is the term for a general increase in awareness of the environment — being on the 'qui vive' (alert). Attention refers to selective arousal: focussing on a particular category of stimulus. Imagine waking in the night and hearing what you think might be an intruder: you are highly aroused, but also attending specifically to noises (listening hard). Noradrenaline activity in the brain increases in both these states (there is some argument about whether more of one than the other). Infusing noradrenaline into the brain increases apparent attention in experimental animals. Drugs that block the action of noradrenaline in the brain reduce anxiety; some people take them before they do stressful things like public speaking. So noradrenaline may also be concerned with evoking the emotion we call anxiety, or even fear, an obvious adaptive advantage in conditions of real or likely danger. The brain also has a much smaller adrenaline-containing system, but what that does is much less well understood.

Noradrenaline does more than simply wake you up, increase the power of your senses or make you anxious. One of the things any animal needs to do is to learn fast about situations or circumstances that can spell danger. If you have just seen a bear in a particular part of the forest, you will not go there again in a hurry. If pulling a particular lever results in a shock, rats quickly learn not to do it. Both peripheral and brain noradrenaline can enhance the effectiveness of this type of learning. That is, noradrenaline makes sure you remember circumstances that have unpleasant emotions associated with them. Whether it also does the same for pleasant events (e.g. a joyous occasion) is not so well established but does seem rather likely. The action of noradrenaline on this type of learning may have something to do with the improved signal-to-noise ratio. If a stimulus has greater impact ('salience' as psychologists would say) then it is likely to be learned better. In the conditions of present day Western society, our chances of coming across a bear or anything like it are remote for most of us, yet we bring to our current everyday lives the adaptive

Prophets and saints and seraphim
Lighten the load with a song,
And the heart of a man is a heavy load
For a man to bear along.

> G K Chesterton. (1958) Confessional. In: *Essays and poems.*
> Ed. W Sheed. (Penguin Books, Harmondsworth.)

She had taken all the first steps in the purest confidence, and then she had suddenly found the infinite vista of a multiplied life to be a dark, narrow alley with a dead wall at the end. Instead of leading to the high places of happiness, from which the world would seem to lie below, so that one could look down with a sense of exaltation and advantage, and judge and choose and pity, it (her marriage) led rather downward and earthward, into realms of restriction and depression where the sound of other lives, easier and freer, was heard as from above, and where it served to deepen the feeling of failure.

> Henry James. (1881) *The portrait of a lady.*

Have no doubt it is fear in the land. For what can men do when so many have grown lawless? Who can enjoy the lovely land, who can enjoy the seventy years, and the sun that pours down on the earth, when there is fear in the heart? Who can walk quietly in the shadow of the jacarandas, when their beauty is grown to danger? Who can lie peacefully abed, while the darkness holds some secret? What lovers can lie sweetly under the stars, when menace grows with the measure of their seclusion?

> Alan Paton. (1944) *Cry, the beloved country.*
> (Jonathan Cape, London.)

I must say a word about fear. It is life's only opponent. Only fear can defeat life. It is a clever, treacherous adversary, how well I know it. It has no clemency, respects no law or convention, shows no mercy. It goes for your weakest spot, which it finds with unerring ease.

> Yann Martel. (2002) *Life of Pi.* (Canongate Books Ltd, Edinburgh.)

mechanisms inherited from our feral past. And we still use them, though our emergencies are less likely to be the threat of predation, but more often a dispute at work or home, a crisis or disappointment in our lives, a sudden call on our time or resources that we find difficult to meet, a near-miss in car accident. The design of our emergency system is so good that it is still doing its job, in conditions that are so different from those for which it was originally evolved.

There is another sort of learning, rather a special one, that is also altered by noradrenaline. Males of many species battle to get their genes transmitted, that is, to get females pregnant. None more so than male mice. When a pregnant female mouse mates, she 'remembers' the scent of her male. Females live in the territory of their mates, so they ought not to smell a stranger male. If they do, it must mean he has taken over the patch, and the female aborts (this is good for propagating the new male's genes, she becomes fertile again). But take away her noradrenaline and she cannot 'remember' his smell (the apostrophes indicate that this probably is not a memory in the usual sense), and so she aborts even if she smells her mate, a highly maladaptive reaction.

There is a game I like to play with my students. Cambridge University is difficult to get into. After a rather prolonged process, the day comes when the letters are posted to all applicants telling them whether they have a place. Ask any student, even two or more years later, where he/she was when the letter arrived and they will tell you, and exactly what happened in the few minutes afterwards. The event is printed on their brain like a little movie; they can relive the moment. They may remember it for the rest of their lives, for all I know. But what happened the previous day, or even the next, is completely forgotten. I cannot tell you whether this enduring memory is the result of a noradrenaline rush in their brains as the letter arrived, but I would like to think so, it fits so well what we know about noradrenaline. You will have similar memories; and people often share them. For example, in the UK, they remember where they were when they heard about the death of Princess Diana in 1997. In the US, it is the World Trade Center disaster or, for an older generation, President Kennedy's assassination. Incidentally, the brain can also store very bad personal memories in perhaps the same way, and one result may be post-traumatic stress disorder (PTSD), but that is another story (see

Arousal, Attention and Stress

To begin, let us grant, on the basis of much evidence, that a general pattern of sympathetic discharge is characteristic of emotional states. Given such a state of arousal, it is suggested that one labels, interprets, and identifies this state in terms of the characteristics of the precipitating situation and one's apperceptive mass. This suggests, then, that an emotional state may be considered a function of a state of physiological arousal and a cognition appropriate to this state of arousal. The cognition, in a sense, exerts a steering function. Cognition arising from the immediate situation as interpreted by past experience provide the framework within which one understands and labels one's feelings. It is the cognition that determines whether the state of physiological arousal will be labeled 'anger', 'joy', or whatever.

S Schachter. (1975) Cognition and peripheralist — Centralist controversies in motivation and emotion. In: *Handbook of psychobiology*. Eds. M Gazzaniga and C Blakemore, pp. 529–562. (Academic Press, New York.)

Many theories of selective attention are based on the notion of 'filtering out' input signals, either early or late. But there is a variety of evidence suggesting that such filtering does not occur. I have favored the notion, posited by others, that brain mechanisms of attention were originally derived from evolutionary pressure on an animal to select one out of a set of appropriate actions. An animal that is hungry or being threatened has to select an object or an action from many possible ones. It is obvious that the ability to choose quickly one action pattern to be carried out to the exclusion of others confers considerable selective advantage. Possessing such an ability makes it possible to achieve a goal that would otherwise be interfered with by the attempt to undertake two incompatible actions simultaneously. Survival may depend critically on this ability.

G Edelman. (1992) *Bright air, brilliant fire*. (Allen Lane, London.)

Chapter 12). I have always wondered whether those who do not get into Cambridge remember their letter in quite the same way.

Emergency responses are not all we need, for our lives are filled not so much with acute events (though they do occur) but rather with persistent stress. A job that is demanding, but over which we feel we have little control; an unsatisfactory relationship, from which there seems no resolution or escape; a loved one who is ill or otherwise endangered; a bereavement; the loss of a friend; all these are the stuff of life's slings and arrows. In animals, too, persistent demands are the rule: the constant fear of predation, the struggle to get enough food or water, the threats from other members of the group competing for scarce resources. We need a way of coping with these sorts of stress as well as with sudden emergencies.

Luckily we have one. It is back to the adrenal gland, but this time to the outer ball of cells that make up the adrenal cortex. This is a classical hormone-producing gland, and it secretes several steroid hormones. The one we are interested in is cortisol (also called hydrocortisone); in the rat, cortisol is replaced by corticosterone, a very similar compound with almost identical properties to cortisol. Some species (e.g., guinea pigs) secrete both cortisol and corticosterone. Cortisol is one of the few hormones essential for life. Complete failure of the adrenal cortex with consequent loss of cortisol (Addison's disease) was once fatal, though it is now easily treated by giving the patient the missing hormones. In normal people, the activity of the adrenal cortex varies widely during the day: in the early morning, your adrenal is producing rapid pulses of cortisol (about one per ninety minutes) so your blood levels of cortisol are quite high. As the day wears on, so your adrenal slows down, so that by the time you are thinking of going to bed, you have very little cortisol in your blood. This is a good example of a daily rhythm (called a diurnal rhythm: see Chapter 11); it is not peculiar to the adrenal, but cortisol has a particularly steep one. Think of it as a sort of daily tide of hormone. Rats, who are active at night, have the opposite rhythm: their corticosterone is highest as the night begins (and when they wake up). If you change their lighting, so that they are in the dark during your day, and in light as you sleep, then their corticosterone rhythm changes accordingly. So does yours if you fly across the world from East to West (or vice-versa) and enter a new time zone, and have to reset your sleep and wake pattern. But this takes a few days, which may be one reason why you

Corticoids and Stress

From the work of Hans Selye to the present time, we have been aware of the delicate balance between the protective effects of adrenal steroids secreted in response to stressful experiences, and the negative consequences that these same hormones have for many processes. While, on the one hand, excess adrenal steroids suppress immune defense mechanisms and cause such negative consequences as neural damage, muscular atrophy, and calcium loss from bone, the insufficiency of adrenal steroids makes the organism much more vulnerable to inflammatory disturbances and autoimmune responses, fever, and damage from catecholamine metabolites, as well as increasing fear responding and anxiety.

> B S McEwen. (1995) Adrenal steroid actions on the brain.
> Dissecting the fine line between protection and damage.
> In: *Neurobiological and clinical consequences of stress.*
> *From normal adaptation to PTSD.* Eds. M J Friedman,
> D S Charney, A Y Deutch, pp. 135–147.
> (Lippincot-Raven, Philadelphia.)

It makes its approach in so slow and insidious a manner that the patient can hardly fix a date to his earliest feeling of that languor which is shortly to become so extreme. The countenance gets pale, the whites of the eyes become pearly, the general frame flabby rather than wasted.... The leading and characteristic features of the morbid state are, anaemia, general languor and debility, feebleness of the hearts action, irritability of the stomach, and a peculiar change of colour of the skin, occurring in connection with a diseased condition of the supra-renal capsules. In some cases... a few weeks prove sufficient to break up the powers of the constitution, or even to destroy life, the result, I believe, being determined by the more or less speedy development of the organic lesion.

> Thomas Addison. (1855) On the constitutional and local
> effects of disease of the supra-renal capsules.

Increased glucocorticoids secretion is a key feature of the stress response, serving to mobilise energy substrates, inhibit non-vital processes and restore stress effector systems. However, chronic glucocorticoids excess (in Cushing's disease or during pharmacotherapy) is associated with a broad spectrum of deleterious effects including diabetes mellitus, reproductive failure, hypertension, get the state called 'jet-lag'. You need your internal and external rhythms to be in sync. This will be discussed more in Chapter 11.

But the really interesting fact is that cortisol alters its level not only as the day passes, but in response to what happens during that day. The adrenal gland is highly responsive to stress. Expose a rat to the scent of a cat, or to cold, or to anything painful and within a few minutes the level of corticosterone (I am going to call this 'corticoid', so I can use it for both corticosterone and cortisol) goes shooting up. So does yours and mine if we are faced with equivalent stressors. A job interview; an aggressive encounter; the strain of looking after a dependent relative; an illness, all these stressors result in very marked increases in corticoid levels. Unlike noradrenaline, the corticoid response can last for days or weeks. This increased corticoid level is an essential part of coping.

Some people take corticoids for other (medical) reasons. Perhaps one day they become ill, say they get pneumonia. If they do not increase their dose, they become very ill indeed, in fact, they begin to show all the signs of adrenal failure, even though they have taken their normal amount of hormone. So you really need your extra cortisol in times of need. It is embarrassing to have to admit, in this new millennium, that we do not exactly know why you need more cortisol during illness (and, presumably, other stresses as well). Somehow, the body 'knows' what it needs: so that, for instance, if you habitually secreted cortisol at stress levels without being stressed, you would again become ill, though in this case you would be suffering from Cushing's disease — a condition in which the adrenals produce much too much cortisol. The point here is that there is no correct amount of cortisol: your needs are dependent on what goes on around you, including time of day, and the appearance of stressful events in your life. Your adrenal cortex produces what you need at the time — a good example of homeostasis, and how this is a relative, not an absolute, term. But you do need to regulate cortisol according to your current needs. There are those who think the concept of homeostasis is no longer sufficient to describe such adaptive changes. They prefer 'allostasis,' which is less dependent on feedback (an essential ingredient of homeostasis) and allows for forward planning in anticipation of future needs, rather than just is response to current ones. 'Allostatic load' is thus a 'cost' of such adaptations. I think that homeostasis, understood properly, accounts for allostasis as well.

osteoporosis, immunosuppression, myopathy, growth impairment and, not least, affective and cognitive dysfunction.

J R Seckl, T Olsson. (1995) Glucocorticoid
hypersecretion and age-impaired hippocampus:
cause or effect? *Journal of Endocrinology* **145**, pp. 201–211.

We propose that (1) the physiological function of stress-induced increases in glucocorticoid (cortisol) levels is to protect not against the source of stress itself, but against the normal defense reactions that are activated by stress; and (2) the glucocorticoids accomplish this function by turning off those defense reactions, thus preventing them from overshooting and themselves threatening homeostasis.

A Munck, P Guyre, N Holbrook. (1984) Physiological actions of
glucocorticoids in stress and their relation to pharmacological
actions. *Endocrinology Reviews* **5**, pp. 25–42.

Your adrenal gland, buried deep in the abdomen just above the kidneys (hence its name), cannot know the time of day or that you are stressed, without being told by something else. The coded message that keeps it producing the right amounts of cortisol comes from the pituitary gland, lying just below the brain. The pituitary's message is encoded as a large peptide hormone called ACTH (adrenocorticotropic hormone: such a mouthful that not even medics say it). ACTH stimulates the adrenal: inject some, and there follows a brisk surge of cortisol in about 10–15 minutes. So you can get too much or too little cortisol if your pituitary does not work properly. ACTH has nothing much else to do except regulate the adrenal cortex. It is the command signal, as far as the adrenal is concerned. Note that a peptide signal has resulted in a steroid hormone being secreted; just what peptides do, they communicate. ACTH production is highest in the morning, lowest in the evening, and increases rapidly in response to stress, as you would expect.

But what tells the pituitary what time of day it is or if you are stressed? It is also buried (under your brain) and needs its own instructions, which it then passes on to the adrenal. The only organ that can tell the time of day, or know if you are under unusual demand (another term for stress) is your brain. So the brain controls the pituitary but the way it exerts this control is altogether crucial. At this point, it is important to point out that the pituitary is, in fact, two glands. The front part (anterior pituitary) is the one that secretes a number of big peptide hormones, including ACTH, and is controlled by a special set of blood vessels that deliver peptides to it from the overlying hypothalamus (recall Chapter 2).

It took until the 1970s before the molecule that acted as the chemical signal from the brain regulating ACTH was identified. It will be no surprise to you that it turned out to be another peptide, about the same size as ACTH. It is called CRF (corticotropin releasing factor) and its discovery was even more important than it appeared at the time. CRF is one of a whole collection of peptides that the hypothalamus secretes into the special system of blood vessels linking it with the anterior pituitary (discussed in Chapter 2). The precise mix (and amounts) of all these peptides determines from moment to moment, from day to day, what hormones will be released into the general bloodstream from the anterior pituitary. Not all

Allostasis

Allostasis, because it involves the whole brain and body rather than simply local feedbacks, is a far more complex form of regulation than homeostasis, yet it offers definite advantages. One is that it permits fine matching of resources to needs. In homeostasis, negative feedback mechanisms, uninformed as to need, force a parameter to a specific 'setpoint'. If blood pressure were actually determined in this way, that is set to an average, 'normal', value, it would almost invariable be too high or too low for whatever was going on at the moment. Allostasis provides for continuous re-evaluation of need and for continuous readjustment of all parameters toward new setpoints. This makes the most use of the organism's resources.

Another advantage of allostasis is its design for anticipating altered need and achieve the necessary adjustments in advance. In homeostasis, when increased need creates an 'error' signal, negative feedback mechanisms may try to correct the error, but by then the required resources may be unavailable and the time needed for corrections may be too long. Errors corrected by negative feedback can get dangerously large. . . . If one is called upon to leap into action from a sitting position, blood pressure to the head tends to fall as blood drain to the lower body. . . . The most advantageous time for resetting is *before* one leaves the chair.

P Sterling, J Eyer. (1988) Allostasis: A new paradigm to explain arousal pathology. In: *Handbook of life stress, cognition and health.* Eds. S Fisher, J Reason. (Wiley, Chichester.)

these controlling molecules activate the anterior pituitary; some inhibit it, so there are 'no-go' as well as 'go' codes. CRF is a 'go' code, and it causes a particular set of cells in the anterior pituitary to release large amounts of ACTH. CRF is quite a big peptide (41 amino-acids), and, as you would expect, the pituitary cells are sensitive to it because they have receptors for CRF. Because of the private, and focussed, anatomical delivery system (the special blood vessels) between brain and pituitary, only a rather small amount of CRF is needed to release quite a large amount of ACTH.

Stress, sensed either directly by the hypothalamus or relayed to it by other parts of the limbic system, causes the hypothalamus to release CRF into these blood vessels, which then activate ACTH, which then stimulates the adrenal cortex to secrete cortisol (corticosterone in the rat). This chain of command molecules is so arranged that each step amplifies the previous one, you need a little CRF to release a larger amount of ACTH, which then releases even more cortisol. As you might expect, since the response to stress is so universal, CRF is not the only peptide to regulate ACTH. There are quite a few others, including angiotensin (which is otherwise concerned with salt and water intake as mentioned in Chapter 6), and vasopressin, a small (8 amino acids) peptide, which we will consider in more detail later on, since it may be particularly important in the response to persistent stress. The mix of all these peptides in the blood vessels supplying the anterior pituitary is a sort of chemical sentence; the exact message ('you are stressed') has a different structure according to the context. But CRF is perhaps the most emphatic part of the signal.

The discovery of CRF (and the other 'releasing' peptides) in the hypothalamus was stupendous in its time. It showed that there was a chemical code (or series of codes) by which the brain commanded the exact mix of hormones from the anterior pituitary that circumstances demanded; but more was to come. For a decade or so, this was thought to be a peculiar, if fascinating, property of the pituitary, something that was the private interest of a rather small band of neuroendocrinologists. This comfortable notion was blown sky-high by the discovery that peptides such as CRF were not only released onto the anterior pituitary, but also found within nerve cells and fibres in the brain itself, in other words, CRF was a neurotransmitter, as well as a releasing factor. There were particularly

. . . He went in trepidation about the world, holding himself in, avoiding every conceivable object of danger. He watched the others riding bicycles in Market Street and swarming up the Martello Tower, and wading out into the middle of one of the streams, looking for fish, and caught his breath for them, terrified by their physical ease and struck dumb by the pressure of his need to warn them, warn them. Your own fault, he would have said, listen, listen, it will be your own fault, you are to blame, nobody will help you.

Susan Hill. (1971) *The albatross.* (Hamish Hamilton, London.)

Long years are not life; healthy years are life.

R Burton. *The anatomy of melancholy*

Shukhov went to sleep fully content. He'd had many strokes of luck that day: they hadn't put him in the cells; they hadn't sent the team to the settlement; he'd inched a bowl of kasha at dinner; the team leader had fixed the rates well; he'd built a wall and enjoyed doing it; he'd smuggled a bit of hacksaw-blade through; he'd earned something from Tsezar in the evening; he'd bought that tobacco. And he hadn't fallen ill. He'd got over it. A day without a dark cloud. Almost a happy day.
There were three thousand six hundred and fifty three days like that in his stretch. From the first clang of the rail to the last clang of the rail.
The three extra days were for leap years.

A Solzchenitsyn. (1963) *One day in the life of Ivan Denisovich.* (Gollancz, London.)

To have one's heart frozen and one's world destroyed in a moment — that was what it had meant. She could not draw a long breath or make a free movement in the world that was left. She could breathe only in the world she had brought back through memory. It had been, and it was gone. When she looked about this house where she had grown up, she felt so alien that she dreaded to touch anything. Even in her own bed, she lay tense, on her guard against something that was trying to snatch away her beautiful memories, to make her believe they were illusions and had never been anything else.

Willa Cather. (1935) *Lucy Gayheart.* (Alfred A Knopf, New York.)

high amounts of CRF in the limbic system, though nerve cells were found containing CRF in other parts, including the cerebral cortex. What was CRF doing in the rest of the limbic system? Not acting on the pituitary, for sure. Suddenly, hypothalamic peptides like CRF were mainstream neuroscience.

A good way to test the effects of a peptide on the brain is to infuse a small amount (peptides are very potent) into the brain ventricles, the spaces inside it that are full of cerebrospinal fluid. In one sense, this is not a very realistic experiment, because the infused peptide rapidly diffuses into most of the brain, unlike the natural condition, in which peptide is released locally from particular nerve endings. However, it does mean that if one gets an interesting effect, one can then go on and do more focussed experiments. Infusing CRF into the brain results in an extraordinary and extremely interesting result: the animal seems to become very anxious. There are various accepted ways of testing for anxiety in animals (much used by drug companies looking for new tranquillisers), and CRF is highly active in them all. Why is this so interesting?

Because here we have a behavioural action which is part of the stress response (anxiety or fear), induced by the very same peptide (chemical code) that releases ACTH from the anterior pituitary. It seems that CRF can invoke not only the hormonal, but also the behavioural response to a stressful situation. It does not stop there. If we measure an animal's heart rate and blood pressure, we see that both go up after CRF infusions. This is a direct action of CRF on the centres in the brainstem that control cardiovascular activity, independent of its ability to induce anxiety.

We can now see that 'CRF' is a misnomer: not because CRF does not do what its name implies, but because it does much more than that. Restricting its name to just one action (that on the pituitary) undervalues its biological importance. It is the same with several other hypothalamic peptides. The reason for this is the same as for CRF; they were first discovered as controllers of the pituitary, and only later was it realised that they had other, closely-related, functions. In the case of CRF, a single 41 amino acid peptide encodes a complete response to a stress (any stress). Behaviour (anxiety), hormones (cortisol) and cardiovascular activity (increased heart rate etc.) are all part of the biologically-effective response to a challenge or demand, and all are invoked by CRF. This triad of responses is by now a familiar theme: it is the means whereby any animal

The intellect of man is forced to choose
Perfection of the life, or of the work,
And if it take the second must refuse
A heavenly mansion, raging in the dark.

When all that story's finished, what's the news?
In luck or out the toil has left its mark;
That old perplexity an empty purse,
Or the day's vanity, the night's remorse.

W B Yeats. (1865–1939) *The choice.*

The day may dawn when fair play, love for one's fellow men, respect for
justice and freedom, will enable tormented generations to march forth
serene and triumphant from the hideous epoch in which we have to dwell.
Meanwhile, never flinch, never weary, never despair.

R Jenkins. (2001) *Churchill's last commons*
speech. (Churchill Macmillans, London.)

or person deals with a demand. In this case, it is a generalised response to most demands, irrespective of their precise nature. The brain has a chemical 'word' meaning 'stress'.

So the hypothalamus, the pituitary and the adrenal cortex form a functional chain (thus called the HPA axis) which is highly responsive to stress in general. There have been those who thought that the activity of the HPA axis was a sufficient and complete explanation of stress and the effects it has. Hans Selye, an Austro-Hungarian scientist who spent much of his life in Canada, was the foremost proponent of this idea. He proposed a 'general adaptation syndrome' which had a number of phases. The first was the acute response: you reacted to the onset of the stress by increasing your cortisol levels. Then came a period when your adrenals continued to enable you to deal with the stress; however, if this phase went on too long, you could develop one or other of a number of stress-related illnesses (gastric ulcer, immune failure and so on), the adrenals might begin to fail, and the stressed individual would either become very ill indeed or even die. There are two important points about Selye's ideas: the first, no longer so persuasive, is that stress equals adrenal corticoids. Nowadays we think that stress is more complex and the response to it more varied than Selye thought to be the case. Though, to be fair, his views, like those of any good scientist, changed somewhat over the course of his very productive life. The second is still very relevant: that responding to stress carries a penalty; even though one may apparently cope with it successfully, there may be a cost. Much of this cost may be due to too much corticoid, rather than (as Selye thought) too little. The cost may be considerable, as we will see later (Chapter 12).

Until recently, the parts of the brain responding to stress had to be inferred by looking at what happened in the body. For example, because the pituitary secreted more ACTH, and we knew CRF stimulated ACTH, it was assumed that the nerve cells that produced CRF were more active. But we could not know whether there were any other brain areas that were specially reactive to stress. There was no way of knowing where to look. It would be too naïve to think that only CRF was activated: and, anyway, how do the CRF cells know the individual is stressed? One way was to try to record changes in electrical activity, but this can be done on only a few cells at a time, and the problem of where to stick the electrode remained.

Psychological Reactions to Stress in Man

Historical changes in the meaning of a word are common in ordinary conversation as well as in the technical prose of scientific communities. It is not surprising, therefore, that both the sense and the referential meanings of the English words that name emotions have undergone serious transformations. John Bunyan, for example, understood fear to be an adaptive feeling because it ensured civil behavior and permitted one to love the Deity. Contemporary psychiatrists and psychologists, in agreement with the larger community, regard fear as maladaptive because it restricts freedom of action.

J Kagan, J Schulkin. (1995) On the concepts of fear.
Harvard Review of Psychiatry **3**, pp. 231–234.

Perhaps there are no more vivid memories than those which are stored in the brains of soldiers who have experienced excruciatingly horrible combat situations. Witness the account . . . of a 50-year-old Viet Nam veteran who cannot hear a clap of thunder, see an Oriental woman, or touch a bamboo placemat without re-experiencing the sight of his decapitated friend. Even though this occurred in a faraway place more than 28 years ago, the memory is still vivid in every detail and continues to produce the same state of hyperarousal and fear as it did on that fateful day.

W A Falls and M Davies. (1995) Behavioral and physiological analysis of
fear inhibition. In: *Neurobiological and clinical consequences of stress:*
From normal adaptation to PTSD. Eds. M J Friedman, D S Charney,
A Y Deutch, pp. 177–202. (Lippincot-Raven, Philadelphia.)

The Miss Haversham syndrome appears to be confined to the female sex. The usual setting is that of a young woman of exceptional beauty, domineering and intelligent, of aristocratic or well-to-do parentage. Then, at a climactic point in the personal history, comes some catastrophic disappointment: a bereavement, or a callous rebuff. From this moment, the victim chooses to opt out of life. Time stands still, and this is reflected both in her material entourage and in the realm of her body-image. . . . In the case of Queen Victoria, widowed in 1861, . . . everything remained as it had been at the time of her beloved husband's death. . . . Prince Albert's clothing was laid and pressed and ready on the bed each evening, with basins filled with fresh water as though he were still living. . . . (this) was carried out with scrupulous regularity for nearly 40 years.

M Critchley. (1979) The Miss Haversham syndrome.
In: *The divine banquet of the brain.* (Raven Press, New York.)

However, an answer was at hand, though, as often happens in brain research, it came from a very different area of science.

It has long been known that damage to DNA can cause cells to become cancerous. About 30 years ago, the exciting discovery was made that changes (mutations) in certain genes were closely associated with the development of cancer. These genes were ones that were known to be involved in some way with the growth and division of cells. Since cancer is a disorder of growth, this is what you would expect. Viruses can induce cancer in some (perhaps all) species, and it was found that one way they did this was to alter the structure of a gene called v-fos ('v' stands for viral, 'os' for osteogenic sarcoma, the kind of cancer that was produced). Of course, this meant that there must be a 'normal' gene corresponding to v-fos, and indeed there is: it is called c-fos (the 'c' means 'cellular' to indicate that it is a normal constituent of cells). All cells contain the c-fos gene, but it is only active ('expressed') when the cell is growing or about to divide. Anything that stimulates a cell to divide, therefore, activates c-fos, and it is therefore a sign of activity. You can tell when the c-fos gene is active by looking for its protein (the c-fos protein); this will only be present in the cell when the c-fos gene is expressed.

Now, conventional wisdom has it that adult nerve cells do not grow or divide. In fact, this is not entirely true, and there are exceptions that are important for our story, and to which we will return. But it is true for most nerve cells. So there is not a lot of point, you may think, in looking for c-fos expression in the nerve cells of the brain. To do so would, in scientific parlance, be counter-intuitive. Though most counter-intuitive experiments are simply wrong, occasionally (and perhaps more often than we would care to admit) they turn out to be brilliant (some call them 'Friday afternoon' experiments). In the middle 1980's, a group of American scientists looked for c-fos protein in nerve cells in culture: they found that when they added substances (like neurotransmitters) that were known to activate these cells, then they also began to express c-fos, even though they did not divide. It was not long before the intact brain was shown to express c-fos, but only in nerve cells that were stimulated. So we have a way of mapping patterns of nerve cell activity in the brain and we can use this to see which parts of the brain respond to stress.

It is clear from scientific observations that PTSD and its symptoms are present across cultures, with the only differences being the culturally specific expression of symptoms and the indigenous ways in which sufferers deal with them. Studies have shown that cross-cultural similarities and consistencies greatly outweigh cultural and ethnic differences.

> T Elbert, M Schauer. (2002) Burnt into memory.
> *Nature* **419**, pp. 883.

Life, as irritating pub philosophers say, is not fair. Research has consistently found that the higher a person's occupational grade or status (and, therefore, the higher their pay) the better their mental health, physical health and longevity. The galling truth is that the fat cats are less likely to get sick or die prematurely than those lower down the greasy pole. Sorry, but there is not an ounce of *Schadenfreude* to be had here.

> Paul Martin. (1997) *The sickening mind.* (Harper Collins, London.)

Suppose we put a rat into a plastic tube (equipped with plenty of air holes) for half an hour or so. This is not at all painful, but it is unpleasant. A rat does not like its movements to be constrained any more than you would. So it shows all the physiological signs of stress: there are increases in heart rate, blood pressure and corticoid levels in the blood. Examine its brain half an hour or so later for c-fos. You will find clumps of cells with lots of c-fos mRNA and protein, whereas in an unstressed rat there is hardly any. Nearly all of these nerve cells are in the limbic system, emphasising the central role of the limbic system in responding to stress. But there is also increased c-fos in the nerve cells of the brainstem containing noradrenaline (just as well, or our theory that noradrenaline is important for stress takes a tumble) and serotonin, as well as those known to be important for controlling heart rate etc. We have a map of the stressed brain. It is a specific map (many nerve cells are not activated) but a dispersed one (the active cells are scattered round the brain). By looking at these groups of nerve cells in more detail, we may be able to understand better which part of the brain does what.

It gets even more interesting. If we put our rat into the restraining tube every day, after a few days we notice a change in his behaviour. He no longer struggles as much, though he clearly still does not like it. But his heart rate goes up rather less, and returns to normal quicker than it did on the first occasion. His levels of blood corticosterone are less than they were, though they are still raised above normal. In other words, he has begun to adapt to the repeated stress. Now look again at the brain, the pattern of c-fos expression has also changed. It has not disappeared: some parts that were highly activated after the first stress now show hardly any c-fos, but others still show plenty. We now have a brain map of adaptation; and one that shows that different parts of the brain play distinct roles in this process. You can do the same experiment using a more biologically-meaningful stress such as your rat having to face a larger and rather aggressive second rat, and you will get roughly the same effect. Localised but dispersed c-fos expression in the brain on the first occasion, but a different pattern as your little rat copes with the daily experience of having to deal with a bigger confrere (as it must do in the wild). It is a sort of social learning.

It is no use pretending, all stories in science have messy parts. Those are the ones that we cannot explain (scientists tend to use the phrase 'not fully understood' to mean 'we have no clue'). The messy bit about the c-fos story

She would scold him — frightfully, loudly, scornfully, and worse than all, continually. But of this he had so much habitually, that anything added might be borne also — if only he could be sure that the scoldings would go on in private. . . . But to be scolded publicly was the great evil which he dreaded beyond all evils. . . .When that voice was heard aloud along the corridors of the palace. . . and when he was compelled to creep forth from his study, at the sound of that summons, with distressed face, and shaking hands, and short hurrying steps — a being to be pitied even by a deacon — . . . than, at such moments as that, he would feel that any submission was better than the misery he suffered.

Anthony Trollope. (1867) *The last chronicle of Barset.*

(Penguin Books, Harmondsworth.)

The world's a stage. The trifling entrance fee
Is paid (by proxy) to the registrar.
The Orchestra is very loud and free
But plays no music in particular.
They do not print a programme, that I know.
The cast is large. There isn't any plot.
The acting of the piece is far below
The very worst of modernistic rot.

Hilaire Belloc. (1870–1953)

They lived too many to a room. There was no sanitation. The streets reeked of shit. Children died of mild colds or slight rashes. Children died on beds made from two kitchen chairs pushed together. They died on floors. Many people believed that filth and starvation and disease were what the immigrant got for his moral degeneracy.

E L Doctorow. (1976) *Ragtime.* (Pan Books, London.)

They left the busy scene, and went into an obscure part of the town, where Scrooge had never penetrated before, though he recognised its situation, and its bad repute. The ways were foul and narrow; the shops and houses wretched; the people half-naked, drunken, slipshod, ugly. Alleys and archways, like so many cesspools, disgorged their offences of smell, and is that we do not really know what c-fos does in stress. The c-fos protein (usually called Fos) regulates DNA. That is, when the c-fos gene is activated, its Fos protein goes back into the nucleus of the nerve cell, and binds to specific regions of DNA. It does this to regulate the expression of other genes, so that Fos is one of a large number of 'transcription regulators.' The problem with this is that we do not know which of the genes important for stress it is regulating. Some may be directly concerned with organising the stress response, but others may not. The trail goes rather cold at this point. An obvious possibility is that Fos and similar proteins regulate the amount of CRF and other peptides in the brain: this still is not certain.

Peptides in the limbic system are clearly very important in encoding the response to stress. What do they encode? In the hypothalamus, they ensure that our physiological systems (hormones, cardiovascular system) are in a stress-ready state. In other parts of the limbic system they induce other, equally important, parts of this state. For example, CRF infused into the amygdala, a nut-shaped part of the limbic system lying deep beneath the lower part of the cerebral cortex (discussed more in Chapter 10), makes an animal more anxious: an essential behavioural ingredient of being stressed. This is also a great example of the same peptide doing different, but related, things in different parts of the limbic system, physiological actions in the hypothalamus, but behavioural (emotional) ones in the amygdala. Two coding processes are interacting: a chemical code (in this case, CRF) and an anatomical one (hypothalamus vs. amygdala).

Peptides also change as an animal adapts to a continuing stress. In the hypothalamus, many of the nerve cells that contain CRF also contain a second peptide, vasopressin (much smaller). If you were to measure the amounts of CRF and vasopressin in the hypothalamus after an initial stress, you would find large amounts of CRF but rather little vasopressin. But after a few days of repeated stress, the picture changes: now there is less CRF but much more vasopressin. The two peptides act together on similar (but not identical) targets. This altered peptide code represents part of adaptation. The hypothalamus has recognised that the stress is a repetitive or chronic one, and has adjusted its code accordingly. What tells it? One signal is cortisol. It is greatly increased by stress, as we have seen, and this continuous signal tells the hypothalamus that the stress is persistent, and results in changes in expression of the CRF and vasopressin genes.

dirt, and life upon the straggling streets; and the whole quarter reeked with crime, with filth, and misery.

Charles Dickens. *A Christmas Carol.*

He was a tall blonde from Michigan, probably about twenty, although it is never easy to guess ages of marines at Khe Sanh since nothing like youth ever lasted in their faces for very long. It was the eyes: because they were always either strained or blazed-out or simply blank, they never had anything to do with what the rest of the face was doing, and it gave everyone the look of extreme fatigue or even a glancing madness.

Michael Herr. (1977) *Dispatches.* (Alfred A Knopf, New York.)

When my father came down he was quiet. . . he was tired, his eyes were red and inflamed, and his cheeks sunken and dark with fatigue. His whole appearance was one of unspoken reproach. I would have bled rather than hurt him, rather than have him condemn me. . . . His head turned and his eyes flared at me with hate and disgust. I felt myself colouring and burning. His punishment was no longer physical, but when it appeared, it was more implacable than his occasional blows. I was terrified with fear and love of him; of when he had hit my brothers and I had screamed at their helplessness, at the break in their dignity, tearing at my chair when he beat them. . . . He had a miner's indifference to the physical, a savage complacency, that (linked) his silent approach on me with a long association of childhood meanings.

David Storey. (1960) *Flight into Camden.*
(Longmans, Green, London.)

So we are beginning to understand the brain chemistry of adaptation, successful adaptation, we suppose. An intriguing thought is that this may also tell us something about unsuccessful adaptation, the cost we mentioned earlier. Before we pay more attention to the costs of adapting to stress, we should go for a walk in the hypothalamus.

We take with us a friendly neuroanatomist. We shall need to become, for a while, one of those creatures in animated films that take tours of the human body. In we go, into the special world of the base of the forebrain, just above the pituitary. Immediately we see all around us bundles of cables that we recognise as nerve fibres. Some seem to be passing right through the space in which we now stand, the hypothalamus itself. But others run between great clumps of what look like surreal trees; surreal because they form three dimensional floating groves, rather than the terrestrial ones we are accustomed to in real life. Each grove is a group of nerve cells, what anatomists call a 'nucleus' and we splash our way towards one, for the tissue we are in is quite wet. It is large, and we push our way through the first of the 'trees' into its centre, and peer out of the other side of our thicket. We spy a thin, flat three-dimensional lake. Our companion, the neuroanatomist, tells us that this is a ventricle, a fluid-filled space that lies between the hypothalami of the two sides, right in the middle of the brain; dimly we see the shore of the opposite hypothalamus. If we look in other directions, we see more bundles of fibres and, distantly, other great clumps of bushy nerve cells, floating round bodies in the hypothalamic firmament.

Then he tells us that our clump is called the 'paraventricular nucleus' (PVN, for short) because it lies so close to the ventricle. A neutral name, telling us nothing about what it might do. The anatomist invites us to look more closely at the groups of neurons that make up the PVN. All around are tree-like nerve cells. But we can see they are not all the same. Just like a real orchard, there are clusters within this three-dimensional orchard of similar types of 'tree' (nerve cells). Here is one of 'apple' trees, there another of 'pears', over the way, a bunch of 'plums.' The cells of the PVN are not all the same. There is an internal organisation. What we take for fruit are, in fact, different neurochemicals. Just as fruit distinguishes trees, so their content of neurotransmitters is a good way of classifying nerve cells. We see a cluster of huge neurons in one corner: the neuroanatomist tells us that they are called, naturally enough, magnocellular neurons

All About the Hypothalamus

... Numerous foci are present in the hypothalamus from which quite characteristic behavioral patterns can be elicited on electro-stimulation, including eating, drinking, grooming, fear, attack, rage and reproductive behavior. All of these behavioral patterns are related to the maintenance of the internal milieu (homeostasis), to the maintenance of the integrity of the individual or to the preservation of the species. In fact, the entire hypothalamus can be defined as a center which generates integrated somatomotor, visceromotor and endocrine responses directly aimed at the survival of the individual and of the species.

> R Nieuwenhuys. (1996) The greater limbic system, the emotional motor system and the brain. In: *Progress in brain research.* Eds. G Holstege, R Bandler, C B Saper, **107**, pp. 551–580. (Elsevier Science.)

People tend to stay away from the hypothalamus. Most brain scientists... prefer the sunny expanses of the cerebral cortex to the dark, claustrophobic regions at the base of the brain. They think of the hypothalamus — though they would never admit this to you — as haunted by animal spirits and the ghosts of primal urges. They suspect that it houses, not the usual shiny hardware of cognition, but some witches' brew of slimy, pulsating neurons adrift in a broth of mind-altering chemicals.

S LeVay. (1993) *The sexual brain.* (MIT Press, Cambridge, Massachusetts.)

Stimuli that are interpreted by the brain as extreme or threatening, regardless of their modality, elicit an immediate stereotypic response characterized by enhanced cognition, affective immobility, vigilance, autonomic arousal and a global catabolic state. The brain's ability to mobilize this so-called stress response is paralleled by activation of corticotropin-releasing hormone (in several nuclei, including the hypothalamus, amygdala and locus ceruleus, and stimulation of the locus ceruleus norepinephrine (noradrenaline) system in the brain stem. These systems perpetuate one another, interact with several other transmitter systems in the brain and directly activate the hypothalamic-pituitary-adrenal axis and the three components of the autonomic nervous system, namely the sympatho-adrenal, the cranio-sacral parasympathetic and the enteric nervous systems.

> K E Habib P W Gold, G P Chrousos. (2001) Neuroendocrinology of stress. *Endocrinology and Metabolic Clinics of North America* **30**, pp. 695–728.

('big nerve cells'); we are not much impressed by the imagination of neuroanatomists. But there are other clusters of much smaller cells. Each has its own collection of neurochemicals. We also notice bundle of fibres entering and leaving each cluster; each group of fibres seems to come and go in different directions. We ask the neuroanatomist, our guide, why he has chosen the PVN, of all nuclei in the hypothalamus, for us to visit. He sits on a nearby nerve cell, and tells us the following story.

You are, he says, in the middle of an extraordinary structure. This is the control centre of the stress response. Within its cells are myriad codes, many of them different peptides, that specify one or another way of responding to stress. He points to a clump of cells just over our heads, and we can see that this contains CRF, but also some vasopressin. But there are other types of nerve cell, each containing its own mix of peptides. And we see that, unlike the trees in our terrestrial orchard, these 'trees' not only send off nerve fibres to other places, they also receive them. We are sitting in the middle of a three-dimensional electro-chemical computer, rather than an orchard. Some of the incoming fibres, we notice, carry a substance we recognise as noradrenaline, and peering deeply into the brainstem, we see they come from those clumps of nerve cells that specialise in this neurochemical. We recall its role in stress. Floating around in the cells of the PVN are big structures that our neuroanatomist tells us are the receptor molecules for cortisol. As we watch, molecules of cortisol arrive, attach themselves to these receptors, and are whisked off to the nerve cells' nucleus; we can see them sticking to those familiar coiled structures we recognise as DNA. Genes begin to buzz. There is lots of information coming into the PVN.

And plenty going out. Fibres passing down towards the pituitary, and to the amygdala, and to the brain stem. The PVN is indeed a control centre, sending peptide-encoded messages to other parts of the limbic system as well as direct instructions to the pituitary and the brainstem. The neuroanatomist points to the those big neurons (the magnocellular ones) and shows us that they are actually pumping peptides (including vasopressin) directly into the bloodstream of the body, just like any other hormone-producing gland. So the PVN can send 'private' peptide messages to the anterior pituitary, but more general ones via the bloodstream. What a busy, versatile structure! It is beginning to make sense: inputs from systems (such as noradrenaline and cortisol) that are responsive to stress,

. . . A man is likely to find the prospect of worldly ruin ghastly enough to drive him to the most uninviting means of escape. He will probably prefer any private scorn that will save him from public infamy. . . to the humiliation and hardship of new servitude in old age. . . . . But though a man may be willing to escape through a sewer, a sewer with an outlet into the dry air is not always at hand.

George Eliot. (1866) *Felix Holt.*

The land was open here and bare and the people looked bent and small under the sky, and they walked as if they were pushing against a current, their bodies bending and straining forward. First there was a man pulling a two-wheeled cart, and beside him walked his woman and behind, painfully, their eyes on the cart, keeping up with it, trying not to be lost and left behind, came the old people, the man walking with a stick, the woman shading her eyes, her face soft and folded with age, but gaunt with weariness. The cart was piled high with mattresses and blankets, the pots tied on behind clinked cheerfully. The younger women opened her worn black purse and took out a large piece of dry bread. She did not stop walking. She carved off a strip of the bread and handed it to the man. He shook his head; he could not pull the cart with one hand, and they must keep walking.

Martha Gellhorn. (1940) *A stricken field.*

(Virago Modern Classics, London.)

There is, sometimes in thunder, another person who thinks for you, takes in one's mental porch furniture, shuts and bolts the mind's window against what seems less appalling as a threat than as some distortion of celestial privacy, a shattering insanity in heaven, a form of disgrace forbidden mortals to observe too closely: but there is always a door left open in the mind — as men have been known in great thunderstorms to leave their real doors open for Jesus to walk in — for the entrance and the reception of the unprecedented, the fearful acceptance of the thunderbolt that never falls on oneself, for the lightning that always hits the next stress, for the disaster that so rarely strikes at the disastrous likely hour. . .

Malcolm Lowry. (1947) *Under the volcano.*

(Penguin Modern Classics, London.)

outputs to structures (pituitary, amygdala, brainstem) that are essential for the response that may save our life when we are stressed. Time to leave the hypothalamus, and take a broader view.

The path through life is a rugged one. Although we have developed, through ages of evolution and selection, the means to defend ourselves against stress, indeed, would never have arrived as a species without being able to do so — we pay a price. Everything we do has a cost. Reproduction carries a cost, so does going out to get our food (particularly if, as in primeval times, we had to find it, chase it, and kill it; but even today, we have to pay something). Fighting off an infection carries a cost: we are left weakened for a time. Defending ourselves against stress carries a cost: the hope is that our brain can calculate the relative risks of the penalties we may have to pay by either not adapting adequately or paying whatever price adaptation will cost, and make the right choice. But any brain, any biological system, is not infallible. It makes mistakes. It can afford to do so, provided it gets enough right to tip the balance in favour of the survival of the species. But individuals may go to the wall. We now know enough about the consequences of stress to realise that not everyone copes with it adequately; and even those who seem to cope may pay a steep price.

Persistently high cortisol has curious effects. It dampens down your immune system (it is used for this clinically), it delays wound healing, it reduces inflammation. Not very helpful during stress, you would think, which can include increased chances of wounds and infections. Yet, as we have seen, we need extra cortisol in times of stress. One way round this apparent dilemma is the idea that higher cortisol stops you overreacting to stress. There is not a great deal of hard evidence for this, but it remains a popular notion. But there is increasing evidence that persistently high cortisol may be bad for the brain.

Imagine walking along a cliff path, when a sudden gust of wind blows you towards the edge. Whether you go over or not depends on several things, including the strength of the gust, but also how near you are to the edge at the time. Now apply this to the brain, or rather, to some agent (a toxin, a lack of oxygen as in a stroke) to the brain. Whether your brain is damaged depends also on many things, the severity of the attack and so on. But high cortisol seems to push the brain nearer the brink; it's called

Pain took hold. First a fluttering as of doves in her stomach, then a kind of burning, followed by a spread of thin wires to other parts of her body. Once the wires of liquid pain were in place, they jelled and began to throb. She tried concentrating on the throbs, identifying them as waves, hammer strokes, razor edges or small explosions. Soon even the variety of the pain bored her and there was nothing to do, for it was joined by a fatigue so great she could not make a fist or a fight the taste of oil at the back of her tongue.
Toni Morison. (1980) *Sula*. (Chatto and Windus, London.)

Most people do not wish to remember suffering. My concern is not to forget it. It is not merciful to forget; to obliterate the live sore of remembrance with creeping, bloodless scar tissue. For me, always the unabated rawness, the fresh profitable spur of pain.
Han Suyin. (1952) *A many-splendoured thing.*
(Jonathan Cape, London.)

'endangerment'. Raise cortisol levels and agents that would be resisted now provoke damage, or a small amount of damage becomes larger. Cortisol pushes the brain nearer the edge.

Cortisol may even damage the brain by itself. We return to this topic later (Chapter 12), but here let us simply note that high cortisol can interfere with certain forms of memory, and even induce depressed mood. Experimentally, high cortisol can damage nerve cells directly, or increase their sensitivity to substances like amyloid, an abnormal protein that is suspected of contributing to the brain damage seen in Alzheimer's disease. And now to something extraordinary: certain parts of your brain go on making new nerve cells throughout life. This is astonishing because it was always thought that this process stopped either at or shortly after birth. In your hippocampus, for example, a region known to be important for memory, new nerve cells are being made all the time. Is this important? We do not know yet. But what we do know is that high cortisol suppresses this activity.

Cortisol levels may have more sinister consequences or implications. A few weeks after experiencing some disaster in their lives (usually a loss of some sort), a small proportion of people become depressed. We now know that those with higher cortisol levels, from whatever cause, have a greater risk of reacting in this way. We will discuss this in more detail in Chapter 12, but it represents another 'cost' of adaptation and example of 'endangerment'.

Age increases the brain's susceptibility to damage. Cortisol goes up slightly if at all with age but what goes down is another steroid from the adrenal called DHEA (dehydroepiandrosterone). DHEA is very low at birth, goes up rapidly to very high levels during later childhood, adolescence and in young adults. Then, remorselessly, it goes down, down, down, every year, every decade, so that by the time you're 70 or so it is about a quarter of what it was at 20. Does this matter? Many people (particularly in the US) take DHEA as an anti-aging pill. The interesting thing is that DHEA can restrain the action of cortisol. So if you have low DHEA, your brain may react more to your cortisol (in effect, it is more potent) and stress may have a greater effect. DHEA reduces some sorts of brain damage, and prevents cortisol interfering with those new nerve cells in the hippocampus. Is this why older brains are more vulnerable to damage?

During the early days and weeks of her solitude Frances had come to realise that grief like illness is unstable; it ebbs and flows in tides, it steals away to a distance and then comes roaring back, it torments by deception. On some mornings, she would wake and Steven's presence was so distant and yet so reassuring that she thought herself purged; he seemed both absent and present, she felt close to him and at the same time freed, she thought that at last she was walking alone. And then, within hours she would be back once more in that dark trough: incredulous, raging, ground into her misery.

Penelope Lively. (1983) *Perfect happiness.*
(William Heinemann, London.)

I stopped going out; I stopped wanting to go out. That happens very easily. It's as if you had always done that — lived in a few rooms and gone from one to another. The light is a different colour every hour and the shadows fall differently and make different patterns. You feel peaceful, but when you try to think it's as if you're face to face with a high, dark wall. Really all you want is night, and to lie in the dark and pull the sheet over your head and sleep, and before you know where you are it is night — that's one good thing. You pull the sheet over your head and think, 'He got sick of me,' and 'Never, not ever, never.' And then you go to sleep. You sleep very quickly when you are like that and you don't dream either. It's as if you were dead.

Jean Rhys. (1943) *Voyage in the dark.* (Constable, London.)

*Seventeen years ago you said
Something that sounded like Good-bye;
And everybody thinks that you are dead,
But I.*

*So I, as I grow stiff and cold
To this and that say Good-bye too;
And everybody sees that I am old
But you.*

Is this why younger people withstand stress better than older ones? For example, elderly people who are burgled (a huge stress) have a markedly increased chance of dying before they otherwise would. We do not really know yet, but it is worth finding out. By the way, DHEA is also reduced by stress.

But it is important to remember that cortisol is not always the villain. Not only do we need extra cortisol to survive stress, as we saw, but this cortisol may act on the brain to improve memory for dangerous or unpleasant events, rather like noradrenaline. It is interesting that the two molecules, so different, act together. They seem to need each other to be able to affect memory. A chemical syntax for stress. Your limbic system tries to ensure that the balance between the benefits and the costs of adaptation to stress come out in your favour. Most of the time, it succeeds. Sometimes, it does not.

And one fine morning in a sunny lane
Some boy and girl will meet and kiss and swear
That nobody can love their way again
While over there
You will have smiled, I shall have touched your hair.

Charlotte Mew. (1869–1928) *A Quoi Bon Dire.*

Chapter 5

The Weight-Watcher in the Brain

The helicopter takes us to this uninhabited valley, lush and distant. We land in a clearing, and our pilot helps us unload several packages for our four day stay. It only takes a few minutes, and with a cheerful wave he takes off, leaving us with the intense silence you only get in utterly remote parts of the world. We unpack, checking that we have no phone or any other sort of communication. After all, we want to be alone for the next few days. Then we notice that there does not appear to be any food. Surely this was not planned? No matter, we say to each other in the euphoria of a new experience: we will live off the land. After all, our forebears did just this. The valley looks verdant and fertile, and we can hear the noise of running water nearby.

It is only after we have put up our little tent, and arranged our deliberately meagre belongings, that we begin to feel hungry. We look around for something to eat. There is not anything remotely edible. Plenty of trees, but we cannot really eat leaves. We recall that certain monkeys can, but they have specially developed guts to deal with high bulk, low calorie food. Neither can we eat grass, as ruminants do: they have specially-designed guts as well. But even they spend much of their waking life looking for vegetation to eat; the calorie yield is so low. Fruit or berries? There is no obvious fruit around, and the few red berries give a warning rather than an appetising signal. We realise that in the primeval world food does not lie around. You have to go and get it. Know where to look. Find it. Catch it. Even compete for it.

How different from the world we have so recently left. We begin to have nostalgic thoughts about fridges, or walking down to the local supermarket, or opening a tin. In our world, food does lie around. But only

Regulating Body Weight

It is now clear that factors influencing food intake play a much greater role for weight maintenance than changes in energy expenditure, as the former can reverse, whereas the latter can only attenuate the effects of previous differences between energy intake and expenditure. Human beings' great tolerance for substantial daily variations in energy expenditure and food intake makes it very difficult to establish which among the many known regulatory effects are likely to play dominant roles.

A Astrup and J P Flatt. (1996) Metabolic determinant of body weight regulation: In: *Regulation of body weight; Biological and behavioural mechanisms.* Eds. C Bouchard and G A Bray. (John Wiley and Sons, London.)

. . .Hunger is neither a necessary nor a sufficient condition for eating. People can refrain from eating in the presence of hunger and can apparently consume food in the absence of hunger. . . .

It could be supposed that energy intake and energy expenditure are controlled in harmony to regulate body weight. In practice, it is difficult to demonstrate such reciprocal function. It seems likely that we are dealing with two systems that are only loosely and imperfectly coupled.

J E Blundell. (1996) Food intake and weight regulation. In: *Regulation of body weight; Biological and behavioural mechanisms.* Eds. C Bouchard and G A Bray. (John Wiley and Sons Ltd, London.)

Food intake in humans and almost all animals occurs in bouts or meals. Meals are the basic unit of analysis because to understand meal size and number would be to understand food intake. What physiological signals initiate meals? What maintains meals? What ends them?

James Gibbs. (1994) The physiological control of food intake. *Contemporary Nutrition*, Vol 19.

because we have arranged things that way. Cultivation and domestication have resulted in food being concentrated in fields or farmyards, in yields being increased by genetic engineering (though for most of recorded history, people did not realise this was what they were doing), and in food becoming comparatively cheap. Getting food now involves reduced amounts of physical effort; no more chasing after game that does not want to be caught. We need to use fewer resources to get food, including the money to buy it, and hence the amount of work needed to provide that money. We now live in a world stacked with cheap, palatable, easy to prepare, food. Rather, the 'developed' world lives that way. In other parts, it is still a different story.

Wild animals also live in a food-scarce world. For them, there is no well-stocked fridge, or the convenience of a nearby supermarket. Those that eat meat often have to wait days for a decent meal, and then gorge themselves so that they can make do throughout the almost inevitable wait until the next kill. Whatever extra skill or physique predators may develop is usually matched by opposing developments in their prey. The majority of hunts by lions end in failure. The energy expended in these hunts, whether successful or not, is considerable. A wild animal has to balance expending this resource against the likelihood of making a kill, or the possible risk of going without food for an extended period. Species that live off vegetation also pay a price as they spend much of their time feeding, since the nutritional value of vegetable food is usually less than animal food. But they are also subject to the vagaries of season or climate, and spending so much time with your head down looking for food is not the best way to avoid becoming food yourself.

So sitting in our now-not-so idyllic valley, we face the same problems as our ancestors. How do we obtain sufficient energy in a world in which this is hard to come by? Luckily, we know the helicopter will come back in a few days, and that even if we fail to find anything to eat, we will still be alive, though possibly possessing a more elegant shape. We will survive because the body has well-developed means for combating starvation. The scarcity and inconsistency of the primeval food supply makes this essential. No good having the most elaborate body if it fails after a few days without refuelling. The body therefore needs to 'know' when there is not enough energy supply (food); it also needs to know

Heaped up on the floor, to form a kind of throne, were turkeys, geese, game, poultry, brawn, great joints of meat, plum-puddings, barrels of oysters, red-hot chestnuts, cherry-cheeked apples, juicy oranges, luscious pears, immense twelve-cakes, and seething bowls of punch, that made the chamber dim with their delicious steam. In easy state upon this couch, there sat a jolly giant, glorious to see; who bore a glowing torch, in shape not unlike Plenty's horn, and held it up, high up, to shed its light on Scrooge, as he came peering round the door.

Charles Dickens. *A Christmas carol.*

He began to eat the cabbage with what was left of the soup. A potato had found its way into one of the bowls, . . .a medium-sized spud, frost-bitten, hard and sweetish. There wasn't much fish, just a few stray bits of bare backbone. But you must chew every bone, every fin, to suck the juice out of them, for the juice is healthy. Today was red-letter day for him: two helpings for dinner, two helpings for supper. . . .

He supped without bread. A double helping and bread — that was going too far. The bread would do for tomorrow. The belly is a rascal. It doesn't remember how well you treated it yesterday, it'll cry out for more tomorrow.

A Solzehenitsyn. (1963) *One day in the life of Ivan Denisovich.* (Gollancz, London.)

. . . Mr Luce, her worthy husband, a tall, lean, grizzled, well-brushed gentleman who wore a gold eye-glass and carried his hat a little too much on the back of his head. . . . went every day to the American banker's, where he found a post office that was almost as sociable and colloquial an institution as in an American country town. He passed an hour (in fine weather) in a chair in the Champs-Elysees, and he dined uncommonly well at his own table, seated above a waxed floor which was Mrs Luce's happiness to believe had a finer polish than any other in the French capital. Occasionally, he dined with a friend or two at the Café Anglais, where his talent for ordering a dinner was a source of felicity to his companions and an object of admiration even to the head-waiter of the establishment. These were his only known pastimes, but they had beguiled his hours for upwards of half a century. . . .

Henry James. (1881) *The portrait of a lady.*

when the body stores of energy are sufficient. Because of our biological past, we bring into the present world of plenty a body adapted for a world of scarcity, and one that is superbly equipped to detect shortage and to deal with it in a way that maximises survival. But it is not so bothered about excess. Having too much food is an unusual situation in the 'real' world. The only animals that are commonly persistently fat are those who share our environment: the domesticated species. Some wild species put on temporary fat in times of plenty (eg. the summer) as a precaution for the lean times ahead (winter). Other animals, such as gerbils, stay slim in their natural habitat, but become obese and diabetic in captivity, when food becomes easy to get.

The body does not 'know' anything about your energy supply, or whether you need food, or whether you have enough stored energy; but the brain does. And it does a very good job. As we sit on a grassy hillock in our picturesque but apparently food-free valley, dreamily thinking about hamburgers, we recall that our body weight has, for the most part, remained quite steady for the last ten years or so, as is the case for most (but not all) people. We reflect on how this can come about: after all, we have not weighed ourselves every day, nor paid much attention to how much we eat, only eating enough to be reasonably satisfied after each meal; occasionally gorging ourselves (a night out, perhaps), or even missing a meal (too rushed for breakfast). Nevertheless, despite lack of conscious thought our weight is maintained, except in those who diet. Furthermore, some are persistently fatter than others. Our brain is good at keeping our body weight reasonably constant, regardless of day-to-day alterations in food intake.

A moment's thought will show you that achieving this is not a simple matter. We remember, with increasing fondness, the good breakfast we had in the base camp before we left for the valley. We ate as much as we cared to, as we had the day before, and the day before that. But after a while, something stopped us eating. Had we been asked why we stopped, we would have said we were 'full' or 'had had enough'. In other words, we were satiated. Now, it is quite impossible that the body could, in the 30 minutes or so we were at breakfast, estimate how much our energy stores would change as the result of our breakfast. Yet something stopped us eating. So there must be a short-term 'satiation' signal which is responsible

The smell of wine and sweet chicken meat. The waiter bringing sprouts and baked potatoes. . . . O that thing called food. . . if I ever had money I'd have all my friends to a place of mine in the country where we would sit to a table an Irish mile long with our fists greasy with the lashings of beef and turkey and our women coming from the fire groaning under the weight of the wild berries and plover plucked from the sky, and the bulls' heads for sport. . . . O have you ever heard of oats. Or spuds fit to put heathen desires in ye for the rest of your life. Mary leave some chicken for me.

J P Donleavy. (1955) *The ginger man.* (Corgi Books, London.)

It is always easier to eat things if you know what they are called or, better, if you know what they are made of. There was no cosmological structure in Mahalingam's meal, at least none that could make sense to a Western mind. To begin with what looked like beef rissoles in black sauce and find them to be piercingly sweet cakes in honey was disconcerting. I mean, a Western banquet recapitulates the history of the earth from primal broth through sea beasts to land predators and flying creatures and ends with evidence of human culture in cheese and artful puddings.

Anthony Burgess. (1980) *Earthly powers.*

(Hutchinson and Co, London.)

for the ending of a meal. Then a second mechanism kicks in: one that determines the interval between this meal and the next when we become hungry again. This can quite easily use energy stores as a marker, since the interval allows two processes to occur: our food to be converted into storable energy, and a reassessment of the amount of energy in those stores. This enables us to compensate for a big meal by extending the interval to the next, or eating again sooner if we have had an unusually light breakfast. The brain has to arrange that the 'satiation' system and the 'interval' system work together in such a way that our body weight remains approximately the same. Experiments show that it can: children, for example, compensate for extra calories at one meal by taking fewer at the next. But the two mechanisms are quite different, and making sure the two together achieve the desired steady state (body weight) is a complex computational problem. How does the brain do it?

Let's start with ending a meal. The obvious answer is that a full stomach signals satiation: hence the usual way of saying you are no longer hungry. Obvious, but not sufficient. Those with their stomach removed, or partially removed, still stop eating, though reducing the size of the stomach surgically is used to treat extreme obesity. A famous experiment, in which swallowed food was diverted from the stomach back into the outside world through a fistula, proved the same point. However, allow the food (particularly fat) to enter the next part of the intestinal tract and you get a different result: the meal is likely to end. Some signal from the small intestine evidently tells the brain you have had a meal. It is not distention, either, because simply distending the gut won't do. But it is not the only signal. As you eat your breakfast, your blood glucose increases. In response to this, you secrete more insulin, the hormone that allows you to make use of the increased glucose, and which is missing in the juvenile form of diabetes (type 1 diabetes). There is good evidence that your brain senses changes in blood glucose, and also in insulin, and that this may play a part in satiety. As you break down the protein in your food, levels of amino acids, which are the building blocks of proteins, increase in the blood. These, too, may signal to the brain that you have eaten. And your liver, which is busily converting your food to useful compounds, also sends its own signals to the brain. Regulating food intake is so important that the brain gets multiple chemical messages about the food you eat. In general, the

Leptin

The discovery of (leptin), a singular event in my life, was absolutely exhilarating. The realization that nature had happened upon such a simple and elegant solution for regulating weight was the closest thing I have ever had to a religious experience.... It is as yet unclear whether I will succeed in understanding how a single molecule can influence a complex behavior.

J Friedman. (2001) In: *Neuroscience*. Exploring the brain.
2nd ed. Eds. M F Bear, B W Connors, M A Paradiso.
(Lippincott William and Wilkins, Baltimore.)

The discovery of leptin marks an important milestone in our understanding of metabolic physiology.... It is likely that the most important physiological role of leptin is as a signal for the switch between starved and fed states. Although some leptin is thought to prevent obesity, most obesity occurs in the presence of increased leptin levels.

R S Ahima and J S Flier. (2000) Leptin.
Annual Review of Physiology **62**, pp. 413–437.

... Leptin signals the brain that energy stores are sufficient. As starvation has been a recurrent threat to survival throughout evolution, numerous physiological systems have developed to defend against it.... With continuous leptin deficiency, the brain perceives starvation, promoting increased food intake, efficient metabolism and obesity. Thus defects in leptin production, delivery or response would be expected to create a 'starvation signal' in the midst of plenty ...

J K Elmquist *et al.* (1998) Unraveling the central nervous system pathways
underlying responses to leptin. *Nature Neuroscience* **1**, pp. 445–450.

What is causing this dramatic rise in overweight among the population? Although research advances have highlighted the importance of molecular genetic factors in determining individual susceptibility to obesity, the landmark discoveries of leptin, uncoupling proteins and neuropeptides involved in body weight regulation cannot explain the obesity epidemic. Our genes have not changed substantially during the past two decades. The culprit is an environment which promotes behaviors that cause obesity. To stop and ultimately reverse the obesity epidemic we must 'cure' this environment.

J O Hill and J C Peters. (1998) Environmental contributions
to the obesity epidemic. *Science* **280**, pp. 1371–1373.

more information the brain has, the more accurate its control. The body makes sure that the brain has plenty of information about food intake.

But it is not enough. If, in the longer-term, food intake is to match energy stores, then some way of measuring these stores is needed. If you force-feed an animal so that it gains weight, and then let it choose what it eats, it will eat less for a while until its weight has returned to its previous value. The same happens if you starve an animal, though now, of course, it eats more for a while. This is another example of a 'set-point', the characteristic feature of a homeostatic process. And the set-point seems to depend on the brain knowing how much fat we have, the so-called 'lipostatic' hypothesis. For years this remained a hypothesis, though one increasingly supported by a number of experiments. Some of these showed that there was a factor in the blood that regulated appetite and body weight, though no one knew what it was or where it came from.

It took until the 1990s for the mystery to be revealed. When it came, the answer contained a number of surprises. The signal itself turned out to be a largish peptide, which was called 'leptin' ('leptos' is Greek for 'slim'). Injections of leptin greatly reduced food intake in rats. Whilst it was exciting to have discovered a new hormone controlling appetite, this was not the only surprise. For leptin comes from fat cells. The more fat you have, the more leptin you make, and so the less you eat. Here, then, was the signal telling your brain how fat you are, or, to put it in a more biological way, how much energy you have in your energy stores. Fat is by far the most important energy store. But leptin levels do not change much after an individual meal: so leptin is not a major player in defining satiation. It is a longer-term regulator of appetite, and hence body weight. Just what you need to ensure your weight remains reasonably stable over long periods.

By now, you must be thinking that the discovery of leptin goes against the general idea that the body defends itself against starvation rather than over-feeding. Not so. In fact, the absence of the leptin signal is a major indication of sub-optimal energy stores, another way of saying starvation. Adequate leptin levels signal that these stores are sufficient. Sufficient for what? Reproduction for one. Under-weight rats and mice do not reproduce; neither do under-weight women. You can restore fertility to skinny rats and mice by giving them leptin; the brain thinks they have put on weight.

Obesity

Is the current prevalence of obesity a legacy of the evolutionary development or our physiological system coupled with an aggressive environment? Two scenarios can be envisaged: one in which energy expenditure is high and food is scarce (or periodically scarce), and the other in which energy expenditure is low and food is abundant. It can be argued that the first situation prevailed during most of the course of human evolution; the latter situation has occurred only in the last 50 to 60 years. Consequently, biological processes concerning food intake and energy conservation are well adapted to the first situation and very poorly adapted to the second (the present) situation.

J E Blundell. (1996) Food intake and weight regulation. In: *Regulation of body weight; biological and behavioural mechanisms.* Eds. C Bouchard and G A Bray. (John Wiley and Sons Ltd, London.)

Adolescent obesity represents the most prevalent nutritional problem among American adolescents between the ages of 12–17 yr. Currently, at least 27% of children and 21% of adolescents are obese. This represents a 54% increase in child obesity and a 39% increase in adolescent obesity during the last two decades.

B McCarty and L Mellin. (1996) Obesity. In: *Adolescent nutrition. Assessment and management.* Ed. Rickert VI. (Chapman and Hall, New York.)

On the simplest levels, obesity can only arise when energy intake exceeds energy expenditure. Our current environment is characterized by an essentially unlimited supply of convenient, relatively inexpensive, highly palatable, energy-dense foods, coupled with a life-style requiring only low levels of physical activity for subsistence. Such an environment promotes high energy intake and low energy expenditure. Under these circumstances, obesity occurs . . . because, while the body has excellent physiological defenses against the depletion of body energy stores, it has weak defenses against the accumulation of excess energy stores when food is abundant.

J O Hill and J C Peters. (1998) Environmental contributions to the obesity epidemic. *Science* **280**, pp. 1371–1373.

In the United States of the 1990s, signs of health consciousness are everywhere — except at people's waistlines. . . . Statistics suggest that this health awareness is paying off. . . blood pressure and blood cholesterol

Young rats that are underweight do not pass through puberty but giving them leptin allows them to do so. There is also a relation between minimal body weight and puberty in humans. It is all part of the adaptive process. Reproduction is such a severe metabolic demand that to attempt it if you do not have enough energy stored would be adaptively crazy. It is also a lesson to us that dividing adaptation into separate 'boxes' (eating, drinking, reproduction and so on) may not reflect how the body sees it, or how the biological factors that enable us to survive actually work. This is particularly true for the systems regulating body weight and fertility, as we will see. But there is no doubt that leptin is a major controller of body weight in humans. People who have a rare gene that produces abnormal leptin, or another (equally rare) gene that causes abnormalities in the receptor molecule that detects the presence of leptin are grossly obese; they also tend to be infertile.

The body may also produce a peptide that starts us eating. Unsurprisingly, it comes from the stomach, another organ whose capacity as a major secretor of hormones has only relatively recently been established (though there were hints for years). Ghrelin is the rather unattractive name for a peptide from the stomach that acts on the brain to increase appetite. Exactly what it does is still being sorted out, but it may be a major player in initiation of eating. That is not the only thing it does. One of its action (and why it was first discovered) is to cause the pituitary gland to secrete growth hormone, a big peptide that, as it name implies, promotes growth. Growth hormone is also part of our defence against starvation, as we will see later in this chapter. But events over the past few decades suggest that what we in the West really need is a defence against obesity.

Obesity is the last thing on our minds as we contemplate a hungry day or so, and try to think of ways of getting something to eat in our picturesque valley, but it is very much on the minds of health care professionals in the US and Europe. Obesity is officially defined as having a body mass index (BMI) of 30 or over. You calculate your BMI by dividing your weight (in kilograms) by your height (in metres) squared. Most people have a BMI of around 20. The proportion of people with a BMI of 30 or more has increased dramatically in the US over the past 20 years or so. About 25–30% of all adults are currently classified as obese, and the EU countries are fast catching up. This is an obesity epidemic though note levels have been dropping, while rates of coronary heart disease mortality have declined by more than half. Given these trends, you might expect to see a trim, well-toned population, but you don't. . . . Currently, 22.5% of the US population is considered to be clinically obese — compared with only 14.5% in the 1980s. . . what's more, this 'obesity epidemic', as many public health experts call it , affects all demographic groups, including children.

> G Taubes. (1998) As obesity rates rise, experts struggle to explain why. *Science* **280**, pp. 1367–1368.

Recently, there has been a surge of interest in understanding the mechanisms controlling energy homeostasis, as it has become increasingly recognized that an estimated 33 billion dollars a year are spent on weight loss measures that are largely futile.

> B Hamilton. (1996) A new role for a fat actor. *Nature Medicine* **2**, pp. 272–173.

Socially. . . obesity is a disaster. . People who are overweight are depressed, they have lower than average income, a higher divorce rate and commit suicide more often. Obesity is probably the single most important reason why, in spite of all the advances in medicine and sanitation, we are not living much longer than people a hundred years ago.

> S R Bloom. (2003) The fat controller. *New Scientist*, 9 August 2003, pp. 38–41.

that the definition of obesity is an arbitrary one (BMI > 30). Who knows, it may change (upwards?) in future years. The chances of being obese increase with age, though obesity in children and adolescents is an increasingly serious problem. What is more, an obese child is likely to be an obese adult. The chances also increase if you are female. Obesity carries significant health risks such as increased heart disease, maturity-onset (type 2) diabetes, high blood pressure, joint damage, and reduced fertility. There are significant social risks as well: for example, obese women tend to be less well-educated, poorer, and less likely to marry even after adjusting for other socioeconomic factors (such as social class, family income, social group etc.). In the US, there is also a genetic risk associated with 'race': blacks (particularly female) are more likely to be obese than 'whites', again even after taking account of other factors (e.g. poverty).

It is striking that only in 'developed' countries is poverty a risk factor for obesity. You will not find many obese poor in Africa or India. This is because poverty is relative, not absolute, as Karl Marx pointed out. The poor in the third world are likely to be undernourished; the poor in the rich countries have to make do with cheap food which is high in fat content and carbohydrate. In earlier times, such as Victorian England or early twentieth-century United States when food was relatively more expensive and incomes much lower, obesity was a sign of prosperity and social success. It still is in some other societies. How fascinating that obesity has changed in the West from something to be desired to one that proclaims relative poverty. Yet, the fundamental brain processes regulating weight have not changed. It is the social control of these processes that has altered.

Scientists struggle to explain this epidemic of obesity, let alone do anything about it. The currently fashionable explanation (more a theory than an explanation) is that we bring to our world of plenty a body genetically adept at defending itself against starvation, but with no previous need to bother about over-feeding. Animals eat when they can, and as much as they can. The next meal may be a long way away. So, we presume, did primeval man (or even medieval man, unless he was a lord). If there are enforced periods of starvation, a common event in the natural world, then an array of physiological adaptations exist to defend the body against

Back home a momentous change was coming over the United States. There was a new President, William Howard Taft, and he took office weighing three hundred and thirty-two pounds. All over the country men began to look at themselves. They were used to drinking great quantities of beer. They customarily devoured loaves of bread and ate prodigiously of the sausage meats of poured offal that lay on the lunch counters of the saloons. The august Pierpont Morgan would routinely consume seven- or eight-course dinners. He ate breakfasts of steaks and chops, eggs, pancakes, broiled fish, rolls and butter, fresh fruit and cream. The consumption of food was a sacrament of success. A man who carried a great stomach before him was thought to be in his prime.

E L Doctorow. (1976) *Ragtime*. (Pan Books, London.)

He comes into Mindy's one evening with a female character who is so fat it is necessary to push three tables together to give her room for her lap, and it seems that this character is Miss Violette Shumberger. She weighs maybe two hundred and fifty pounds, but she is by no means an old Judy, and by no means bad-looking. She has a face the size of a town clock and enough chins for a fire-escape, but she has a nice smile and pretty teeth, and a laugh that is so hearty it knocks the whipped cream off an order of strawberry shortcake on a table fifty feet away and arouses the indignation of a customer by the name of Goldstein who is about to consume same.

Damon Runyon. (1956) *A piece of pie (Guys and dolls)*.
(Penguin Books, London.)

The immense accretion of flesh which had descended on her in middle life like a flood of lava on a doomed city had changed her from a plump active little woman with a neatly-turned foot and ankle into something as vast and august as a natural phenomenon. She had accepted this submergence as philosophically as all her other trials, and now, in extreme old age, was rewarded by presenting to her mirror an almost unwrinkled expanse of firm pink and white flesh, in the centre of which the traces of a small face survived as if awaiting excavation.

Edith Wharton. (1920) *The age of innocence*.
(Penguin Books, London.)

reduced energy supplies; but there was no need to take account of excess energy stores — they rarely if ever happened. There may be other factors. Palatability is one. Modern techniques in food manufacture are designed to make food more appetising. How often have you, at the end of a large meal, incapable of another mouthful, accepted that Belgian chocolate? Rats are the same: give them a varied and highly palatable diet, something they rarely encounter in their natural state, and they become over-weight.

As we trudge gloomily in the direction of the sound of running water, hoping perhaps for a small lake in which there might be fish, we are acutely conscious that being hungry is an overwhelming and unpleasant experience. Which suggests to us that the brain, or at least part of it, has a central role in determining when we eat, what we eat, and why we stop eating. We have already mentioned some of the signals that the body sends to it about our nutritional state. But what does the brain do with all this information?

Real progress started in the 1940–1950s. Experimental damage to the hypothalamus was found to result in rats becoming obese. In retrospect (always easy), it is not too surprising that the hypothalamus regulates body weight. After all, it is the part of the brain that monitors what goes on in our bodies (the internal environment) and it has the means for correcting internal imbalances. Though rats with hypothalamic damage become fat, they do not go on eating until they explode; their body weight stabilises at a much higher level than in control rats without such damage. There are rare cases of hypothalamic tumours in man resulting in obesity. But why do these rats become obese? The obvious answer is that they overeat, and they do. They eat more at each meal then normal animals, and they may also eat again (that is, become hungry) sooner than normal.

But there are some puzzles. When you (or a rat) are very hungry, you will eat things you might otherwise refuse. Cattle do this: they eat whatever they can get when they are ravenous but choose only the more delectable grass as they become more satisfied. There are awful stories of people, walled up in caves, who ate their own hands. So you would confidently expect rats with hypothalamic damage to be less choosy about what they eat. And you would be wrong. In fact, they are more easily put off food by making it bitter than are normal rats. Not at all what you (or the scientists doing the experiments) expected.

Amit's uncle Mr Ganguly was an extremely taciturn man whose energies went entirely into eating. His jowls worked vigorously, swiftly, almost twice a second. . . while his mild, bland, bovine eyes looked at his hosts and fellow-guests who were doing the talking. His wife was a fat, highly emotional woman who wore a great deal of sindoor in her hair and had a very large bindi of equally brilliant red in the middle of her forehead. She was a shocking gossip and in between extracting fine fishbones from her large paan-stained mouth she impaled the reputations of all her neighbours and any of her relatives who were not present. Embezzlement, drunkenness, gangsterism, incest: whatever could be stated was stated and whatever could not was implied.

Vikram Seth. (1993) *A suitable boy.* (Phoenix House, London.)

We don't eat just because we are hungry, or because we need food: we eat because we are bored, sad, anxious, angry; and we give food to others to placate them, welcome them, control them. . . . We don't not eat because we are not hungry: we starve ourselves out of psychological disturbance, and because everywhere we look thin is beautiful and powerful.

Nicci Gerrard. (2003) The politics of thin.
The Observer, 5 January 2003.

Then it was discovered that damaging the hypothalamus right next to the area that caused obesity resulted in rats that would not eat. In fact, they had to be hand-fed for a time if they were to survive. Eventually they started eating on their own, but only if their diet was semi-liquid and rather palatable. And they did not regain all their lost weight. There seemed to be two 'centres' in the hypothalamus. One that regulated eating, the other that was responsible for satiety. And there the story stuck for quite a few years.

Until, in 1960, a landmark experiment was carried out. Sebastian Grossman knew which part of the hypothalamus was implicated by the experimental work. It was the middle bit, called the medial hypothalamus. Instead of damaging it, or even electrically stimulating it (this has the opposite effect) he infused either noradrenaline or acetylcholine into the same area, and watched what happened. Both noradrenaline and acetylcholine (they are distant cousins in a chemical sense) were known to be chemical transmitters in the hypothalamus. The extraordinary result was that Grossman's rats ate after noradrenaline infusions, but drank after acetylcholine.

It was extraordinary because, for the first time, here was clear evidence for chemical coding of ingestion in the hypothalamus. Up to this point, separation of function had been based on anatomical differences. One part of the hypothalamus did one thing, another did another. But here was an example of the same population of nerve cells (not necessarily the same cells) being selectively activated chemically and causing opposite, but equally important, adaptive behaviours. In the years that have followed, this experiment has been repeated in various ways dozens of times, always with similar results. Does it mean that noradrenaline 'codes' for feeding and acetylcholine for drinking? There are big problems with this interpretation. Neither chemical is actually limited to the hypothalamus, in fact, the nerve cells that make noradrenaline (and much of the acetylcholine) lie in other parts of the brain (Chapters 3 and 4). So the code, if there is one, is not very specific. There was the persistent notion that the brain might have a more dedicated chemical code for eating. This idea had to wait for the surge of work on peptides in the 1970s and onwards. In particular, until a peptide called neuropeptide Y was infused into the brain.

Dinner for six persons	*Dinner for six servants*
Caviare	*Boiled beef, carrots, potatoes*
White soup	*Pancakes*

Stewed carp
Oyster patties

Veal rissoles
Fricandeau of Beef

Snipe

Plum pudding
Compote of fruit

Celery salad

Angels on horseback

> Mrs Isabella Beeton. (1901) *The book of household management*. (Ward, Lock and Co., London.)

...There is a strong case for judging individual advantage in terms of the capabilities that a person has, that is, the substantive freedoms he or she enjoys to lead the kind of life he or she has reason to value. In this perspective, poverty must be seen as the deprivation of basic capabilities rather than merely as lowness of incomes, which is the standard criterion of identification of poverty. The perspective of capability-poverty does not involve any denial of the sensible view that low income is clearly one of the major causes of poverty, since lack of income can be a principal reason for a person's capability deprivation.

> Amartya Sen. (1999) *Development as freedom*. (Oxford University Press, Oxford.)

The name, wholly unromantic, derives from the letters given as codes to the individual amino acids that make up a peptide. Neuropeptide Y consists of a chain of 36 amino acids: and, as it happens, the chain begins and ends with the amino acid tyrosine. The letter assigned to tyrosine is 'Y'; hence its name. There are several other peptides with similar structures; one is found in the pancreas, others in the gut. Infuse a tiny amount of neuropeptide Y (called NPY for short) into the brain, and the animal eats and eats. If you infuse NPY every day, it puts on lots of weight. NPY is the most powerful appetite stimulant known. What is more, animals infused with it tend to prefer carbohydrate to other types of food. Now you can explore the brain to see whereabouts NPY has its action. No surprise here, it is the medial hypothalamus. Does this prove that NPY is a code for 'eating' in the brain? Certainly not. You need another set of experiments.

You need to show that the medial hypothalamus contains NPY and the receptors that respond to it: it does. Now you need to show that when an animal is deprived of food, NPY levels go up: they do. Finally, you need to show that when you block the action of NPY in the hypothalamus, a food-deprived animal no longer eats: that is what happens. Does NPY respond to the signals from the body that alter appetite? It does: leptin decreases NPY, but insulin increases it. The two signals have opposite effects on appetite. Even more interestingly, infusing NPY into the hypothalamus increases insulin. There is, it seems, a two-way signalling system between brain and body regulating energy intake. So NPY is not just an 'eating' peptide, it also helps the body prepare for food; in other words, it codes for the co-ordinated behaviour and hormonal changes that represent the adaptive response to the need for food. It puts you in eating mode.

Now we will try another experiment. Let us put a male rat into a large cage containing some food, but also a sexy female rat. The male goes for the female, ignoring the food. Now do it again, but this time infuse a tiny amount of NPY into the male's hypothalamus. This time he switches to the food, and ignores the female. NPY not only increases eating, it also changes the priority an animal gives to food over other possible rewards. The real world, unlike the laboratory, is full of alternative avenues of action. What an animal (or even you) will do depends on many things,

The Brain and Eating

Rats do not nibble continuously. Rather, they choose to arrange their feeding in an unmistakable sequence of discrete bouts, just as humans do... one of the great themes of Curt Richter's life-work (is) the physiological mysteries so forcefully presented by the rhythmic nature of many behavioral phenomena.... Sharply intensified activity always precedes and follows each meal; the very brief meals are always separated by intermeal intervals of approximately 3 hours.... within a few minutes of meal initiation, ingested food stops feeding behavior for hours, generating a fast, total and enduring abolition of the behavior. If the phenomenon were not so familiar to each of us, it would seem amazing.

> J Gibbs, G P Smith D Greenberg. (1993) Cholecystokinin: A neuroendocrine key to feeding behavior. In: *Hormonally induced changes in mind and brain*, pp. 51–67. (Academic Press, Amsterdam.)

The current intense interest in the hypothalamic circuitry of food intake is reminiscent of the interest in hypothalamic centers of motivation in the 1950s. The main difference is that excitatory and inhibitory centers have been replaced by excitatory and inhibitory peptides.

> A A Ammar *et al.* (2000) NPY-leptin: Opposing effects on appetitive and consummatory ingestive behavior and sexual behavior. *American Journal of Physiology* **278**, pp. 1627–1633.

The fact that rats eat less and lose weight when their diet tastes bad has never been surprising, but the many studies demonstrating that rats become obese on tasty diets have been a thorn in the side of homeostatic theories of food intake, particularly those that incorporate a setpoint for body weight.

> E Satinoff. (1983) A re-evaluation of the concept of the homeostatic organization of temperature regulation. In: *Handbook of behavioral neurobiology*. Eds. E Satinoff and P Teitelbaum, **6**, pp. 443–472. (Plenum Press, New York.)

(The) evidence... shows that the orbitofrontal cortex is involved in decoding and representing some primary reinforcers such as taste and touch; in learning and reversing associations of visual and other stimuli to these primary reinforcers; and in controlling and correcting reward-related and punishment-related behavior, and thus in emotion.

> E T Rolls. (2000) The orbitofrontal cortex and reward. *Cerebral Cortex* **10**, pp. 284–294.

but particularly on current physiological need. Many peptides, like NPY, have two actions: they increase (or decrease) one category of behaviour, but they also decrease (or increase) others. You think you are making a choice: your limbic system — or, rather, the peptides currently being released in it — is actually making it for you. Suppose you infuse NPY into our male rat in the absence of food but in the presence of the sexy female: he mates with his usual gusto. So preference really is being altered by this chemical code.

Eating is such an important activity that it would be odd if it were controlled by only one peptide. You eat for many reasons. And you eat different things, sometimes preferring carbohydrate, at another time fat; your body has the ability to signal its needs to the brain. So there are several other peptides that also stimulate eating. There is limited evidence that some 'code' for certain types of food: for example, fat (that is coded by a peptide called galanin), and, as we have seen, NPY inclines one towards carbohydrate. Cannabis alters appetite by acting on a special set of receptors, and this may offer a new means of weight control. Another peptide that might interest you is an opiate. Opiates (morphine is an artificial one) stimulate eating (incidentally, they decrease sex). Blocking their action stops NPY from making animals eat. This is one example of the way that these peptides interact. A complex interwoven chain of chemical signals regulates appetite in all its variety. The exact way they all relate to each other is still being worked out. But we now know enough to be sure that peptides in the hypothalamus play a fundamental role in maintaining energy balance by regulating appetite.

Since peptides do more than one thing, sometimes the initial function ascribed to them turns out not to be the most important. One example of this is a peptide called orexin (actually, there are two closely-related ones). Infusing it caused animals to eat, hence its name. It appeared to activate a region of the hypothalamus that was essential for appetite. It all seemed to fit. But it turns out to have more important roles in sleep. Animals with a genetically-abnormal form of orexin or its receptor have narcolepsy: they suddenly drop off into sleep at the wrong time (i.e. during their day, in the middle of doing something else). A similar condition is known in humans. So orexin keeps you awake; and when you are awake, you eat. This shows us that not only do peptides code for

The swift December dusk had come tumbling clownishly after its dull day and, as he stared through the dull square of the window of the schoolroom, he felt his belly crave for its food. He hoped there would be stew for dinner, turnips and carrots and bruised potatoes and fat mutton pieces to be ladled out in thick peppered flour-fattened sauce. Stuff it into you, his belly counselled him.

James Joyce. (1916) *A portrait of the artist as a young man.*

In his first excitement, a prisoner couldn't get anything down his throat. . . . But gradually one's appetite returned; and then a chronically famished state ensued that became almost unbearable. Then, if one managed to get it under control, one's stomach shrank and adapted itself to inadequate food, at which point the meager Lubyanka fare became just right. One needed to have self-control to achieve this, and also needed to stop looking round to see who might be eating something extra. All those extremely dangerous prison conversations about food had to be outlawed. . . .

Alexander Solzhenitsyn. (1974)
The gulag archipelago. (Fontana, London.)

These foreign voices became engraved on our memories as on a blank tape; in the same manner, a famished stomach rapidly assimilates even indigestible food. Their meaning did not help us remember them because for us they had none; yet, much later, we recited them to people who could understand them, and they did have a meaning, tenuous and banal; they were imprecations, curses, or small everyday, often repeated sentences, such as "What time is it?" or "I can't walk," or "Leave me alone". They were fragments torn from the indistinct, the fruit of a useless and unconscious effort to carve a meaning or sense out of the senseless. They were also the mental equivalent of our bodily needs for nourishment, which drove us to search for potato peelings around the kitchens: little more than nothing, better than nothing. Also the undernourished brain suffers from a specific hunger of its own. Or perhaps this useless and paradoxical memory had another significance and purpose: it was the unconscious preparation for 'later', for an improbable survival, in which every shred of experience would become a tessera in a vast mosaic.

Primo Levi. (1986) *The drowned and the saved.*
(Summit Books, New York.)

quite complex patterns of behaviour, but that the brain's way of coding behaviour may not always correspond to our ideas of how behaviour is compartmentalised.

But are there signals in the brain that stop eating? Indeed there are. Tucked under your liver is a little green sac, with a tube connecting it to the small intestine. Just before it enters the intestine, the tube is joined by a second one from the pancreas. The green sac is full of bile: a mixture of pigments and salts. Bile was one of the names for four ancient 'humours' which were supposed to govern our state of health, though, curiously, there wasn't a green bile. Now, let us watch your gallbladder (for that is what the sac is called) as you eat your dinner, particularly if it contains some fat, which is very likely. As your meal enters the small intestine, your gallbladder contracts. This is important: the contents of the gallbladder help you digest your food, acting together with enzymes from the pancreas. But how does the gallbladder know when to discharge its contents? The presence of fat in the small intestine causes it to release a peptide hormone, with the beautiful (if elaborate) name of cholecystokinin (CCK for short; we have met it in an earlier chapter). You will recall that the name means, in Greek, 'activates the gallbladder', and that is exactly what it does. But it does more than that. It also stops you eating. How it does this is something of a mystery, though the most likely explanation is that the released CCK activates nerves from your gut that travel to the brain, and hence the brain knows that food has entered your small intestine. CCK also slows the rate at which your stomach empties, which may also contribute to satiation (also through the nerves from the gut). Your bile, meanwhile, is helping you digest, and giving your faeces their normal brown colour (the green pigment is broken down). One of the signs of a blocked gallbladder duct is very pale faeces.

You might wonder why CCK from the gut does not act directly on the brain. This is because most (but not all) peptides cannot get into the brain from the blood. Some can: leptin is one, insulin is another, but they have to have special transport systems to take them from blood into the brain: a sort of privileged access. CCK does not belong to this club. Why? Perhaps because the brain uses CCK itself, so that extra hormone whooshing in from the blood would cause confusion. What does CCK do in the brain? You have guessed it. It stops animals eating. Infuse

I often had to visit the hospital for my teeth at that time. Whenever I went there I had an attack of nausea at the horrible sight of dozens of people with shiny, almost transparent swollen limbs, as big as barrels. . . . When I asked my dentist what was wrong with them, she said with a sigh, 'Edema.' I asked her what that meant, and she mumbled something which I vaguely linked with food.

These people with edema were mostly peasants. Starvation was much worse in the countryside because there were no guaranteed rations. Government policy was to provide food for the cities first, and commune officials were having to seize grain from peasants by force. . . . As a result, the peasants who had actually grown the food died in the millions all over China.

Jung Chang. (1993) *Wild swans.* (Flamingo, London.)

I shall have lived my life obsessed by the thought of food. My mother stuffed her daughter, her son, and her granddaughter with food because she was always afraid for their futures. Whenever some childhood illness or attack of the flu occurred she felt that all their years to come were in jeopardy. My mother will have spent her life, and taught me to spend mine, in constant fear of tomorrow. Not to eat so much as one can is to invite certain disaster. Anaemic and on the verge of rickets when she left the nun's sewing room, a young girl — my mother — found her insides suddenly swollen with a phenomenal amount of food: a child, For every million sperms in one jet of semen she countered with a million calories for the daughter they produced.

Violette Leduc. (1965) *La batarde. Translated by Derek Coltman.*
(Peter Owen, London.)

They dined at a small dark dingy restaurant nearby run by a member of the resistance. . . no attempt had been made to make this restaurant inviting to the casual diner. . . . But in this shabby room, Hilary had two hours of happiness greater than he had known since he had left Lisa behind in Paris.
To start with, the food was unbelievably luxurious. There was white bread; there were huge steaks an inch thick, dabs of butter melting on top of them. There were meringues filled with whipped cream; there was a

a tiny amount of CCK into the hypothalamus, and even a hungry rat will stop eating. So here we have another marvellous example of the body (this time the gut) and the brain using the same chemical code, together, to fulfil an important adaptive function. In this case, to promote digestion and bring feeding to a close after an adequate meal. Blocking the action of CCK in the brain delays satiation. It seems to be a physiological effect. The presence of the same peptide (CCK) in the gut and the brain, doing related things, is not unique. The gut contains a whole slew of peptides, and many are also found in the brain, particularly in the limbic system. Many of them are now known to act, together, on food intake.

Animals and humans lose their appetite for many reasons. There are peptide codes that direct an animal away from food to sex. For example, the males of some species of deer practically stop eating during the mating season. If you feel ill, particularly if your gut is out of order, then you rapidly lose your appetite, as everyone knows. This makes biological sense. You need not to use a system that is malfunctioning. But this everyday experience has to have a neurological basis. You go off your food because your brain tells you to do so. In fact, animals and humans can stop eating, temporarily, for all sorts of reasons, and behind these reasons lie a variety of chemical codes saying 'stop'. But these codes, important as they are, are not the same as those bringing 'normal' eating to a close, or regulating the interval between meals, or causing you to prefer one sort of food to another. Most people nowadays believe that CCK belongs to the 'specific' class of 'stop' signals, rather than those that are really part of some other process (e.g. illness).

But there are peptides to stop eating when conditions are not suitable. One of those conditions is stress. A stressed animals does not eat, nor should it, because it is fully occupied trying to resolve the stressful conditions, which might be life-threatening. Not a good moment to settle down to a cosy meal. One of the peptides that is closely concerned with stress is CRF (corticotropin releasing factor). CRF also has many behavioural actions (see Chapter 4); one of these is to reduce appetite.

So just as there are many peptides that increase eating, there are quite a few that reduce it. Peptides can also increase eating by blocking those that restrain appetite. There is a rather strange-looking mouse that has *ripe Brie, a perfect claret, a suave Armagnac. Once — but so long ago! — Hilary had understood food. He had treated his palate as a precious instrument of pleasure, and indulged it with esoteric knowledge. But all this was so far away that his consciousness had forgotten its sensations. For so many years now meals had been dull, methodical exercises less pleasurable, in terms of real pleasure, than the movements of the bowel that were their necessary complements.*

Marghanita Laski. (1949) *Little boy lost.*
(Penguin Books, Harmondsworth, UK.)

yellow fur. It is also very fat. Both its fur colour and ample tummy are caused by mutations in the same gene. It is called 'agouti' because the yellow fur reminds some people of the colour of normal guinea pigs. The peptide made by this gene (the agouti-related peptide) blocks a receptor which, in the skin, is responsible for black fur (hence the yellow colour). In the brain the receptor is sensitive to peptides that reduce appetite. Block it, and those peptides can no longer act, and so the mouse eats too much. In fact, this receptor may be the target for a number of peptides regulating body weight, and so has excited the interest of many scientists, as well as a number of drug companies anxious to develop more rational and effective ways of reducing body weight in obese people. A drug that targets this receptor might be just what is wanted in the fight against the obesity epidemic. It might have other important uses as well, as we will see later, when we come to consider how eating disorders fit into what we know of the way that the brain controls body weight.

Defending ourselves against starvation has been an historically vital attribute. Without it, none of us would be here, for our ancestors would never have survived. Periodic starvation was the rule. It still is for most wild animals. These defence mechanisms, of course, are still needed in many parts of our unequal world even today: famine in Africa is a regular event. Though many may die in a famine, some will survive. Many factors contribute to determining who will live and who will die in a famine (like being very young or very old), but the ability to marshal the body's defences against persistent lack of renewable energy is a vital one. Starvation is rather on our mind as we contemplate our scenic, but apparently inhospitable valley, and wonder how to get a meal. Of course, we are in no danger of dying in the few days before the helicopter returns — humans can live a surprisingly long time without food, particularly if they can drink water — but this is because our bodies have already begun to adapt to lack of food. The emergency response has already started. Our brain has had to devise a survival plan.

It is the hypothalamus that does it. Sensing that energy stores are low, and that replenishment is not taking place, the hypothalamus organises the body's defences. Its strategy is simple: self-preservation. The brain is necessarily a selfish organ, because, unlike the rest of the body, it has no energy reserves. You will not find rolls of fat in the brain, nor even

Food and Reward

The distinction between appetitive behaviour and consummatory act separates behaviour as a whole into two components of entirely different character. The consummatory act is relatively simple; at its most complex, it is a chain of reactions, each of which may be a combination of a taxis and a fixed pattern. But appetitive behaviour is a true purposive activity, offering all the problems of plasticity, adaptiveness, and of a complex integration that that baffle the scientist in his study of behaviour as a whole. . . . It is often stressed that animals are striving towards the attainment of a certain end or goal. . . the striving. . . is typical only of appetitive behaviour and not of consummatory actions. . . . The end of purposive behaviour is not the attainment of an object. . . but the performance of the purposive action. . . . Even psychologists who have watched hundreds of rats running a maze rarely realize that. . . it is not. . . the food the animal is striving towards, but the performance of. . . eating.

N Tinbergen. (1963) *The study of instincts.*
(Oxford University Press, Oxford.)

In the Fall of 1953, we were looking for more information about the reticular activating system, we used electrodes permanently implanted in the brain of a healthy, behaving rat. We discovered, quite to our surprise, that an electrical stimulus applied to the brain in the region of the anterior commissure has an effect tantamount to primary reward.

   . . . Later we found that the same animal could be 'pulled' to any spot in the maze by giving a small electrical stimulus after each response in the right direction. . . . Afterwards, the animal was starved for 24 hours. Food was put in both arms of the T maze. The animal was given two forced runs to each arm. He was stimulated in the left arm. After this, he made 10 runs to the left, *stopping at the point of stimulation and never going on to the food.* . . . The rewarding effects of electrical stimulation are largely confined to this anatomically connected set of structures, the limbic system.

J Olds. (1955) Physiological mechanisms of reward.
In: *Nebraska symposium on motivation.*
Ed. M R Jones. (Nebraska Press.)

One fundamental distinction between core processes of reward. . . is between the affective consequences . . . ('liking') and their motivational consequences muscle (lots of protein) or glycogen, the form in which the rest of the body (particularly the liver) stores carbohydrate. The brain, like a pampered autocrat, needs a constant supply of only one food: glucose. Without it, it stops functioning within a few minutes: a more prolonged deficit means permanent brain damage. All its glucose comes from the blood. So nearly everything that the hypothalamus does during starvation is aimed at keeping blood glucose levels as normal as possible. And it has some powerful tools to do it.

As we have seen, the peptides that code for eating also have other functions, and an important one is to alter levels of hormones in the blood that maintain glucose. They do this in several ways. One way is to activate the pituitary to produce several hormones that break down fat, glycogen and protein to make extra glucose. This includes hormones that have powerful effects on breaking down fat stores. This is one of the reasons you lose weight when you diet and these fat products are an energy source that the body (but not the brain) can use. This spares what glucose there is for the brain. Hormones break down muscle protein to make more glucose so starvation makes you weak. You might think this is not such a good idea after all, you need your muscles to hunt for food, but starvation is an extreme emergency, and survival is the priority. The hypothalamus also regulates the body's autonomic nervous system, and this, the emergency system, swings into action and helps to increase blood glucose. Another thing it does is to decrease the body's temperature, thus conserving energy rather like you turning down the thermostat on your central heating to save fuel.

But it is not all up to the hypothalamus. Like any well-designed structure, the body has parallel systems to help it survive starvation, though they all have the same objective: keeping the brain alive. The pancreas is very sensitive to blood levels of glucose. Whether it does this entirely on its own, or whether the brain has some control over it is still uncertain, but lowered blood glucose does very important things to the pancreas. Firstly, it lowers insulin. Since insulin lowers blood glucose, this is what you want when you are starving; the push-pull interaction between glucose and insulin is a good example of a feedback system responsible for homeostasis.

Against all expectations, we have caught a fish. Fishing is so much easier in adventure films than in real life. Now it is sizzling in the pan, ('wanting'). . . . The neurotransmitter that traditionally has been most touted for mediating sensory pleasure, dopamine, turns out to be neither necessary nor sufficient for generating 'liking'. . . . Naturally this forces consideration of alternative roles for dopamine in reward. . . 'Wanting', unlike 'liking' is particularly influenced by dopamine.

K C Berridge and T E Robinson. (2003) Parsing reward. *Trends in Neuroscience* **26**, pp. 507–513.

and increasingly intolerable hunger is being replaced by almost equally intolerable impatience. Finally, we get to eat it and nothing has ever seemed more delicious and succulent though, if we are honest, the fish does have a rather muddy taste. Can peptides in the hypothalamus be responsible for the unpleasantness of hunger, or the sublime pleasure of eating? It is an important question, for this is why we eat, and why we avoid hunger. Just as in many other contexts in which our survival is at stake, the brain makes us avoid situations or conditions (like hunger) that are bad for us, or represent a state of deficit or danger, and attracts us to the process (such as eating) whereby these states or conditions are remedied. It does this by making sure that a deficit is 'unpleasant' or 'aversive,' whereas the remedy is 'pleasant' or 'rewarding.' Somewhere in the brain there is a mechanism for this. It does not happen by chance, or without reason.

Let us start with reward. One essential question is whether the brain has a single 'reward' system, which can be activated by a number of different events, or whether each motivational or 'survival' system (like eating) has a reward system of its own. On one level, the latter must be true. After all, as we sat in our valley craving food, a long drink of water would not have sufficed. If you are parched with thirst, then eating will not meet your need (indeed, you may find it difficult or impossible to eat at all). But this does not necessarily mean that drinking or eating or sex or anything else has to have its own, private, reward system. What the brain might do is to link your current deficit (say, lack of food) with the general reward system thus ensuing that the most rewarding thing imaginable at that moment is something to eat. The general question of what reward is, and how the brain might encode it, is a subject that has importance for all sorts of adaptive and survival-related behaviour. Indeed, it's essential for such behaviour to operate. But we can most easily discuss it in the context of eating, because eating represents the most frequently studied example of reward.

Food, itself, is not a reward. You have to know what food is. It is the sight of food which raises expectation that food is available or the taste/smell of food in the mouth which is rewarding, but only if you are in the appropriate deficit state (i.e. if your energy stores are low, and thus you are hungry). And the particular quality of the food (both its appearance and its taste/smell) is important as well. We all know that we will accept

Smell

The hypothalamus provides a neural substrate for effector programs which are designed to redress an impending homeostatic imbalance or to ward off a threat to the organism's integrity in response to an actually injurious stimulus. These mechanisms can be activated directly at the hypothalamic level by an imbalance in homeostasis. . . . Originally, in very early vertebrates, these may well have been the only stimuli capable of triggering these behavioral patterns. . . . But, in adult higher animals and man, these simple and basic triggering mechanisms of motivational drives are used only as a method of last resort. . . . In the course of individual existence, some sets of originally neutral stimuli acquire affective connotations by virtue of their association with rewarding or punishing life situations. . . . In this evolutionary history, the olfactory sense seems to have opened the way which freed animal behavior from the rigidity of simple reflex mechanisms represented at the hypothalamic level.

> P Gloor. (1972) Temporal lobe epilepsy: Its possible contribution to the understanding of the functional significance of the amygdala and of its interaction with neocortical-temporal mechanisms. In: *The neurobiology of the amygdala.* Ed. B E Eleftheriou, pp. 423–457. (Plenum Press, New York.)

In many respects, the human nose is a vestigial organ. Aside from its function as a respiratory passage with its perpetual vulnerability to infection, its olfactory activity has waned. . . . Perhaps it was for this reason that Coleridge said that the basic reason for the existence of the nose was to take snuff. It cannot be directly viewed by the subject, though in a mirror-reflection it is perhaps the most conspicuous landmark, and one which immediately comes into view. For this reason, Ambrose Bierce called it "the extreme outpost of the face."

> M Critchley. (1979) Man's attitude to his nose. In: *The divine banquet of the brain.* (Raven Press, New York.)

A . . . species of orchid has evolved which gives off an aroma identical to the sex attractant of the female beetle. In fact, orchid and beetle evolution have produced essentially the same molecule. The male beetles turn out to be exceedingly near-sighted; and the orchids have evolved a configuration of their petals that, to a myopic beetle, resembles the female in a sexual posture. The male beetles enjoy several weeks of orgiastic ecstasy among the orchids, and when eventually the females emerge from the ground, we can imagine a great deal of wounded pride and righteous indignation. Meanwhile, the orchids have been successfully cross-pollinated by the amorous male beetles. . . .

> Carl Sagan. (1977) *The dragons of Eden.* (Hodder and Stoughton, London.)

less preferred foods if we are hungry enough, and if we are stuffed, there are those Belgian chocolates. . . so there is an interaction between the quality of a food stimulus and our current internal state. A sort of gastronomic payoff. This must also be represented in the brain. Finally, there is the experience of reward itself — the pleasure that accompanies a good meal (or, indeed, a slice of muddy-tasting fish if you're hungry enough) which is an emotion. This is why the brain keeps you eating, so that your body can get the calories it needs. This must happen in the brain somewhere. Things that are not intrinsically rewarding may become so, either because they represent reward or because they predict it. Money is a good example. A pound coin is simply a metal disc. It only becomes rewarding because we know that it can be exchanged for food (and other things). So it acquires some of the rewarding properties of food itself. A hungry beggar knows this. A bell sounded before food is presented, if it is done reliably, comes to predict food, and so is itself rewarding, provided you can be reasonably sure that the food will follow. Pavlov's dogs knew this. So does a hungry schoolchild as the dinner bell sounds. This implies that certain types of learning can transform things that were neutral into things that are rewarding. More brain mechanisms. All essential for survival, since rewarding events are usually good for you; so you need to know what they are. Where and how does it all happen?

Now, I really do not expect you to feel sorry for scientists, but do spare a sympathetic thought for those trying to find out whether the brain has a recognisable 'reward' system. Reward is difficult to study. 'Reward', 'motivation' and 'drive' are all words that try to describe part of the process by which we find certain objectives pleasurable, why we will strive to get them, and what happens in our brain when we do. They do not mean exactly the same thing, but they do overlap quite a bit. Since you cannot ask a rat whether something is 'rewarding' (i.e. it finds it pleasurable), you have to try to make it do things that will allow you to infer 'reward'. The classical way to do this, invented by the American psychologist B F Skinner, is to make an animal work for something it wants. He called it 'operant' behaviour. Just like you might work to get food in a 'barter' society, or money in a modern one. Only the rat does something like press a lever, or poke its nose into a hole, or turn left at a T-junction; then it gets some food. If you deprive a rat of food for a few hours, it presses the bar

Adam ate some breakfast. No kipper, he reflected, is ever so good as it smells; how this too earthly contact with flesh and bone spoiled the first happy exhilaration; if only one could live, as Jehovah was said to have done, on the savour of burnt offerings. He lay back for a little in his bed thinking about the smells of food, of the greasy horror of fried fish and the deeply moving smell that came from it; of the intoxicating breath of bakeries and the dullness of buns. . . .

Evelyn Waugh. (1930) *Vile bodies.*
(Penguin Books, Harmondsworth, UK.)

Under the opaque glass of the veranda it had become very hot and sultry. The earth smells and the grass smells were exotic now, like incense, not rainy and fresh. Rachel had edged her deck chair close up against mine. I could feel the nearby weight of her sagging body like a gravitational pull upon my own. She had wound her arm underneath my arm and rather awkwardly taken hold of my hand. So two corpses might ineptly greet each other on resurrection day. Then she began to turn over towards me, her head pressing on my shoulder. I could smell her perspiration and the fresh, clean scent of her hair.

Iris Murdoch. (1973) *The black prince.*
(Chatto and Windus, London.)

For my own part, the smell of spring air — that smell which is more a texture than an odor, a sense of the atmosphere's near-palpability, and yet a smell as well, the smell of things above the threshold of sensory perception but below the level at which a name may be given to that which is perceived. . . .

For myself, this almost sexual sense of renascent possibility transports me back to the south of France, on my first solo visit there at the age of eighteen; it brings with it the smell of wild herbs (with thyme dominant), the silvery underside of wind-stirred olive leaves, the plasticky sheen of new-picked lemons, the texture of a pebbled driveway felt through the rope soles of one's espadrilles; nights spent under a single sheet with the moon huge and proximate.

John Lanchester. (1996) *The debt to pleasure.*
(Henry Holt and Company, New York.)

faster; if the food it gets is not very nice, it will press less vigorously, and so on. If a rat (or even you) will do work to get something, then the assumption is that this 'something' is rewarding. The opposite is also true. If you (or a rat) will work to avoid something, then this 'something' represents punishment, rather than reward. So you can measure 'motivation' (changes in 'hunger') by seeing how often the rat presses the lever to get a standard food after you deprive it of food for a period, or 'reward' by seeing what happens in the brain when the animal presses a lever to be given a certain sort of food, or even when it gets the food itself.

But now comes the problem. Pressing a lever, and so on, is not at all natural for a rat. So you have to train it; it has to learn that pressing the bar a certain number of times (or for a certain time) gets some food. But how can you be sure, when you change the brain and this alters bar-pressing, that what you thought was 'reward' may really be 'learning?' Or, perhaps, the ability to recognise the food? Or assess it's value? Or even the ability to find the lever, or press it? And there are other problems: as we have seen, doings things (lever press) or experiencing things (a bell) that predict reward can make either the action or the experience rewarding: but perhaps our brain studies are revealing this process rather than 'reward' itself? And are we studying 'reward' (the pleasure of food) or the removal of the aversive state of 'non-reward' or deprivation (eg. hunger)? These, of course, are all important ingredients in the survival mechanism, but at this moment we want to know how the brain signals 'reward' in general, and, in particular, for food.

Food is recognised as such by its taste, its smell and its appearance — usually some combination of all three sensations. But the three sensations are processed by different pathways in the brain. So somehow they have to be brought together.

Taste depends on special detectors ('receptors') in the tongue though here we should mention that much of what we think of as 'taste' is actually smell, which is why you think you cannot taste your food as well as usual when you have a cold. You can: it is the smell you have lost. Traditionally there were thought to be only four types of tongue receptors (for sweet, salty, bitter and sour tastes) but this has recently been extended to include other specialised tastes such as one for glutamate (called 'umami') which is why adding monosodium glutamate to food enhances its flavour. The sensation of taste ends up in several parts of the brain.

The smells of that time, the smell of that time. Singapore — hot dishrags and catpiss. Moscow — builder's size and the unflushed stools of the smokers of cheap cigars. Dublin — roasting coffee which turns out to be roasting barley. The whole of 1916 had a mingled smell of unaired rooms, unwashed socks, bloody khaki, musty mufti, the rotting armpits of women's dresses, margarine, cheap gaspers made of floorsweepings, floors swept with the aid of damp tea leaves. It was a very un-American smell, one might say.

Anthony Burgess. (1980) *Earthly powers.*
(Hutchinson and Co., London.)

One destination is the 'taste area' in the cortex; not a part of the limbic system, but the area of the brain where taste may actually enter awareness. Another destination is the amygdala, which seems to be part of the limbic system that classifies the taste as 'pleasant' or 'unpleasant' and can form associations between a particular taste and some consequential event like becoming ill. So you will not eat that food again in a hurry. It is also important for the ability to learn which signals (like a bell), initially neutral, can come to predict food; that is, it has a role in certain forms of learning (conditioning). The bell rings, you salivate. Note however, that different parts of the brain allow you to analyse the taste (cortex) and apply a 'value' to it (amygdala). But the information arriving at the taste cortex does not stop there. It passes forward in the brain to a region right at the front called the orbitofrontal cortex. This lies, as its name suggests, at the base of the frontal lobes, the part of the brain right behind your forehead. It is deeply concerned with emotional states. The orbitofrontal cortex thus gets indirect information about sensation. And not just taste.

Smell is quite different. It is important to remember that smell is a very primitive chemical sense. It has been around a long time in evolutionary terms, and so the areas of the brain that process it were also around long before the new cortex (neocortex) had appeared. Like other 'primitive' systems, the amount of processing that's done by the detectors (in this case, in the nose) is relatively great compared to that done by the brain. The big mystery is how the detectors in the nose do it: that is, allow you to recognise hundreds, perhaps thousands, of different smells. It is now known that an enormous number of genes (about 1000–2000) make these detectors (the detectors themselves are proteins). Moreover, each of these genes can make several different proteins. In some ways, this is like the immune system, which also can make myriads of different proteins called antibodies. Each detector has only a small number of receptor protein molecules on it, so the way that the nose actually encodes a given smell is still not really understood. How does the nose ensure that it has all the right molecules? In some cases it does not: certain people can smell things others can't.

Smell information from the nose goes down a nerve to a bump in the brain called the 'olfactory bulb'. In a rat or a dog this is quite a huge structure that sits at the front of the brain. In humans, it is a tiny thing the

At the end of a few days' crawling Scott learned something of the size of the India which he served; and it astonished him. His carts, as you know, were loaded with wheat, millet, and barley, good food-grains needing only a little grinding. But the people to whom he brought the life-giving stuffs were rice-eaters. They know how to hull rice in their mortars, but knew nothing of the heavy stone querns of the North, and less of the material that the white man convoyed so laboriously. They clamoured for rice — unhusked paddy, such as they were accustomed to — and, when they found that there was none, broke away weeping from the sides of the cart. What was the use of these strange hard grains that choked their throats? They would die. And then and there many of them kept their word. . . . In vain the interpreters interpreted; in vain his two policemen showed by vigorous pantomime what should be done. The starving crept away to their bark and weeds, grubs, leaves, and clay, and left the open sacks untouched.

Rudyard Kipling. (1972) William the conqueror. In: *The second Penguin book of English short stories.* Ed. C Dolley. (Penguin Books, Harmondsworth, UK.)

size of a small pea lying under the frontal lobes. That is why dogs are used as bloodhounds, and we have such a (comparatively) poor sense of smell. From here, smell passes to the cortex, not the new (neo) cortex, but a much older part. This is also where smell may reach awareness: epilepsy (which is abnormal electrical activity) starting here gives rise to a powerful (usually unpleasant) hallucination of smell. And from here? You have guessed it: to the amygdala and the orbitofrontal cortex. So both these areas get both taste and smell information, both vital for eating.

The sight of food involves yet another pathway. The detectors in the eye (the rods and cones) send this information to the thalamus, that great distributor, which sends it on to the (new) cortex at the back of your brain. From here, it passes forward, though successive parcels of cortex, each analysing increasingly complex patterns of the object (its shape, size, colour and so on) until it finally arrives at the part of the cortex lying just over your ears: the temporal lobe. This is thought to be essential for recognition by decoding what the object actually is. Damage here renders you unable to recognise familiar things (like cars, faces, foodstuffs and so on). From here it's the same story: lying just below the temporal cortex is the amygdala, and processed information passes between the temporal cortex and amygdala. And also to the orbitofrontal cortex.

You can begin to see how the brain brings together rather different sets of information about food, carried over quite distinct neural pathways. Next time the waiter sets your dinner before you, spare a quick thought about all those pathways telling you how delicious it is going to be. But can we decide which of these parts of the brain is really concerned with telling us that food is good (the biological decision), that is, it is rewarding (the psychological decision)? We have at least two candidates: the amygdala and the orbitofrontal cortex — that is, if we believe that things like 'reward' are encoded in one anatomically distinct region of brain.

We are looking for part of the brain that does not just signal a sensation, but one that changes its response according to demand state: in other words, that reflects whether or not the animal is hungry. The primary taste cortex does not fit: it responds to taste whatever. But the orbitofrontal cortex is different: its neurons respond to a taste if a monkey is hungry, but not if it is satiated with food of that taste. Furthermore, a hungry monkey will work for electrical stimulation of the same part of the orbitofrontal

Human Culture and Food

Plant and animal domestication meant much more food and hence much denser human populations. The resulting food surpluses, and (in some areas) the animal-based means of transporting those surpluses, were a prerequisite for the development of settled, politically centralized, socially stratified, economically complex, technologically innovative societies. Hence, the availability of domestic plants and animals ultimately explains why empires, literacy, and steel weapons developed earliest in Eurasia and later, or not at all, on other continents.

Jared Diamond. (1998) *Guns, germs and steel.*
(Vintage, London.)

. . . The origin of food taboos must therefore be sought in the fanciful imaginations of particular ancestors. Frazer believed that they were the indirect result and distant repercussion of the cravings and sickly imaginings common amongst pregnant women. He held that this psychological trait, which he elevated to the status of a natural and universal phenomenon, was the ultimate origin of all totemic beliefs and practices. . . .

Both the exchange of women and the exchange of food are means of securing or of displaying the interlocking of social groups with one another.

C Levi-Strauss. (1962) *The savage mind.*
(Weidenfeld and Nicolson, London.)

cortex, but only if it is hungry. Interestingly, there are nerve cells in this area that also respond to smell, particularly if it is associated with the taste of food. And these 'smell' neurons are also sensitive to satiation. Even more interestingly, nerve cells may be quite specific: give a monkey lots of a particular food, and these cells stop responding to the taste/smell of that food; but try a new one, and they respond again. It is the Belgian chocolate effect. Now try the sight of food, and you get much the same result. The 'primary' visual cortex at the back of the brain and even the more specialised cortex in the temporal lobe respond to food irrespective of whether or not the monkey is hungry: but the orbitofrontal cortex does not. It is looking good for the orbitofrontal cortex.

A psychologist friend points out that the amygdala has a strong case as well. There is no doubt that the amygdala plays an important part in eating. Tucked into the temporal lobe, this big ball of nerve cells receives information from all the other parts of the brain concerned with eating, including smell, taste and highly processed visual information from the overlying temporal cortex. Damage the amygdala, and you get an extraordinary set of curious behaviours, called the Kluver-Bucy syndrome after the two scientists who first described it. One of its features is that animals eat things that would not ordinarily eat — meat, in the case of monkeys. And they tend to put any object they come across into their mouths — rather like a very young human child. Another is that they lose the ability to show (and apparently experience) emotions such as fear: recall that the pleasure of eating is an emotional response. The role of the amygdala in fear and aggression is discussed in Chapter 10. But the amygdala is also important for learning to associate food with other sorts of stimuli. For example, that bell which signals food to dogs or schoolchildren: damage the amygdala, and this connection is no longer possible. Recall that the bell itself becomes rewarding, and you begin to see how the amygdala may fit in. Recognising food by its appearance is actually a learned ability (unlike its taste or smell); so knowing that a piece of cheese is good to eat, or even that a tin of spaghetti contains food, may owe a lot to your amygdala.

Whether or not the cells of the amygdala respond differently according to how hungry you are is a bit uncertain. One set of experiments shows a rather small effect: another that there are neurons that respond to the sight

There are certain types of conversations, certain types of self-awareness, which only take place in restaurants, particularly those bearing on the psychodynamics of relationships between couples who. . . I notice often eat out with the specific purpose of monitoring the condition of their affair, as if breaking up were something that, by fixed anthropological principle, can only be done in installments and in public. . . .

John Lanchester. (1996) *The debt to pleasure.*
(Henry Holt and Company, New York.)

But a big dinner, with a hired chef and two borrowed footmen, with Roman punch, roses from Henderson's, and menus on gilt-edged cards, was a different affair, and not to be lightly undertaken. As Mrs Archer remarked, the Roman punch made all the difference; not in itself but by its manifold implications — since it signified either canvas-backs or terrapin, two soups, a hot and a cold sweet, full decolletage with short sleeves, and guests of a proportionate importance.

Edith Wharton. (1920) *The age of innocence.*
(Penguin Books, London.)

We warmed the glass slightly in a candle, filled a third of it, swirled the wine around, nursed it in our hands, held it to the light, breathed it, sipped it, filled our mouths with it and rolled it over the tongue, ringing it on the palate like a coin on a counter, tilted our heads back and let it trickle down the throat
'It is a little, shy wine like a gazelle.'
'Like a leprechaun.'
'Dappled, in a tapestry meadow.'
'Like a flute by still water.'

Evelyn Waugh. (1945) *Brideshead revisited.*

He noticed with surprise and a certain solicitous distress that Miss Emmeline's appetite was poor, that it didn't, in fact, exist. Two spoonfuls of soup, a morsel of fish, no bird, no meat, and three grapes — that was her whole dinner. He looked from time to time at her two sisters; Georgiana and Caroline seemed quite as abstemious. They waved away whatever was offered them with an expression of delicate disgust. . . .

of food, most vigorously when the animal is hungry. If you degrade food (i.e. contaminate it with salt, say) then the amygdala responds to it less — again, the neurons of the amygdala seem to be encoding 'value' (Is this good food?) as well as 'category' (What is this? Is it food?). Scanning humans brains also shows that the amygdala responds to the sight of food more if the person is hungry. So the amygdala may be sensitive both to rewarding stimuli (food) and the 'value' of this reward depends on current need. Just what we would expect.

You will know that people from different cultures have different tastes in food. You acquire your taste in food as you grow up. One of the recent social changes in the UK has been the ease with which people adopt new foods. It wasn't always like this. A previous generation regarded foreign food with suspicion and dislike. Even now, in certain parts of the world, you can find restaurants catering for UK tastes that serve 'British' food. We like what we know. Few Brits will eat sheeps' eyes or chicken feet, though these are delicacies elsewhere. There are heart-rending accounts of people starving to death in a famine rather than eat the strange foods provided by an earlier generation of foreign aid agencies. Rats are the same. They are very wary of new food. They need to be: eating something they have not tried before can be a fatal business. But damage their amygdala, and they eat it with gusto. A warning system has been disabled.

You also need to know when what you eat makes you ill. Everyone has a similar story. In my case, it is chicken tandoori, which I used to love. Now I never choose it. Why? Years ago I had it for supper one night in India, and became ill about 30 minutes later. Now, this was not due to the chicken tandoori, but the fish I had had for lunch (6 hours before). I know this. Or rather, my cortex does (it's medically trained). My limbic system does not. It associates illness with the chicken tandoori, and warns me off it. No amount of logic can change this. I have hardly ever ordered this lovely dish since, but I continue to enjoy fish. Rats are the same; you can induce a mild gastric illness by giving them an injection of lithium chloride. Do this after they have just eaten a distinctive food, and next time (after they have recovered) they avoid it — this is sometimes called 'bait-shyness' or, scientifically, 'conditioned taste aversion.' Just like me and the chicken tandoori. But damage their amygdala, and they no longer seem bothered. They have lost the association between illness and

"Pray, don't talk to me of eating," said Emmeline, drooping like a sensitive plant. "We find it so coarse, so unspiritual, my sisters and I. One can't think of one's soul while one is eating."

Aldous Huxley. (1921) *Crome yellow.*
(Penguin Books, Harmondsworth, UK.)

The King bade us sit down, and presently his servants set before us dishes of such meats as we had never seen before in all our lives. My famished companions ate ravenously; but my stomach revolted at the sight of this food and, in spite of my hunger, I could not eat a single mouthful. As things turned out, however, my abstinence saved my life. For as soon as they had swallowed a few morsels my comrades began to lose their intelligence and to act like gluttonous maniacs; so that after a few hours of incessant guzzling they were little better than savages.

Whilst my companions were thus feeding, the naked men brought in a vessel filled with a strange ointment, with which they anointed their victims' bodies. The change my companions suffered was astonishing; their eyes sank into their heads and their bellies grew horribly distended, so that the more they swelled the more insatiable their appetites became.

Translated by N J Dawood. (1954). *The thousand and one nights.*
The fourth voyage of Sindbad the sailor.
(Penguin Books, Harmondsworth, UK.)

preceding food, something all animals need to learn fast. Another warning system lost. So the amygdala functions not only to tell you what to eat, but what not to eat.

Can we reconcile the roles of the orbitofrontal cortex and the amygdala in eating? First, we should remember that, whilst the amygdalae of rats and monkeys (and of humans) are recognisably similar (though not identical) their orbitofrontal cortices are very different. Rats do not have much orbitofrontal cortex (though it's not absent) whereas primates have lots. So one possibility is that some of the functions of the amygdala in rats has been taken over, or at least supervised, by the orbitofrontal cortex in primates. So we might have to be careful about exact comparisons between experiments in rats and primates. Another is that the two structures are interconnected, so it may be that the 'reward centre' is not a centre at all, but more of a system. One way of separating the amygdala and orbitofrontal cortex might be to say that the amygdala is more concerned with persistent, longer term aspects of food (i.e. what food is, what food you like, what you avoid, what you associate with food) whereas the orbitofrontal cortex is important for moment to moment decisions (Shall I eat now? What shall I eat? Is this particular food good to eat?). So they work together, as we know they must.

There is experimental evidence that damaging the dopamine system in the brain alters reward, so here is another part of the brain to add to our reward system. We begin to see that the very idea of what a 'reward' is turns out to be much more complex than we originally thought. Does dopamine play any special role in reward?

Nearly all the brain's dopamine comes from rather few cells lying in the upper brainstem: from here, dopamine fibres travel to very restricted parts of the brain (Chapter 3). If you give an animal a drug that blocks the action of dopamine, it finds things less rewarding than it otherwise would. The same result occurs if you destroy the brain's dopamine system. Such animals don't eat, even though they are foods-deprived; they do not drink, even though they are dehydrated, they do not mate in situations when they otherwise would. They do not do much at all. Do the reverse experiment, and increase dopamine using suitable drugs: the opposite occurs. They eat more, or more often, than they would, mate when previously they had been uninterested and so on. If you electrically stimulate the brain's dopamine system, animals also find this very rewarding. The electrical stimulus seems to have replaced the more natural reward, and the experimenter has maybe short-circuited the reward pathway.

One idea, then, is that all rewards are signalled as such by a puff of dopamine in the brain. This assumes that the current motivational (demand) state connects a category of stimuli (either an object or doing something with it) to the dopamine system, thus causing the brain to release dopamine when the object appears. Simple. The idea gets more attractive. People take some drugs because they are highly rewarding. These drugs includes amphetamine, cocaine and crack. Guess which brain system these drugs activate? Dopamine — of course. Even addictive (demand-creating, reward-providing) drugs such as morphine and heroin may act indirectly on the dopamine system. It is beginning to look good for dopamine. Perhaps misers count their gold because it activates their dopamine; computer nerds activate theirs by playing games; perhaps listening to music or watching a beautiful sunset, are simply other ways of giving yourself a dopamine high. Follow this line of argument to its conclusion: life is mostly trying to maximise your dopamine activity. You find this ridiculous? Is it all that simple?

No it is not. If you think for a moment, it is clear that activating dopamine is unlikely to represent 'reward'. Dopamine can only be detected by the brain because the released dopamine acts on a number of other nerve cells. If they did not exist, changes in dopamine activity wouldn't matter. These activated 'receptor' cells are more likely to represent 'reward' than dopamine itself. Of course, changes in dopamine might be essential for reward to occur. A direct way of measuring what dopamine does is to record the electrical activity in the dopamine cells during the process of receiving a reward, such as a drink of fruit juice. These cells lie is a small, tight, bunch in the upper midbrain. Sure enough, a monkey's dopamine cells respond when it gets a drink of juice. It seems to signal reward. However, now let us flash a light just before the monkey gets its drink. At first, the dopamine cells seem uninterested: but as the monkey learns to associate the light with the food, the appearance of the light activates dopamine. Hurrah! Just what we would expect, because we know that stimuli (light) predicting reward (food) themselves become rewarding. But wait, we have just noticed something peculiar:

the dopamine cells are responding to the light all right, but no longer to the fruit juice. . . . . . . Now that is a real puzzle. Is the juice no longer rewarding? No: if we stop giving it, the monkey stops responding to the light (psychologists call this 'extinction'). So the juice is still rewarding, but dopamine no longer responds to it.

One idea is that dopamine neurons encode *predictions* about rewards. When *nothing* unexpected happens, the juice keeps coming, the system is quiet. Dopamine activity only changes, and you only learn, when something *unexpected* happens — either the appearance of an unexpected reward, or the failed appearance of an expected one. This *error* signal then instructs or 'teaches' other brain areas, so they can learn about the reward.

So our search for the reward system in the brain has taken us on quite a journey, and we still cannot really decide whether there is one reward system or many. But amongst all the names of brain areas that have a claim on this most central of brain activities you will have noticed a conspicuous omission. No mention at all of the hypothalamus. Now, it is an extraordinary fact that those working today on the brain and reward seem curiously uninterested in the hypothalamus (unlike an earlier generation of neuroscientists). Yet, as we saw earlier in this chapter, there are elaborate neurochemical codes in the hypothalamus, or acting on the hypothalamus from the body, that control when we stop eating, and when we start again: the essential regulators of energy stores and body weight. We also saw that these codes operate by making us hungry, or satiated, with all that this means in terms of reward (the pleasure of eating) and its converse, punishment (hunger itself). There must be some connection between this physiological control system and that encoding reward. There is plenty of anatomical evidence for such a connection between the amygdala and the hypothalamus, as well as others to and from the orbitofrontal cortex and so on. But nobody knows how information about physiological deficits (coded in the hypothalamus) gets translated into activity in the reward system. And, if truth be told, nobody is doing anything much about it.

By the time the helicopter returns we are all looking rather trimmer than when we arrived, though we have managed to eat something now and again. Once we get back to the world we left behind only four days ago, we know that we will quickly return to our previous body weight. For most people, body weight is defended: deviations in direction are quite quickly corrected. The hypothalamus can be relied upon. But not for everyone. Eating disorders, particularly in young people, seem to have increased dramatically in the past couple of decades. Curiously, obesity is not classed as an eating disorder perhaps for social rather than logical reasons though the risks it carries suggest otherwise. Are these disorders another example of maladaptation to an environment for which evolutionary defences are not well-developed?

Anorexia nervosa was only recognised as a discrete condition in the late 19th century, though it took longer for it to be accepted as a disorder. Voluntary food restriction (fasting) has been known since the dawn of recorded history, particularly as part of religious observance. There has been a very marked increase in anorexia during the last twenty or thirty years, overwhelmingly in young women, a fact that has attracted a variety of explanations. Some estimate the current incidence of anorexia nervosa as between 0.5% and 4% (i.e. 1–8 per two hundred) young women, but only about a tenth or less than that in young men. It is a disorder of puberty (though it can occur during the prepubertal or the post-pubertal years), which immediately suggests a hormonal explanation. And it's particularly prevalent in those in whom minimal body weight is an advantage (models, ballet dancers, athletes) which suggests a social factor — though do anorexics become ballet dancers or vice-versa? Anorexic women think of themselves as fat, which suggests a cognitive or 'body-image' disorder, and feminists point to the social pressure on young women to stay slim. Earlier times thought it romantic for young women to look 'wasted' or 'ethereal'. Even today, excessive slimness is prized.

Anorexia is often accompanied by other recognisable psychological conditions, like low self-esteem or depressed mood. Untreated anorexics can starve themselves to death; there is a complete failure of the normal defences against starvation, even though these defences have been honed during the long history of humanity surviving in a food-scarce world. It is ironic that females (rats, anyway) seem to be better than males at coping with food shortage. Bulimia was once thought of as a variant of anorexia, but is now increasingly recognised as a distinct disorder. Bulimics binge, eating huge but infrequent meals, and then often vomit. There are more young female bulimics than males, but the sex ratio isn't quite as extreme as in anorexia.

You might expect that anorexics have disordered satiety or energy store signals. Perhaps their body is fooling them into thinking they are well-fed and fat whereas just the opposite is true. Not so: their leptin levels, for instance, are what you would expect in an underfed, underweight person. The brain ignores the starvation signals the body sends to it. And reproduction is turned off, just as you would expect in times of food shortage. Severely anorexic girls don't menstruate, and even those who do are likely to be sub-fertile. There has been speculation about the role of oestrogens. These hormones certainly reduce appetite experimentally, and castration in animals (or menopause in women) is associated with increased body weight.

The complex behavioural and psychological features of anorexia have been a real problem for those seeking a 'biological' explanation. There must be a brain-state that reflects the anorexic condition, maladaptive as it is. This might be the primary cause, that is, a genetic or neurochemical abnormality is primarily responsible for self-starvation or secondary to a 'social' factor such as peer pressure, adverse family conditions, excessive educational or social demands or even physical abuse. Although the role of serotonin in 'normal' eating has not been found to be particularly prominent, it could play a role in anorexia. Giving anorexics drugs that increase serotonin can be helpful for the associated depression, but is not very effective on food intake (in fact, raising the brain's serotonin in normal people will decrease appetite). But let us not fool ourselves: we do not understand the cause of anorexia, or why it is on the increase (alongside, strangely, increased obesity). The answer may lie in understanding more about how all those peptides in the hypothalamus function in anorexia. Or are there abnormal ones that override those that should protect you against starvation? One thing we can be sure about: the 'social', 'psychological' 'genetic' and 'biological' explanations of anorexia or any other eating disorder are not alternatives, but complementary.

Our rather pathetic performance as food-gatherers in our verdant but strangely unyielding valley might suggest that the modern human brain is not too good as a food-supplier, in an emergency, at least. In fact the exceptional qualities of the human brain are shown to perfection by what we do with our food. The limbic brain in humans is recognisably similar to that of other mammals, and serves much the same purpose. Most of what we know about the signals, hormones and chemicals regulating food intake applies to them as well as to us. So it is not here that we look for distinct human abilities. The point has already been made that we can only understand the function of the human limbic system, and its role in survival, together with the other properties of the rest of the brain — in our case, the cognitive abilities of our huge cerebral cortex. Humans bring their mental versatility to their eating behaviour, as they do to everything else. The limbic system, beavering away to make sure we survive, is not alone.

First, there is how we get food. Humans are omnivores, and eat meat, fruit and vegetables. This is a huge advantage, since it reduced our ancestors' reliance on the hunt. We do not know which part of the brain enables us to be so versatile. It may, actually, be the limbic system: as we have seen, damage to the temporal lobe, which contains the amygdala and associated parts of the limbic cortex, can result in vegetarian animals eating meat. Hunting is much more effective if done by packs, and primitive human societies have well-developed formalised systems for organising hunts and rules for distributing the food after a success. In this, we are not unique. Chimpanzees and even lions can and do hunt cooperatively, and a kill is shared according to defined 'rules' (usually the most dominant animal gets first choice). And chimps will eat both fruit and meat, though the latter is rather a rare treat. So whilst the human brain may be rather better at some of these things, it is hardly a defining quality.

We also cultivate food, and this needs even more brain power. Sowing seeds, developing cultivated strains with better yields, and breeding cattle needs at least an intuitive grasp of some fairly complex biological principles. Cultivated food represents a ready-made store-house, though it brings other problems like how to defend it against others, or what to do if the crops fail or the herd dies. There are some animals that do a sort of primitive cultivation, but nothing like what we do. Even chimps, living alongside us for millennia, have no cultivation system. We only need to take note of the huge expansion in 'scientific' farming that is, farming based on principles learnt through experience over the past centuries, including the use of genetically-engineered crops and animals in this one, to see how the unique potential of the human brain has been applied to a fundamental limbic problem of feeding ourselves adequately. But it is not our limbic system that has allowed all this to happen, it is our cortex. Here, surely we have one exceptional property of the human brain.

Cooking is another. Cooking food, a unique human discovery, has several advantages. It can make indigestible foods digestible (for example, potatoes). It also improves variety and tastiness. France, India, China and some other countries show that culinary technology can rise to the level of supreme art. But it is the cortex that cooks, not the limbic system. The limbic system enjoys the result and, perhaps, tells the cortex if it has got it right and what it would like next.

Many hunting animals run faster than we can, are stronger than us, have sharper claws or better night-vision. But we make tools. Spears to throw, arrows to shoot, traps to set and guns to fire. Not all, of course, to get food, but essential for increasing the efficiency of hunters, that is, decreasing the cost/benefit (energy expenditure/energy gain) ratio. Agricultural tools are equally vital for growing crops only possible if you have the cortex required to see what is needed and to invent them. The development of the hoe, the spade, the plough, the fishing net were all landmarks, invented by the cortex at the behest of the limbic system. Now, other animals also use tools. Chimps 'fish' for termites, some animals even build traps. But none come near the versatility and ingenuity of the human brain to use tools to get food or ensure reliable supplies.

But we also use food as a social instrument. Food is not distributed evenly in our society any more than in those of most other animals. Take a look at that small male baboon hanging around on the edge of his social group, trying hard not to attract the aggressive attentions of the dominant males. He is skinny, his fur is unkempt and his condition contrasts with the glossy, well-fed appearance of the powerful males at the centre of the group (at this point you may find drawing human parallels difficult to resist). Though the persistent stress of avoiding injury no doubt plays its part in his condition, a less-than-optimal food supply does not help. Our history shows the same uneven distribution of food in our own species. The reasons for this are varied, but the upshot is that giving or receiving food has become a way that humans regulate and define their social groups. We have instrumentalised food. We use it as a means of social control and social interaction, deriving, perhaps, from the time when there was not enough food even in the West for everyone. Thus the tribute to

Eating Disorders

Whereas most of us assess ourselves on the basis of our perceived performance in various domains — e.g., relationships, work, parenting, sporting prowess — patients with anorexia nervosa or bulimia nervosa judge their self-worth largely, or even exclusively, in terms of their shape and weight and their ability to control them.

In anorexia nervosa, the pursuit of weight loss is successful in that a very low weight is achieved. . . . In most instances, there is no true anorexia as such. . . . Interest in the outside world . . . declines as patients become underweight, with the result that most become socially withdrawn and isolated. . . .

The combination of undereating and binge eating in bulimia results in bodyweight being generally unremarkable. . . . Most patients with bulimia are distressed by their loss of control over eating and ashamed of it, which makes them easier to engage in treatment that those with anorexia. . . .

Anorexia is the one eating disorder to be associated with a raised mortality rate, the standardised mortality ratio over the first 10 years from presentation being about 10. Most deaths are a direct result of medical complications or due to suicide.

. . . Virtually nothing is known about the individual causal processes involved or how they interact. . . . There is a clear and possibly substantial genetic contribution to both anorexia nervosa and bulimia nervosa. . . . There has been extensive research into the neurobiology of eating disorders. This work has focussed on neuropeptide and monoamine (especially 5-HT) systems thought to be central to the physiology of eating and weight regulation. . . .

Drug treatment does not have an established place in the management of anorexia nervosa. . . . . The gulf between research evidence and service provision needs to be investigated and bridged; too few patients receive evidence-based treatment and too many receive suboptimal or inappropriate therapy.

C G Fairburn and P J Harrison. (2003) Eating disorders.
Lancet **361**, pp. 407–416.

kings and chieftains was often based on gifts of food, and even today we continue the practice, taking bottles of wine to parties, sending chocolates to those we love or presents of food to those we want to influence, doing business over lunch and courting those we fancy over candle-lit suppers. Even in a society where money is the principal means of barter, conditions can quickly change to a more primitive pattern: witness the different social roles of food during periods of rationing in the UK during the second world war. It is highly characteristic of the human brain that it takes a basic 'need' such as food, and develops it into a more complex instrument of social regulation. It is the cortex taking heed of the limbic system, but using this information for a different, more complex purpose than simple survival.

Getting Food

What are the major facts that scientists have discovered about food intake? Name one fact about food intake! Researchers often find this a very difficult question to deal with. Why is this so? Is it because there are no facts (universally agreed statements)? Or is it because we are dealing with a form of *behaviour* which operates according to probabilistic rather than deterministic principles? Whatever the answer to this question, it should be kept in mid that food intake is a form of *behaviour* believed to be under voluntary control. . . a study of food intake should concentrate on the way in which environmental, cognitive, or biological events can be translated into effects upon an act of behaviour.

> J E Blundell. (1996) Food intake and weight regulation. In: *Regulation of body weight; Biological and behavioural mechanisms*. Eds. C Bouchard and G A Bray. (John Wiley and Sons Ltd., London.)

Most species are useless to us as food, for one or more of the following reasons: they are indigestible. . . poisonous. . . low in nutritional value. . . tedious to prepare. . . difficult to gather. . . or dangerous to hunt. . . .
By selecting and growing those few species of plants and animals that we can eat, so that they constitute 90 percent rather than 0.1 percent of the biomass on an acre of land, we obtain far more edible calories per acre. As a result, one acre can feed many more herders and farmers — typically, 10 to 100 times more — than hunter-gatherers. That strength of brute numbers was the first of many military advantages that food-producing tribes gained over hunter-gatherer tribes.

> Jared Diamond. (1998) *Guns, germs and steel*. (Vintage, London.)

Why (do) we heat our food and eat it while it is still hot? There are three alternative explanations. One is that it helps to simulate 'prey temperature'. Although we no longer consume freshly killed meat we nevertheless devour it at much the same temperature as other carnivore species. Their food is hot because it has not yet cooled down; ours is hot because we have re-heated it. Another interpretation is that we have such weak teeth that we are forced to 'tenderize' the meat. . . but this does not explain why we heat up many kinds of food that do not require 'tenderizing'. The third. . . is that, by increasing the temperature of the food, we improve its flavour. . . . This relates back to our ancient primate past. . . Moneys and apes. . . are extremely sensitive to subtleties of varying tastiness in their food. . . . Perhaps we are harking back to this earlier primate fastidiousness.

> Desmond Morris. (1967) *The naked ape*.
> (Jonathan Cape, London.)

Chapter 6

Staying Wet and Salty

As a preclinical medical student, I remember being told by a tutor that the body was 90% water. I also remember not being too sure about how I was supposed to react to this information: am I just a bag of dirty water? By amazement, that just 10% of the molecules in my body could turn me into a human being? It was only after I had seen patients in hospital that I understood what he was trying to say. People with gut diseases, who are unable to retain intestinal fluid, were being kept alive by having fluids dripped into their veins; others with kidney-diseases who spent their days passing huge quantities of urine; casualties who had lost a large amount of blood being revived by a transfusion. I realised that keeping the body's fluid balance in shape was a major responsibility, and that when it went wrong, everything else began to fail. And I also learned that my tutor's statement (despite his air of authority) was wrong: The body is about 70% water. But that is still more than half.

The only animals who do not have to worry too much about their water supply are those who live in it. None of them lives in pure water, and most live in the salty sea. The cells of the body function only when they are surrounded by a solution that has a composition rather similar to sea-water, which is dilute saline (though with a few other very important chemicals in it). So when we left the sea, as our remote ancestors are thought to have done, we took our sea-water with us. We did this by having a relatively impermeable skin, containing our own private bath of sea-like water, in which our cells can flourish. This is called 'extra-cellular' (outside the cells) fluid. The first important point about extracellular fluid (ECF for short) is that we need to keep it rather constant, otherwise our cells will become very unhappy indeed. The second important point is

Thirst

The sensation of thirst is central to our very existence. It is, as Rullier said in 1821. . . 'le sentiment le plus vif et le plus imperieux de la vie'. . The gratification of thirst is universally held to be one of the pleasures of life; the sensation cannot be ignored, and if water be lacking, thirst comes to dominate our thoughts and behaviour; it drives us to the utmost endeavour and achievement. . . or to the depths of despair and degradation.

J T Fitzsimons. (1979) *The physiology of thirst and sodium appetite.*
(Cambridge University Press, Cambridge.)

'Thirst is not a local sensation, as certain physiologists have thought, but on the contrary, it is an expression of a general need to restore the liquids of the economy that have suffered a loss. Again it is for the same reason that bleeding often produces the sensation of thirst'.

C Bernard. (1856) Quoted in *The physiology of thirst and sodium appetite.*
(Cambridge University Press, Cambridge.)

Body fluid homeostasis requires the successful integration of the complementary physiological mechanisms of conservation and behavioral controls of ingestion. The regulation of these diverse homeostatic processes involves the coordination of neural and endocrine signals. . . Another general principle that has emerged from the study of body fluid homeostasis is that the genomic actions of steroids function as longer-term signals that regulate the more rapid behavioral actions of peptides. . . .

The best testimony regarding the generalities and importance of the neuroendocrine principles that govern fluid homeostasis is the increasing evidence that similar processes subserve hunger and energy homeostasis.

S J Fluharty. (2002) Neuroendocrinology of body fluid homeostasis.
In: *Hormones brain and behavior.* Eds. D Pfaff, A P Arnold, S E Fahrbach,
A M Etgen, R T Rubin. (Academic Press, Amsterdam.)

Water has long been a critical problem for poor people. In many places, access to clean water all but defines poverty. The consensus among experts in that 1.4 billion people in the world do not have access to safe water (. . . roughly one in four). . . . If you live in North America or Japan, you use on average 158 gallons of water a day. . . . If you live in Europe, you use about 80 gallons, and if you live in sub-Saharan Africa, 2.5 to 5 gallons.

Bill McKibben. (2003) Our thirsty future.
New York Review of Books **50**, pp. 58–60.

that we live in a rather dry, salt-deficient world, and, try as we may, we persistently leak water (and salt). So keeping the ECF in proper order is a major homeostatic challenge. But we do it all the time, without thinking much about it. Unless some of our regulatory mechanisms break down, when suddenly we realise how important this water and salt business really is.

You can easily test how efficient your body is about controlling its water and salt content by taking a walk in a desert. After a few hours, slogging through the sand and the heat, you begin to be very thirsty. As you plough on, your thirst increases, becoming ever more imperative, until it begins to occupy your every thought. You think you will go crazy unless you get a drink. And you notice that you do not pass much urine, and what you do pass seems very concentrated. Your sweat runs into your eyes, making them smart, and into your mouth, tasting salty. Finally, you reach the oasis, and a cool drink. It is one of the most wonderful experiences of your life. At the subsequent meal, you notice that your food seems to need a lot of salt to make it taste good. Put a little of this food, after you have added the right amount of salt, into a container, and try it again a few days later, when you are back in the normal world. It tastes awful. It is much too salty.

In the desert, our body trades off one important control (keeping cool in the heat of the sun by sweating) against another (losing too much salt and water). Our little experiment has shown us that the body has both physiological ways of combating fluid loss (conservation by reducing urine flow) and the now familiar trick of making us behave in such a way that we restore the deficit. In this case, we are made to want to drink. The brain also ensures that we take in the extra salt we have lost by making us like concentrations of salt that would otherwise be distasteful. If you were to do a similar experiment on an animal, you would find that it, too, would seek out water and salt. It would drink large amounts of quite concentrated salt solution, which under more normal conditions it would refuse to touch. It would go to places that it knew had salty food, or work (in the laboratory) — say by pressing a lever — to get access to salt or salty water. How does the brain make sure you have enough salt and water?

You can actually think of your body as three bags, each inside one another. In the centre bag are the cells. They are also full of fluid, though

'*Water!*'

As in the sea at a moment of desperate crisis his body changed, became able and willing. He scrambled out of the trench on legs that were no longer wooden. . . he came to the edge of the cliff and a solitary gull slipped away from under his feet. . . . He worked himself round on his two feet but the horizon was like itself at every point. . . . He went around again. At last he turned back to the rock itself and climbed down. . . . When he was below the level of the bird droppings he stopped and began to examine the rock foot by foot. . . . He saw water on a flat rock, went to it, put his hands on either side of the puddle, and stuck his tongue in. His lips contracted round his tongue, sucked. The puddle became nothing but a patch of wetness on the rock.

William Golding. (1956) *Pincher Martin.*
(Faber and Faber, London.)

Then to this earthen Bowl did I adjourn
My Lip the secret Well of Life to learn:
And Lip to Lip it murmur'd-
"While you live
Drink! — for once dead you never shall return".

The Rubaiyat of Omar Khayyam.
Translated by Edward Fitzgerald. (Collins, London.)

From time to time M'Crae would leave Eva to rest while he reached out towards the valley of the river to see if any sign of water were there. Time after time he returned with a solemn face which told her he had failed, and every time she was ready to meet him with a smile. It wasn't easy to smile, for though she dared not let him know, she was suffering a good deal, and the little doles of water which he allowed her to take were never enough to quench her thirst. Always in the back of her mind, whatever she might be saying or doing, thirst was the dominant idea. In all her life, she had never been far away from the sweet moisture of Brookland air: but the country through which they now struggled might never have known any moisture but that of the dew for all they could see of it. It was an endless arid plain, so vast and so terribly homogeneous that their progress began it is made up very differently from the ECF. About two-thirds of your body water is inside your cells. It is thus called intracellular fluid (ICF). Round this central bag of cells is the one we have already mentioned: the ECF (about 25% of total body water). The outside bag is the blood (about 7–8% of total body water), then we are at the skin. Now, of course, the body is not made like this. There are blood vessels all over it, and cells too, surrounded by their ECF. But, conceptually (as physiologists like to say), there are three compartments: the blood, the ECF and the ICF. Interestingly, the brain sits inside its own compartment. The major difference between ICF and the other two is that the principal salt in ECF and blood is sodium chloride (common salt) whereas inside the cells it's a range of potassium salts. The big difference between blood and ECF is that blood is full of red cells (hence its colour), but also has quite a lot of protein, which is much lower in ECF. Each compartment has to be regulated. The body has to 'know' when the composition of the fluid in any compartment is disturbed. Let's start with the blood.

The blood carries oxygen, other nutrients and things like white blood cells and antibodies to the cells of the body; it regulates the composition of the ECF (the only way anything can get into the ECF is through the blood) and it does all this by ensuring that each part of the body has an adequate blood flow — that is, a sufficient blood pressure. If this is too low, then the amount of blood (with its oxygen and nutrients etc.) reaching the cells will be too little. What happens when we lose blood: that is, when the normally secure closed blood system springs a leak? We go off to the casualty department, where a young man has been stabbed, and has lost a lot of blood.

Acute loss of blood represents loss of body fluid from one compartment. We notice that the patient looks very pale and feels cold. It is clear that the blood vessels in his skin are tightly contracted, so that blood flow is reduced. Imagine a balloon containing enough water to be fully expanded. Then suppose half of the water leaks out: the balloon partially deflates (the pressure goes down). There are only two ways to restore pressure: either pour in more water, or reduce the size of the balloon by, say, rolling a corner up. Our patient has done the latter; his body has tried to maintain his blood pressure by reducing the volume of his blood system by constricting the blood vessels in his skin (and *to seem like a sort of nightmare in which they were compelled to trudge for ever. . . .*

Francis Brett Young. (1925) *The crescent moon.*
(Penguin Books, Harmondsworth, UK.)

I had to have water. I brought my hand down and quietly undid the hasp. I pulled on the lid. It opened onto a locker. . . (he drinks from a can)

My feelings can perhaps be imagined, but they can hardly be described. To the gurgling beat of my greedy throat, pure delicious, beautiful, crystalline water flowed into my system. Liquid life, it was. I drained that golden cup to the very last drop, sucking at the hole to catch any remaining moisture. I went, "Ahhhhhh!", tossed the can overboard and got another. I opened it the way I had the first and its content vanished just as quickly. That can sailed overboard too, and I opened the next one. . . . I drank four cans, two litres of that most exquisite of nectars, before I stopped. You might think such a rapid intake of water after prolonged thirst might upset my system. Nonsense! I never felt better in my life. . . .

Yann Martel. (2002) *Life of Pi.*
(Canongate Books Ltd, Edinburgh.)

elsewhere, if we could only see inside him). The doctor tells us his blood pressure is 100/50: that means it is varying between 100 and 50 mm mercury; in a normal person of his age it would be about 120/70. But it would be even lower had he not constricted his skin vessels. We feel his pulse, it is about 120 beat per minute. Normally, it would be about 70 in someone lying down. His heart is doing its best to maintain adequate blood flow by working harder, pushing what blood there is round faster. He will not pass much urine over the next few hours, and he repeatedly licks his lips and asks for water. His body is doing its best to hang on to fluid and to replace what has been lost.

Even before the doctor begins to replace the lost blood (by a transfusion) the patient's brain has taken emergency action to keep him alive. How does it know what has gone wrong, and what to do? Your brain monitors your blood vascular system in several ways. There are nerves from some of the arteries (those in the chest, particularly) that act in much the same way as pressure gauges on a tyre. If the pressure drops, they send a message to the brainstem. The brainstem is able to activate the autonomic nervous system, the pathway that controls (amongst other things) the width of your blood vessels, hence the pale skin of the haemorrhaging patient. There are also ways of detecting changes in blood volume (pressure and volume are not the same, though one can affect the other). This information is also carried by nerves, this time from the large veins in your chest and from the atria of the heart, to the brainstem. The brainstem centres not only activate the autonomic nervous system after a haemorrhage, they also send messages to your limbic system. The limbic system makes you thirsty, and sends out urgent hormonal messages from the pituitary gland to your blood vessels (more constriction) and to your kidney. The principal message is a hormone called vasopressin, a small peptide of 8 amino-acids. It constricts blood vessels (not very powerfully) but it causes your kidney to reabsorb as much water as it can, thus retaining every drop possible. So now we know why the patient is pale, why his heart beats faster, and why his urine flow is reduced. But why is he thirsty?

Your brain is not the only structure keeping an eye on your blood pressure. Your kidney is not just an organ that excretes soluble waste products. It has a mechanism for detecting reduced blood pressure or blood volume (it also monitors blood oxygen levels, but that is another story). When these decrease, the kidney releases a big peptide called renin ('ren' is Latin for 'kidney'). Renin is actually an enzyme, and it breaks down another big peptide in the blood to a much smaller one, called angiotensin ('angio', Greek for 'vessel', 'tensin' means 'activate'). Angiotensin (Ang for short) is a remarkable peptide, only 8 aminoacids long. It carries three messages: it helps constrict blood vessels (we have seen this is an essential response to low blood pressure or reduced blood volume), it causes the adrenal gland to secrete a steroid hormone called aldosterone (which in turn acts on the kidney to make it retain salt) and. . . it makes you thirsty. All this in one peptide. A concerted set of instructions to your body that can save your life.

The brain also makes Ang. And it seems to release it under much the same conditions as the kidney. Another example of the brain and a peripheral organ working together and using the same chemical message to ensure an effective adaptation to an emergency. If you infuse a tiny amount of Ang into the brain of a rat, the animal stops whatever it is doing, and dashes off in search of a drink. Motivation in a bottle, one scientist called it. The discovery that Ang worked in the brain was largely the work of James Fitzsimons, a physiologist from Cambridge. If we map the parts of the brain stimulated by Ang, we see activated nerve cells scattered in different parts of the limbic system: some in the hypothalamus, others in the amygdala, some in the brainstem. These nerve cells represent the brain's emergency system or, rather, an emergency system, one that is specialised for water or salt deficits and waiting to spring into action. Other demands require other emergency systems. The important feature of this scattered system is that it all responds to Ang and is responsible for the fact that we behave adaptively (drink) secrete the right hormones (aldosterone and vasopressin) and our autonomic nervous system helps our heart and blood vessels adapt to the emergency. A co-ordinated adaptive response, physiologists call it. Ang is so powerful that drugs inhibiting its action on blood vessels are now a prominent and much-used method of treating high blood pressure.

Dehydration is an ever-present problem for many mammals. Dehydration will increase the concentration of salt in the ECF. If this happens, then water is sucked out of the cells in an attempt to dilute the

ECF back to its normal concentration. So the cells shrink. Detectors in the limbic system (discovered more than 50 years ago, but people are still arguing about exactly where they are) signal this shrinkage, and pass the message on to the hypothalamus. In particular, to two special nuclei that contain huge nerve cells. They are so big because they have to make enough hormone to secrete into the blood. This takes a lot of synthetic machinery, so the cells are enormous (they are called 'magnocellular' or 'big celled' nuclei). Vasopressin is one of these hormones.

The power of vasopressin becomes obvious if you lack it. There is a small town in Vermont, USA called Brattleboro; not one most people will have heard about. But every researcher working on water balance knows its name. Why? Because, about 40 years ago, a laboratory there was breeding rats and noticed that the floor was persistently wet in some of the cages. Their first thought was that the water supply was leaking or that the rats were somehow interfering with the water bottles. Then they realised that the wetness was caused by urine, not water, and that the rats spent much of their day drinking. By chance, these rats had a defective gene associated with the formation of vasopressin. Essentially, their brains were vasopressin-free. Because their kidneys had no vasopressin signal they were unable to retain water and so they passed dilute urine all the time, and had to drink constantly to keep their body water in balance. These Brattleboro rats are now used in many laboratories as a sort of natural 'knockout': that is, a strain that lacks one particular gene.

We should note here that vasopressin is used by the brain as a transmitter in some (normal-sized) nerve cells as well as in the strange magnocellular ones, so some of the deficits these rats show could be due to other parts of the brain malfunctioning. For example, vasopressin in small neurons (quite close to the big ones) is known to be concerned with the response to stress (see Chapter 4). There was some excitement, a few years ago, when it was found that Brattleboro rats could not learn as well as normal ones. Vasopressin as a 'learning' peptide? Could we inject vasopressin and improve memory? Some thought so, until it was shown that, actually, getting up all night (actually during our day, since rats are nocturnal) to pass urine was the reason that these rats were impaired: they were dog-tired! Rats, like many other animals, do not like to urinate in their beds. Once you reduced their urine flow, they learned as well as any other rat.

Humans can also suffer from lack of vasopressin, though it is quite rare. Usually it's a result of damage to the hypothalamus or pituitary by a tumour, or a blow to the head. Such people show similar problems to Brattleboro rats: they pass huge amounts of urine, a condition called diabetes insipidus (this is quite different from the more common diabetes mellitus, caused by lack of insulin) and have to drink equally large amounts of water to keep in balance. They can be cured by giving them a vasopressin-like compound, often as a snuff. But untreated lack of vasopressin is a major problem, and vastly disturbs normal homeostasis, showing just how important this hormone is for regulating water balance. Incidentally, some people with diabetes insipidus gradually recover spontaneously. This is due to the regrowth of the damaged magnocellular neurons. They are one of the few parts of the adult brain that can regrow after damage, a fascination for those trying to understand why most of the rest of the brain cannot repair itself.

Whilst vasopressin deals with dehydration by acting on the kidney, another signal is sent causing the animal to feel thirsty, and drink, thus ensuring that there is increased water intake for the kidneys to act upon. This form of thirst (cell shrinkage) does not seem to depend on Ang, but exactly what happens is still debated. Most people agree that the control centre for dehydration-induced drinking lies in the hypothalamus somewhere, not a surprising conclusion bearing in mind the overall function of this part of the brain in detecting and remedying metabolic imbalances of various sorts. Water from the stomach passes into the blood, where it is joined by that retained by the kidneys; then the blood passes the water to the ECF, which passes it onto the cells.

As well as water, it is a lack of salt we need to worry about or rather, what our bodies are set up to detect most readily, since we, like most other mammals, live in a world in which salt is quite hard to obtain. The scarcity and value of salt was recognised by primitive human tribes, who sometimes used it for bartering. Salt was even thought a suitable present for kings in earlier times. One of the triumphs of the human brain (the cortex) is to have worked out how to supply salt easily and cheaply, so that our problem nowadays is not too little salt, but too much. Low body salt induces animals and people to search for salt (as we saw after our walk in the desert). Unlike thirst, salt appetite develops much more slowly, over hours or even days, so the mechanism is different. But the signals are ones we have already met: aldosterone, and Ang; both make animals seek salt, and they act together. Aldosterone, which comes from the adrenal gland, both stimulates salt appetite and makes the kidney retain salt, so levels in the urine fall. Take too much aldosterone, and you retain too much salt, followed by more water (to dilute the salt) and your blood volume expands. This, in some people, can overload the heart, so that one treatment for heart failure is to give a drug that blocks the action of aldosterone. You might be wondering how Ang from the kidney can get into the brain; after all, the barrier between the blood and the brain keeps out many peptides. But there are special areas in the limbic system where this barrier is incomplete, and Ang acts at two or three of them to stimulate the brain. And the Ang produced by the brain itself plays a role. Inject Ang into the brain, and in a few hours the animal will start to want salt (after the thirst for water has died down).

As you would expect, although the brain may seem preoccupied with the too-little-salt condition, there are also ways of coping with too much salt. At least two hormones (one, intriguingly, from the heart itself) cause you to excrete extra salt in the urine, and are activated when the receptors detect too much salt, or too big a blood volume. The finding, only 20 years ago, that the heart produced a hormone was astonishing at the time, nobody had thought of the heart as a hormone-producing (endocrine) gland. The hormone is called atrial natriuretic factor (or peptide) (ANP, which means 'a hormone from the atrium that causes salt to be excreted'). It acts on the kidney in a way opposite to aldosterone. It causes the kidney to excrete increased amounts of salt. So you are protected against too much as well as too little salt. This 'see-saw' method of making sure you stay in balance is a common one in many hormone systems. Other hormones may also play a role in getting rid of too much salt. One is oxytocin, one of the hormones from the magnocellular nerve cells in the brain that also produce vasopressin. Oxytocin is chemically very similar to vasopressin, but has very different actions (another property of peptides is that if you change the signal ever so slightly then you change the function dramatically). Oxytocin is more familiar as a hormone concerned with milk production and maternal behaviour, and we consider it more in chapter 9. There are those who think it has a major role in salt excretion, though whether this relates to its other actions is still unclear.

Water and salt intake is increased in females during pregnancy and lactation, when the need for both extra salt and water becomes imperative. The curious thing is that some researchers find that oestrogen, a major hormone from the ovary and the placenta during pregnancy, actually seems to decrease water and salt appetite, though there have been those who find the opposite. Nevertheless, pregnancy is accompanied by increased appetite for salt, which is further enhanced during lactation when there is massive loss of both water and salt in the milk. The exact mechanism for these changes, though certainly hormonal, is still not too well understood. Oestrogen, as we have seen, may or may not alter salt intake and progesterone, the other major steroid hormone of pregnancy, does not have much effect on salt appetite. Prolactin may have a role. As its name implies, this peptide hormone from the pituitary plays a big part in lactation in most mammals. But in some other species, it has a different role. For example, when sea-water fish (like salmon) move into fresh-water to breed, prolactin helps them maintain their salt and water balance in their new environment. Other hormones alter during pregnancy, including aldosterone and angiotensin, and they may also contribute to the essential adaptation in salt and water appetite during pregnancy and lactation.

The limbic system of the brain takes very good care to ensure that your blood and ECF (your private sea) stay as they should, whatever the circumstances, and it has multiple ways of doing it. As in a well-designed car or plane, each critical system (the brakes, for example) has several separate systems controlling it, so that should one fail, there are others to cope. Though we have emphasised the importance of sodium chloride (common salt) in the blood and ECF, levels of other substances are also vital. For example, though potassium levels in the blood are only a fraction of sodium levels, too little potassium causes you to become very weak, and too much may stop the heart. No wonder there are so many control systems regulating the composition of the blood and ECF. The limbic system is also sensitive to potassium levels, and many of the hormones that act on sodium can also be used to regulate potassium (eg. aldosterone). Calcium is another essential ingredient of the blood, too little causes tetany (uncontrolled muscle contractions) or even convulsions. There is a special gland, the parathyroid gland in your neck, which is largely dedicated to the control of calcium levels in the blood. In fact, there are four, just to make sure! Very rarely the parathyroids fail (or are removed by mistake): the result is low blood levels of calcium, a dangerous condition. The parathyroids produce a hormone (another peptide) that increases the absorption of calcium from your gut, causes calcium from your bones (the major store of calcium) to enter the blood, and decreases calcium excretion by the kidneys. There is even another hormone (from the nearby thyroid gland) called calcitonin, which has an effect opposite to the peptide from the parathyroids. Another see-saw.

Cholera has been a scourge throughout most of human history. In 19th century England, epidemics of cholera were quite usual. In 1854, there was an outbreak in London. Within a few days, hundreds of people living in the Soho region of the city had died. Thousands fled their homes. London, deserted by those who could get away, took on the appearance of the great plague, two hundred years earlier. The medicine of the time had no answer. But in a nearby street lived Dr John Snow, who had already suspected that cholera was spread through the water supply, though no one believed him. In those days, people got their water from communal pumps. Snow interviewed the families of those who had died. He found that nearly all the deaths had been of people that used a particular pump, the one in Broad Street. He examined the water from the pump, it appeared to be contaminated. The authorities, after some persuading, took the handle off the pump so people could not use it. Within a week or so, the epidemic was over. So began the science of public health, and the realisation that an uncontaminated water supply was important, a lesson that is still being learned today in many parts of the world. Amazingly, John Snow's ideas were not accepted for many years, and the communal pumps remained dangerous.

Cholera is caused by a bacterium transmitted by contaminated food or water. Without treatment, about 50% of those with severe cholera die. But it is not the bacterium that kills them. It is the profuse, painless, watery diarrhoea. Within a few days, they are dead. Why? Because they have lost too much water and salt, not only sodium chloride, but potassium as well, and their heart fails. When this was realised (a 100 years or so after Dr John Snow) it immediately suggested an effective treatment, and a very cheap one — cholera is an illness of the poorer parts of the world.

You simply give cholera patients salts and water (in the right proportions) by mouth — the most severe cases may need them intravenously. And nearly all these people recover. You do not even need to treat the infection itself. Surely no clearer demonstration of the importance of salt and water regulation, and of the impact that physiological knowledge can have on people's lives.

Trying not to think too much about cholera, we go for lunch. We sit together in the café, and watch others. We notice that nearly everyone has a drink with their meal; so do we. So we do not just drink when we are dehydrated, or have taken too much salt. We drink for many other reasons, and meal-time drinking (psychologists call it prandial drinking) is common in humans and many other animals. Eating dry food is particularly liable to induce prandial drinking, which recalls the now discredited idea that all drinking was the result of a dry mouth. But we would not expect the brain to control prandial drinking in the same way as the sorts we have been discussing. Dehydration and salt loss are emergencies, or at the very least, require an important regulatory mechanism to be activated. Prandial drinking is not, though it may play a significant part in digestion or the subsequent metabolism of ingested food. The point is that a similar behaviour (drinking in this case) has different biological functions, and the way the brain controls the behaviour will depend on the function, not on the form of the behaviour.

Many animals and humans drink when water is available, irrespective of whether they are thirsty or in need of water replenishment. This 'anticipatory' drinking is yet another form of the behaviour, and will have its own controls. Clearly, it can be very useful for adaptation to a water-scarce environment. Drink now, you never know when water will be available again. Though if you drink too much, your limbic system will detect that you are over-hydrated and arrange that you excrete the excess water. Some animals (and even some humans) drink more when they are stressed. Again, the brain mechanisms responsible will be very different from those responding to dehydration or salt loss. We should not confuse the appearance of a behaviour with its biological significance. The motivation to drink will vary according to the circumstances in which it occurs, but drinking itself will look much the same. This implies that there are a number of ways the brain drives us to drink — the same applies to many other behaviours. All drinking may look the same to you, but not to your brain.

Although the 'dry mouth' theory as the cause for thirst has been replaced by the notion that the urge to drink arises in the brain (specifically in the limbic system), this does not mean that the sensations accompanying drinking play no role. Indeed, much evidence suggests that the rewarding effect of drinking (that blissful feeling when you took that cool draught at the end of your walk in the desert) relies highly on sensation from the mouth and pharynx. But if you bypass absorption of water (by leading it out of the stomach through a tube), drinking is still rewarding in the thirsty animal. There is argument about how much of a role 'taste' really plays in drinking water. After all, pure water has very little taste, though, of course, water in the real world often does. And we humans increase that taste by flavouring our water with all kinds of additives (e.g. fruit juice), a good example of how humans modulate the basics of adaptively important reward systems. The rewarding aspect of drinking is dependent on different parts of the brain from those that control thirst itself, or that monitor deficits in either salt or water. It does look as if the brain may have separate ways of making drinking 'rewarding' from the way it regulates the body's physiological state. In other words, as in all behaviours important for survival, one part of your limbic system signals that there is a deficit, another makes you want to do whatever counters that deficit. Chapter 5 discussed this is more detail for eating; the same principles apply to drinking.

Your walk through the desert is finished. Prompted by the signals from your blood, ECF and kidneys, all processed by your limbic system, you gratefully take the proffered glass of cool water, and down it goes. And another. Then you stop: you have had enough. Why do you stop? It is a problem for physiologists to explain: you stop well before your gut has had much of a chance to absorb the water, so you do not stop because your blood, ECF etc. are back to normal. It is still rather a puzzle, though the sensations from your mouth may play a part, as may the distention of your gut by the water you drink. But unless there is a rather clever way of increasing the amount of sensation you need for satiety according to your actual deficit (and this has never been shown, though it might occur), it is difficult to account for the quite accurate amounts of water people and animals drink in accordance with their current need. However, the brain seems to know. If you infuse some angiotensin into the brain of a rat, as we have seen, the rat becomes very thirsty. If you do not allow that rat to drink, then a new pattern of gene expression appears in the hypothalamus. But allow the rat to drink and it does not happen. It may be that this gene expression represents 'thirst'.

Sources of water have been prized since before recorded history began, and, like all valuable resources, they have been fought over. They still are. Disputes about ownership of rivers are still rife. But once again, the human cerebral cortex has helped the limbic system out. We are so used to turning on a tap at any time of the day or in any season that we forget what a remarkable (and recent) luxury this is, though one still lacking in many parts of the world. The invention of reliable, clean and cheap water supplies is one of the human brain's greatest and most beneficial achievements. First came the concept, the idea that reliable water was important. Then followed the invention of pumps and pipes to deliver it and filters to keep it clean. Every other species, including our near relatives the great apes, has to depend on natural, unreliable and rather scarce sources of water. Only we arrange things differently, though I guess you could argue the case for beavers. Methods of producing salt cheaply have revolutionised the way we control access to this essential substance, though we have risked falling into the same trap as for food. Too much rather than too little, though we do seem rather better at defending ourselves against excess salt than excess food. Easy access to water and salt has made the job of the limbic system much easier in everyday life, for Westerners at least. But, as we have seen already, it is not the limbic system that provides these solutions to an ancient problem. It is the cerebral cortex, acting at the behest of the older limbic system. As in the case for other technologies, this one occasionally goes wrong — the Broad Street pump is just one example. But overall, it has taken human beings out of the struggle for daily salt and water, at least in the better developed parts of the world. But your limbic system keeps you in balance and is still permanently on guard, in case of emergencies.

Chapter 7

Keeping Warm, Staying Cool

Sitting comfortably in your room, you idly turn the pages of this book. The window is half open, and one of those zephyr-like breezes that poets are so fond of wafts gently around you. Suddenly, we know not why, the temperature drops by 10°C. Deeply absorbed though you are, within a few moments you have noticed the change. You look up, frowning slightly, because you find what is happening not very pleasant. You shiver a little, wrapping your arms round yourself. After a few moments you go in search of a sweater, and then close the window. You notice that your hands have gone rather pale and cold in the interim. You might not notice that your heart rate has gone up a few beats.

You have just demonstrated another fundamental adaptive response. Like the other responses discussed in this book, this one has several important features. It is essential for life in the real world. You have to defend your body temperature against the demands of the environment. In this case, a cold challenge. You have an elaborate and very effective system for detecting such a challenge, and something making you respond to it. Your response is a mixture of bodily reactions — shivering, alterations in blood flow to your hands, and behaviour — closing the window, pulling on a sweater. If you were hooked up to a machine that recorded both your heart rate and the levels of hormones in your blood (such as noradrenaline), you would be able to see that both were going up. Later other hormones, such as those from the thyroid gland, might go up as well. Your body has gone into defensive mode. It is doing its best to keep you warm.

Keeping warm is a basic need for mammals. Nearly all mammals maintain their body temperature at around 37°C, though some species vary this by a degree or so. The extraordinary and rather embarrassing fact is

Temperature Regulation

Thermal homeostasis in humans and other mammals is maintained 24 hrs per day from soon after birth until death, with relatively little aberration. Moreover, under most environmental conditions (i.e., barring extreme thermal stress, drug overdose, severe trauma etc.), thermoregulatory systems rarely experience sudden failure or show 'life-threatening' deficits.

> C J Gordon. (1993) *Temperature regulation in laboratory rodents.*
> (Cambridge University Press, Cambridge.)

All (neuronal) models [of temperature regulation] start from two undisputed facts: (a) The thermoregulatory system of mammals is characterized by multiple inputs and multiple outputs. . . . (b) The multiple inputs, which may have opposing values are integrated into a common efferent signal to the effector systems. Heat production and heat loss effector systems are never activated simultaneously. . . .

> C Jessen. (1990) Thermal afferents in the control of body temperature.
> In: *International encyclopedia of pharmacology and therapeutics.*
> Eds. E Schonbaum, P Lomax, pp. 53–183.
> (Pergamon Press, New York)

A homeostatic regulation implies regulated level of some variable that is sensed by the central nervous system. In control system terminology, that regulated level is called a 'setpoint'. In thermoregulation, that implies a set, or reference, or optimal body temperature against which actual body temperature is compared. If there is a discrepancy between the two, an error signal is generated which activates heat loss or heat production mechanisms to return actual body temperature closer to set temperature. The comparator, or signal mixer that compares the two, in other words the thermostat, has been localized in the hypothalamus. . . .

> E Satinoff. (1983) A re-evaluation of the concept of the homeostatic
> organization of temperature regulation. In: *Handbook of behavioral*
> *neurobiology.* Eds. E Satinoff, P Teitelbaum, **6**, pp. 443–472.
> (Plenum Press, New York.)

Deep hibernation. . . is homeostasis in slow motion.

> C P Lyman. (1990) Pharmacological aspects of mammalian hibernation.
> In: *Thermoregulation. Physiology and biochemistry.* Eds. E Schonbaum,
> P Lomax, pp. 415–436. (Pergamon Press, New York.)

that we do not really know why there has been such evolutionary pressure for 37°C; why not 42°? Or 25°? There have been a number of theories (of course), but none is really entirely convincing. Most of them argue either that 37°C is the optimum for chemical reactions in the body to take place, or that 37°C is the easiest body temperature to maintain in an ambient one of around 25°C, which is the average air temperature in regions where mammals are thought to have evolved. The reason why mammals need to keep their internal temperature (usually called 'core temperature') constant is rather easier to understand. The mammalian body is a vast collection of chemical reactions, most of them depending on enzymes. Enzymes act as catalysts: that is, they enable other chemical reactions to occur. For example, a series of enzymes breaks down your food, and then builds up the products into the proteins, fats and carbohydrates you need. Other enzymes make your brain work, or your kidneys function. The important point is that all these reactions are heat-sensitive. Keeping your core temperature constant (within limits) keeps everything else constant, predictable and reliable. If you do not believe this, come with me to the jungle, and watch a passing crocodile. Crocodiles are 'cold-blooded' reptiles. They cannot regulate their body temperature like mammals. In the cold, they cool off, and this makes them sluggish and unable to function properly. So they and many other cold-blooded animals (called 'poikilotherms') start their day by basking in the morning sun. Only when they warm up can they get on with life. Warm up a crocodile, and you have a very frisky reptile and a rather tricky situation on your hands. Mammals do not have to warm up, but need to defend their body temperature against the vagaries of the environment.

Keeping cool is equally important. Just as your body cannot function if it gets too cold, it starts to fail if it overheats. The need to keep body temperature between rather strict limits is one of the best examples of homeostasis. Like other examples of homeostasis, these limits can be changed, or the defence mechanisms strengthened in situations where the demand is persistent — a protracted period in either a very cold or a very hot environment — by the process of adaptation or acclimatisation. Survival may thus depend on how good you are at defending your body temperature against a challenge, or how well you can adapt to a persistent change in external temperature.

When icicles hang by the wall,
And Dick the shepherd blows his nail,
And Tom bears logs into the hall,
And milk comes frozen home in pail,
When blood is nipped and ways be foul,
Then nightly sings the staring owl,
Too-wit, too-woo! A merry note,
While greasy Joan doth keel the pot.

William Shakespeare. *From: Love's labour's lost.*

Wet weather was the worst; the cold, damp, clammy wet, that wrapped him up like a moist greatcoat — the only kind of greatcoat Toby owned, or would have added to his comfort by dispensing with. Wet days, when the rain came slowly, thickly, obstinately down; when the street's throat, like his own, was choked with mist; when smoking umbrellas passed and repassed, spinning round and round like so many teetotums, as they knocked against each other on the crowded footway, throwing off a little whirlpool of uncomfortable sprinklings; when gutter brawled water-spouts were full and noisy; when the wet from the projecting stones and ledges of the church fell drip, drip, drip, on Toby, making the wisp of straw on which he stood mere mud in no time. . . .

Charles Dickens. *The chimes.*

We were between two and three thousand feet above sea-level, it was mid-winter and the cold was unspeakable. The temperature was not exceptionally low, on many nights it did not even freeze, and the wintry sun often shone for an hour in the middle of the day; but if it was not really cold, I assure you that it seemed so. Sometimes there were shrieking winds that tore your cap off and twisted your hair in all directions, sometimes there were mists that poured into the trench like a liquid and seemed to penetrate your bones; frequently it rained, and even a quarter of an hour's rain was enough to make conditions intolerable. . . . For days together clothes, boots, blankets, and rifles were more or less coated with mud. I had brought as many thick clothes as I could carry, but many of the men were terribly under-clad. . . . One icy night I made a list in my diary of the clothes I was wearing. It is of some interest as showing the amount of

I am going to assume that your house has central heating. Let's begin by examining a simple system. There is a temperature sensor in the hallway, this you set to the temperature you need. Both the information about the actual temperature in the hall and the one you have set go to an electronic controller. This does a very simple operation: it compares the two values. If the incoming temperature is lower than the one you have set (this is the set-point) then the heat system is activated. The boiler lights up, the water is heated and at the same time a pump is activated to push the hot water round your radiators. If the incoming temperature is higher than the set point, the reverse occurs. So the temperature of your hall oscillates between being slightly too high and slightly too low. The size of the oscillations will depend on how good your system is in detecting changes in temperature, and how quickly your heating system can respond. Note some features of this system: it has a detector (the sensor in the hall), a set-point (a dial you turn), a comparator (a mechanism for comparing what is with what should be) and an effector (the boiler/pump). Notice that, in this system, you have to ensure that the temperature of the hallway is set such that the rooms you really care about (the living room, bedrooms and so on) — the hall does not really matter — are kept at the temperature you want. Note also that if the outside temperature gets higher than the one you want for your house, there is not much your system can do. You need air conditioning. This, of course, can operate in the same way, though in reverse mode. A more sophisticated system might incorporate individual room controls, so you can set each room to maintain the actual temperature you want for that room (using both heating and air conditioning), without having to use the hall as an estimate (some call this a 'proxy') for the temperature you want in the parts of the house you actually live in.

Now let us see if the body has a central heating system. It is a fact that staying warm is a prime problem for most mammals. Not many places in the world are hotter than 37°C for most of the time (and many never get near this temperature). The average temperature of the earth is about 23°C. Interestingly, earliest man seems to have evolved in those areas with rather higher temperatures (Africa, India, South America etc.) and only later moved into the cooler areas. Perhaps after additional mechanisms for staying warm had been developed? The need to keep *clothes the human body can carry. I was wearing a thick vest and pants, a flannel shirt, two pullovers, a woollen jacket, a pigskin jacket, corduroy breeches, puttees, thick socks, boots and a woollen cap. Nevertheless, I was shivering like a jelly.*

> George Orwell. (1938) *Homage to Catalonia.*
> (Secker and Warburg, London).

Work. Bitter winter mornings, the knife-winds slicing through his clothes, frostbitten on the high city scaffolds, blood in his veins like ice. Work. Blistering high days of summer, the shirt sticking to a man's back, sweat running into his eyes like vinegar, thighs and legs scalded as if he had pissed his trousers, burning the skin.

> Christy Brown. (1970) *Down all the days.*
> (Secker and Warburg, London.)

The wind whipped down into the town from the cold stone churches on the Pentland hills and when you left the kitchen to go to the dunny the dogs threw themselves, yellow-eyed and broken-toothed, against their chains. It was cold out there and a draught as thin as a knife blade blew through the trapdoor at the back of the can and froze your bum and shrivelled your balls.

> Peter Carey. (1985) *Illywhacker.*
> (Faber and Faber, London.)

Now the ice lays its smooth claws on the sill,
The sun looks from the hill
Helmed in his winter casket,
And sweeps his arctic sword across the sky.

> Edwin Muir. (1887–1959) *Scotland's winter.*

By midnight the wind was straight out of the west and he heard the moan leap to bellowing, a terrible wind out of the catalog of winds. A wind related to the Blue Norther, the frigid Blaast and the Landlash. A cousin to the Bull's-eye squall that started in a small cloud with a ruddy corner, mother-in-law to the Vinds-gnyr of the Norse sagas, the three-day Nor'easters of maritime New England. An uncle wind to the Alaskan warm might explain why about 70% of energy intake in mammals is converted into heat. Not very efficient but, perhaps, rather necessary.

The problem facing your body is a good deal more dramatic than that in your house. If your house cools down too much, it does not collapse. But if your 'core' temperature (that is, the temperature of your organs, particularly of your brain) varies by more than about 3–4°C, you are in trouble. If the temperature is too low: hypothermia, followed by death if it is not quickly treated. If the temperature is too high: heat stroke, with similar fatal consequences. So the body's regulatory system needs to be that much better than your central heating.

The importance of temperature control is reflected in the numbers of temperature sensors (detectors) you have. Your body is littered with them. They are in your viscera, your brain and in your skin. Actually, your body does not care too much about your skin temperature, though, of course, the skin can burn or freeze like any other part. But the skin functions rather well even when it is hot or cold, unlike other parts of your body. Its temperature sensors are there not to protect it, but to tell the rest of the body (particularly the brain) what it is like outside (i.e., a 'proxy'). The skin carries information about the current external temperature, and signals any change. You have two sets of detectors. One (cold sensors) begin to signal when the external temperature drops below about 25°C — most of the time for most of us. The second set (the hot sensors) are active at about 30°C and above. However, do a simple experiment. Come in from the cold and dip your hand in lukewarm water: it feels quite hot. Do the same on a hot summer's day, and the water feels rather cool. Similarly, a light breeze might make you feel 'cold' in the summer, but not in the winter. So your skin temperature sensors are not 'absolute' but relative. They detect changes in external temperature relative to current skin temperature.

The sensors in your viscera (gut, heart) are there to monitor 'core' temperature. If this changes, then it means something different: the defence mechanisms have begun to fail, and action is needed. It is the temperature of your organs that the body cares about, because changes here will cause malfunction. But the temperature sensors in your brain are the really important ones. They do two things: they allow the brain itself to sample the internal body (core) temperature, mainly by detecting changes in blood temperature, and they also act as a protective mechanism for the brain itself,

Williwaw and Ireland's wild Doinionn. Stepsister to the Koshava that assaults the Yugoslavian plains with Russian snow, the Steppenwind, and the violent Buran from the great steppes of central Asia, the Cricetz, the frigid Viugas and Purgas of Siberia, and from the north of Russia the ferocious Myatel. A blood brother of the prairie Blizzard, the Canadian arctic screamer known simply as Northwind, and the Pittarak smoking down off Greenland's ice fields. This nameless wind scraping the Rock with an edge like steel.

E Annie Proulx. (1993) *The shipping news.*
(Fourth Estate, London.)

because the brain is very sensitive indeed to changes in its temperature, as you might expect of an organ that is performing thousands of heat-sensitive chemical procedures every second. But why does the brain need to know about core temperature? Because it is the controller that ensures your body keeps its temperature constant despite every pressure to change it.

A clever experiment shows us just what the brain can do and where it does it. A thermistor is a tiny tube that can be heated to a precise temperature. If we put a thermistor into the front part of the hypothalamus, it will cool or warm only this part of the brain (depending on the temperature of the thermistor). A thermistor at 33°C causes the animal to shiver and, if it is able, to move to a warmer part of its environment. A warm thermistor (say 39°C) has the opposite effect: the animal pants, (or sweats, if it can) and moves to a cooler area. The hypothalamus, an area of the brain that we know is specialised for monitoring the internal state of the body, also monitors core temperature. Furthermore, it has within it the means for adapting to excessive cold or too much heat. Damage to this part of the brain prevents animals responding in the normal way to either a hot or cold environment. It is important to mention that other parts of the brain also have temperature sensors — the hypothalamus is not the whole story. But the hypothalamus contains both a comparator, and the activating mechanism for regulating body temperature, just like the electronic box in your central heating. But how does it actually regulate body temperature? Is there a boiler and a pump?

Let's put a small rodent, like a hamster, in a cold room and watch what happens. We are using several instruments, including a camera very sensitive to heat emissions (infra-red). The hamster fluffs out its coat. After a little while, we notice that it begins to shiver, as we might expect. Then, to our amazement, the camera suddenly shows 'hot-spots' scattered over the hamster's body, on its back, in its abdomen, in its chest. It is as if the little animal had suddenly switched on its central heating. Which is exactly what has happened.

Fluffing its coat (pilo-erection) increases the insulation round the hamster, and reduces heat loss, just as if it had put on an extra layer of clothing. Many furry animals do this in the cold. Shivering increases the heat production by muscles, and hence helps warming; actually it is more effective in larger animals than little ones like hamsters. The remarkable

But instead of death came (fever and) delirium. An assembly of corpulent animals with long snouts sat gravely round his bed, like so many doctors at the bedside of a dying man. They swayed their heads backwards and forwards, then, like dogs round a bone, threw themselves down on their knees all round the bed. . . . Luca was terrified by these snouts, which were long and flexible, grey and dry and cracked, with occasional bristles. . . . At the end of each bristle there was kind of sucker with quivering eyelashes all around it, and, in the middle. . . an eye. . . staring at him. . . . In the meantime, there began to be visible, on the wall near the door, a number of green excrescences shaped like crooked fingers. . . . Now there was a wide-brimmed hat flying about in the air. . . . Other hats followed it through the pallid room, as though thrown by a skilful hand. . . . All these hats fell on the plant, covering it. . . . And then, all of a sudden, the whole hat-laden plant detached itself from the crack in the wall and., like an enormous lizard covered in armour from head to tail, started. . . running up and down the wall.

A Moravia. (1960) *Two adolescents*. Translated by A Davidson.
(Penguin Books, London).

Ironically, the characteristics that most strongly distinguish us from other animals, especially other primates, are seldom mentioned or considered in most of the commentaries we see. One such is our ability to run on two legs. Unlike our closest relatives, we do not merely scurry along for short distances with the help of our knuckles — we can race flat out for miles using only our legs and feet. A second characteristic is our nudity, our essentially furless bodies, tufted for the most part on the head and in the interstices of the limbs and torso. A third characteristic is our ability to sweat profusely. Our boastful phrases "sweat like a pig" or "sweat like a horse" are essentially meaningless, since we sweat much more than either of these animals. Running, sweating, and nudity were born of the African savanna, perhaps at the time that our ancestors moved out of the forests to become the slim and graceful Australopithicines. Out in the African sun, away from the trees, we needed to keep cool, hence our sweating, naked bodies, and we needed to protect the overactive brains that since have done so much damage to our planet, hence our thatches of hair.

E M Thomas. (2002) Nature and the art of running.
New York Review of Books **49**, pp. 31–32.

adaptation of many smaller mammals is that they carry their own central heating. It's called brown adipose tissue (brown fat) or BAT for short. It looks different from the more usual white fat (the kind you and I have, and that we see when we eat meat from larger animals like cows). White fat plays a role in resistance to cold by acting as an insulator (so fat people feel the cold less than thin ones). But BAT is special. Pilo-erection, shivering and BAT heat production (called 'non-shivering thermogenesis') are all activated by the autonomic nervous system, that set of nerve fibres that is so closely concerned with dealing with emergencies (increasing your blood pressure and heart rate when you are frightened etc.). Your autonomic system constricts the blood vessels in the skin when it is cold, so that blood is not cooled by contact with the icy air. Which is why you get that pale and pinched look on cold days. But BAT is different from white fat. Not only is it brown, it is packed with energy, and this energy is released (as heat) when the hamster faces severe cold. BAT produces its heat by a chemical reaction triggered by the autonomic nervous system and by increased amounts of adrenaline in the blood. There is BAT in the places it is important to keep warm: the neck (the brain), the chest, round the kidneys, on the back. It is amazingly effective.

The reason that small mammals need such a system is that they lose heat faster than large ones, because their surface area relative to their volume is greater. This is even more pronounced in young animals, so new-borns have plenty of BAT which gradually gets less as they grow older (and bigger). So do big primates like ourselves have BAT? Hardly any, though young adults have some. But babies have lots more, and it is an important way that they keep up their body temperature, though they have other methods as well, such as behavioural ones like snuggling up to their mother.

So far, we have been thinking about what happens when an animal (or human) is suddenly exposed to cold. But this is not the way it usually occurs. Coldness is associated with particular seasons, and they arrive slowly, with plenty of warning, and last for quite a time. Under these conditions, adaptation can occur in advance of the challenge; for example, many animals grow extra thick coats as winter approaches, only to shed them again in the spring. They use the changing daylengths to warn them of imminent winter, implying that hair growth is regulated not only by ambient temperature, but also by the system that measures the duration of the day (or night, in fact). This process, dependent on the pineal gland, is considered in more detail elsewhere in this book (Chapter 11); here we note that adaptation uses many cues, and several separate mechanisms to ensure maximal effectiveness. Some animals that live in very cold (eg. arctic) conditions also have genetic adaptations: for example, reindeer have a special sort of haemoglobin that continues to release oxygen in the blood even at low temperatures — ordinary haemoglobin is rather cold-sensitive, and would stop working. Prolonged cold also activates extra hormonal responses, of which the thyroid gland is the most important.

The thyroid lies in the neck, and makes several related hormones that include thyroxine. The thyroid needs iodine to makes its hormone thyroxine; hence iodine deficiency results in thyroxine deficiency. In such cases, the thyroid may attempt to compensate by growing larger, with a resulting swelling in the neck (a goitre), which is very obvious. Certain parts of the world have very low levels of iodine in the water and soil; one such location in the UK (near Derby) used to cause so many people to have underactive thyroids with associated goitres that this condition was called 'Derbyshire neck'. Nowadays, iodine is added to water.

Thyroxine acts to regulate the rate at which the body's metabolism works. So an injection of this hormone will stimulate oxygen consumption and increase the heat produced by the tissues. You can think of the thyroid as a regulator of the energy production of the body, like increasing the fuel flow to an engine or turning up your boiler. Persistent cold stimulates the thyroid. As well as increasing general heat production, this also helps activate BAT in species that have this tissue. The thyroid gland, like many other hormone-producing glands, is controlled by the pituitary, which in turn is controlled by the hypothalamus. Chemical signals (peptides) provide the link between the hypothalamus and pituitary, and pituitary and thyroid. The hypothalamus produces a tiny peptide (called thyrotropin or TRH), which passes down the special blood vessels linking it to the pituitary (see Chapter 2) and causes the pituitary to produce much larger amounts of another, also much larger, peptide called thyroid-stimulating hormone (TSH). TSH, in turn, kick-starts the thyroid. You can see that the whole control system (for thyroid as well as the autonomic nerves) starts in the hypothalamus, where the core temperature detector lies. People with too little thyroid hormone complain about being cold, those with too much sweat a lot and complain of the heat. To you and me, the temperature seems fine.

Other hormones are also activated by cold. Insulin and glucagon, two hormones from the pancreas, increase; they help heat production, but also are involved in the increased appetite that many animals show in the cold. After all, if your thyroid is making you burn more calories, you need more fuel. The adrenal gland, as well as making more adrenaline, also makes more cortisol (or similar hormones) in the cold. If this is prevented, then animals cannot maintain their body temperature in either hot or cold environments. So a whole array of adaptations help an animal to keep warm when the cold season arrives. Something else happens as well. If you keep an animal in the cold for a few days, and then remove it to normal temperatures, when you next expose it to the cold (reasonably soon) then it adapts much better and much faster. This is called acclimatisation, and it occurs in response to both cold and heat. It is familiar to those who go on holiday to hot countries. For the first few days you feel rather overwhelmed, but then things get better. Those who prefer a cold holiday will notice something similar. Acclimatised animals (or people) can withstand high (or low) temperatures which might well prove fatal to naïve individuals. The exact mechanism is not really very well understood.

So our little rat or hamster enters winter well prepared. It turns out to be a harsh one. The rat copes rather well, growing a thicker coat and spending much of its time snuggled up to its fellows in its burrow, built to provide at least partial insulation against the freezing cold, emerging from time to time to get the food it needs (which may be difficult), but using up its stored body fat for energy as well. Behavioural adaptations such as these are as important as the physiological ones (hormonal changes and BAT). Nevertheless, many rats (but not all) may die. But something odd has happened to the hamster. It seems to have disappeared for weeks. Using our tiny camera, we peek into its nest. There it is, deeply asleep. For days and days, hardly stirring, never coming up for food. We take its temperature. To our amazement, it is only about 3–4°C above that of the outside, well below what it was during the summer. We notice it is hardly breathing. Is this a terminal state of adaptive failure? Is this impending death? Not at all, it's hibernation.

Recall, for a moment, Cannon's dictum about preparing for either 'fight' or 'flight' when faced with an emergency. Cannon really had in mind something like the appearance of another aggressive individual, but we can apply the same idea to coping with cold. The rat is fighting the environment. It is using its array of adaptive behaviours and bodily responses to tide it over the cold spell. The hamster, however, uses 'flight': that is, it opts out of winter by putting itself into a state of suspended life. It simply continues to exist (but no more than that) until reactivated by the warmer air of the spring. Hibernation removes the need to feed, to put much resource into maintaining body temperature and, of course, helps it avoid becoming prey to hungry predators during times of food scarcity. It is clearly a successful survival strategy, because many species living in cold climates hibernate, such as dormice, hedgehogs, ground squirrels and bats, as well as larger animals like polar bears. So why do not they all? Rats never seem to hibernate, however cold it is. We do not know. But I suspect if we looked carefully, we would find that rats had some quality, either behavioural or physiological which hibernating species do not possess. As we see in so many other contexts, there is more than one way to adapt. Even those species that can hibernate do not always do so. Their adaptive response to cold is a flexible one, just what you would expect for maximal survival. What actually triggers hibernation remains something of a mystery. Simply putting hamsters into the cold is not very effective, but all attempts to identify another factor (changes in hormones, daylength and so on) have not been very successful.

Time to get back to the brain. In particular, the human brain. At the beginning of this chapter we saw how you reacted to a sudden drop in temperature because you found it unpleasant being cold. Being uncomfortable and being in danger are not at all the same. In this case, as in so many others, your brain ensures you dislike a situation which may, unknown to you, hold danger. The danger, in this case, of hypothermia. Discomfort is not something we tolerate for long, unless there are special (and overriding) circumstances, so you reduced yours by closing the window and so on, thus (unwittingly) counteracting the threat to your body temperature. Animals do the same: put a rat into the cold, and he will press a bar (if he has been taught how) to turn on a warm lamp for a few seconds; then again when it goes off, and so on. As we have seen, animals given a choice of environments will move to one that is temperate, and avoid either extreme heat or extreme cold. They are, as we say, motivated to stay warm in the cold, cool in the heat. Neither you or the rat do these things because you 'know' that your body temperature is under attack; you do it because your brain ensures that being too cold or too hot is 'unpleasant' and you act to reduce or remove the unpleasantness. In so doing, you may have saved your life. Cooling the hypothalamus makes rats work for heat, so whilst the actual feeling of unpleasantness may or may not result from the activity of nerve cells in the hypothalamus, the temperature sensors in this part of the brain can access those parts of the brain that signal 'unpleasantness'. In this, the human limbic system seems very like that of other mammals.

But the human limbic system is surrounded by the human cerebral cortex, a very different structure, and one that, unlike the limbic system, shows huge development in man compared even to close relatives like apes, let alone little rodents like rats or hamsters. Whilst the strategy of keeping warm is the same for man and rat, the tactics are very different. Primeval man had no fur coat, so he had to think of using the pelts of other animals, and clothing was invented. Adapting clothes to the prevailing conditions may be superficially similar to a cat shedding its winter coat, but it is actually different. Changing clothes is an intentional act. You do it when you want to. But your dog moults when the daylength changes, over which it has no control. You can change your clothes very quickly making adaptation that much more sensitive. Animals do it very slowly. You can regulate the clothes you wear rather precisely but an animal cannot. There is even a unit called the 'clo': 1 clo equals a quarter inch thickness of clothing. Humans being humans, clothing has taken on all sorts of other functions, particularly as a social signal. We have to be careful to distinguish the thermoregulatory role of clothing (the limbic function) from its social role (the cortical function). Social rank and role, gender, sexual attractiveness, social affiliations, nationality, political statements — all and more are signalled by clothing. As so often, the human cerebral cortex has hijacked a fundamental survival technique for other purposes — though some, like sexual signals, are 'limbic' in themselves. But compare the clothing now worn by those in polar regions with that only 100 years ago, and you will see that the ingenuity of the cortical brain continues to be applied to the limbic imperative of survival. Man-made materials provide protection no other animal can match, though we should recall that mammals have colonised most of the hostile parts of the world. So the basic biological equipment is not that bad. The difference is that one species (man) can travel practically anywhere, changing his clothes as he goes, whereas other mammalian species may be more limited. Though some (for example foxes and the ubiquitous rat) are surprisingly versatile.

And we can regulate our environment. The discovery of fire, long recognised as a seminal event in human history, provided, amongst other things, a tractable source of heat. Building shelters from the wet and the cold allowed man to become at least partly independent of natural shelters such as caves — both random and scarce. Humans are, of course, not alone in this: many animals build shelters or nests, some of considerable complexity. But the human brain has allowed this process — building a shelter — to be taken to heights without parallel in the animal world. Our nearest biological neighbours, the great apes, despite their impressive brains, are still building temporary shelters each night in trees, as they have always done. We build blocks of flats, or rows of houses that last for hundreds of years, and heat them artificially. We constantly change the materials we use, or the design of our dwellings. Houses built today are not the same as 200 years ago, let alone 1000 years. Apes build their nests like their great-great-great-grandparents, and always will. Just as clothes have taken on other functions, so have buildings. Cathedrals, theatres, fortifications and hospitals have functions removed from the original idea of a dwelling, a protection against the cold (and from others). The ability to construct cites depends on the planning and inventive capacity of our cortex, and the motor skills of our hands which also depend upon the brain's cortex to function, but the original need was dictated by our limbic system.

Your body has to have defences against overheating as well as the cold. A rise in core temperature of more than a few degrees can damage many organs. In males, the formation of semen by the testes is very sensitive to heat, which is why males hang their testicles in external bags called the scrotum, and why (in some species) warming the scrotum causes the animal to pant even though the rest of the body stays cool. But the brain is disturbed by overheating most of all. So you have some extremely effective ways of staying at around 37°C even in the heat. The body seems to be able to withstand short-term increases in core temperature (though this may not apply to the brain, as we'll see); vigorous exercise can result in body temperatures of around 40°C or more for short spells. However, as soon as your hypothalamus detects either an increase in core temperature or information from the skin that the external temperature has gone up, it acts to increase heat loss. You begin to sweat, a very human activity. Not many other animals have sweat glands (perhaps because they have fur). Sweating cools you because water uses heat when it evaporates. But you pay a price, you lose water and salt, not necessarily a good idea in a hot and arid environment. This is probably why small animals do not sweat. It is estimated that a desert animal (like a jerboa) would lose about 20% of its body weight per hour at an ambient temperature of 40°C if it tried to maintain its body temperature by sweating. Human athletes can sweat their entire plasma volume during a marathon. In the heat, it is the hypothalamus that signals we are losing water. So we get thirsty, and a whole series of hormonal and other responses that act to conserve water. Later, other mechanisms increase your salt appetite and reduce loss of salt in urine. These actions are discussed elsewhere in this book (Chapter 6). The point here is that adapting to a hot environment is not just a matter of regulating body heat. It requires a co-ordinated series of responses that act on other functions, such as water loss, as well.

It does seem, however, that humans have inherited a better set of physiological methods of staying cool than keeping warm, perhaps because of our ancestral origin from the warmer parts of the world. Effective ways for naked, hairless man to stay warm really had to wait for his cortex to invent artificial shelters, fire and the idea of wearing clothes. As in so many other survival stories in man, the limbic system defines the need, the cortex provides the solution.

What about animals that cannot sweat? Some pant: this is also an effective way of losing heat. Others spread saliva on their fur; as it evaporates, they cool. Many animals (including you) dilate the blood vessels in the skin (which is why we go very pink in the heat); this increases the loss of heat from blood to the air, provided that the latter is less than blood temperature. Desert-living animals show the most marked adaptations to heat. They have extreme ways of conserving water (gerbils, otherwise known as desert rats, hardly urinate at all). Camels (and donkeys) can drink huge amounts of water very rapidly, so they make maximum use of whatever water is available. Camels also pack all their fat into a single hump, so that their body insulation is minimal. Incidentally, they do not store water in their hump; and they actually sweat. Many desert animals are pale (reflects heat) and their fur may act as an insulator against the rays of the sun. But many also use behavioural methods to avoid overheating, spending the hot part of the day in burrows, and only coming out during the cooler night. The real danger is that the brain overheats, so the brain has some rather special ways of staying cool.

It is extraordinary that if the body's core temperature increases, the brain stays cooler. There seems to be some way that the brain is selectively cooled. In some species, there is a curious arrangement of blood vessels at the base of the brain (the carotid rete) which may act as a heat exchanger. Humans do not have one. Another possible cooling system lies in the nose. Species that live in the tropics often have enlarged bones in their nose covered with blood vessels. These may also act as a heat exchanger with inspired air, and deliver cooler blood to the brain. Should all this prove insufficient, and brain temperature rise by about 4°C, heat-stroke follows. The brain begins to fail, blood floods into the gut, toxins are released, irreversible brain damage and death may follow. But the cells of the brain and other tissues have one last defence mechanism against overheating. They make a series of special proteins called 'heat shock proteins'.

To understand what these heat shock proteins do, we have to recall that proteins are long ribbons of amino-acids. Like everyday ribbons made out of material, they can fold. But the exact way they fold is critical. If a protein is not folded correctly, it will not function properly. So much effort is currently being put into studying how proteins fold. Normally, this is determined by the sequence of amino-acids. But heat disrupts protein folding (it is called 'denaturing') which is one good reason why over-heating is so bad for you.

If you expose a dish of cells to higher than normal temperature, they make lots of heat shock protein. These proteins have an interesting role: they keep other proteins properly folded. Sometimes they are picturesquely called 'molecular chaperones'. So desert-living animals have large amounts of heat shock proteins. These proteins have important roles in keeping certain other proteins folded (or unfolded) under more normal circumstances as well, but this was a later discovery, so their name persists. It is not really clear whether heat shock proteins are a last ditch defence, or a hangover from an earlier age when most cells were on their own. Bacteria have heat shock proteins, hence those famous bugs that can live in volcanic hot springs (geysers).

There is no doubt that the regulation of body temperature is an excellent example of homeostasis. But homeostasis does not necessarily mean constancy. Your body temperature may be carefully regulated, but it is not constant. It is higher in the evening than the morning. As you fall asleep, your body temperature drops to its lowest level. Some people think the brain is the chief beneficiary of the nightly cooling-off period. As well as a daily rhythm, you have 7-day, 30-day and annual rhythms in body temperature. In women, there is a well-known peak in body temperature near the middle of the menstrual cycle, related to ovulation, which has been used to indicate fertility. Why this peak happens is completely obscure. Rats stressed by being put into unfamiliar environments increase their body temperature. Whether this helps them cope is unknown. But the change we will be most familiar with is fever.

William Osler (1849–1919), a celebrated medical teacher who worked in Canada, the USA and England (Oxford), characterised the three scourges of mankind as famine, war and fever. It was not fever that usually killed people, but the associated infection — though the body temperature of feverish young children can rise to dangerous levels. Characteristically, body temperature rises by a few degrees during an infection, most markedly in the evening (it's called 'pyrexia'). We take aspirin or phenacetin (called acetaminophen in the US), which brings our body temperature down again and makes us feel better. But the evidence suggests that moderate fever actually improves survival, so this may be a short-sighted strategy (except in cases where the fever itself is very high). But why does an infection cause pyrexia, and why is aspirin so effective? This brings us back to the brain.

A constant theme of this book is that the limbic system, the major player in your brain's survival plan, uses chemical signals to communicate. So is there a special set of neurochemicals that are concerned with body temperature? Fever is produced by a two-stage process. The invading organism (say, a bacterium) contains a substance called lipopolysaccharide or 'LPS'. The body responds to LPS by releasing a number of chemicals of its own. These include a peptide called IL1 (interleukin 1, so-called because white blood cells or 'leucocytes' can produce it). IL1 in the blood acts on the brain to release another set of chemicals, the prostaglandins (in the hypothalamus). It is prostaglandins that cause your body temperature to rise. Aspirin reduces the amounts of prostaglandin, and hence lowers your body temperature. Interestingly, the brain may have its own 'aspirin' (though a very different molecule) to keep your temperature from going too high and it may be deficient in children. Equally interestingly, IL1 (which is found in the brain as well as in the blood) may cause you to feel 'ill' as well as being a pyrogen (raising temperature), and hence be a chemical 'code' for illness behaviour — an important adaptation for combating infection and other illnesses. People who are 'ill' show a characteristic set of behaviours and symptoms (for example, they lose their appetite, and IL1 reduces food intake), and experience a consistent set of emotions, all part of the process of 'coping' with the illness or recruiting help from others. Ill people feel miserable, and IL1 has been suggested to induce a depressive state of mind. Ill people also have higher levels of cortisol, and IL1 releases ACTH from the pituitary, which in turn stimulates the secretion of cortisol. IL1 may be a limbic code for 'being' and 'feeling' ill.

But many other chemicals in the brain can alter body temperature, most famously serotonin. Small amounts of serotonin infused into the brain increases body temperature, and is why the drug ecstasy (MDMA) can be fatal. Ecstasy releases serotonin in the brain, and can cause a rapid and uncontrolled rise in temperature (hyper-pyrexia). Serotonin does many other things in the brain, so it is difficult to think of it as a very specific temperature controller (Chapter 3). However, under emergency conditions, (e.g. stress) it may well play a part. The related neurochemicals noradrenaline and dopamine are also able to alter temperature, but the list does not end there. More than thirty peptides can either raise or lower body temperature after being infused into the brain. The obvious candidate for a special role might be TRH, the little peptide that alters thyroid function and might have a controlling action of its own. Unfortunately, the evidence is not that strong. It may be that you need to regulate your temperature in so many different circumstances that you need lots of separate chemical controllers.

Mammals, with their need to regulate their body temperature so closely, seem vulnerable in a changeable and indifferent world. The fact that they survive and prosper in the freezing cold, the howling gales, the burning heat is a tribute to the efficiency of their on-board, highly sophisticated and versatile thermostat buried deep in the limbic system of the brain.

The subjective feelings of sickness, in the form of malaise, lassitude, fatigue, numbness, coldness, muscle and joint aches, and reduced appetite, are well known by everyone who has experienced an episode of viral or bacterial infection.... The psychological and behavioural components of sickness represent, together with the fever response and the associated neuroendocrine changes, a highly organized strategy of the organism to fight infection. This strategy, referred to as 'sickness behaviour' is triggered by the pro-inflammatory cytokines that are produced by (white blood cells) in contact with the invading micro-organisms.

J P Kinsman, P Parnet, R Dantzer. (2002) Cytokine-induced sickness behaviour: Mechanisms and implications. *Trends in Neurosciences*, pp. 154–159.

Chapter 8

The Sexual Brain

Nobody, the American scientist Frank Beach once memorably declared, ever died from lack of sex. Beach made substantial contributions to our understanding of the way that hormones control sexual behaviour, but in this case he was articulating a real problem. If sex is not essential for the individual, how does the brain make it into an imperative demand? The 'why' is rather easier: if we did not bother with sex, there would be no human race to think about it. But sex is a biologically and socially costly business. We spend a great deal of time doing things that is related to it, or to parenthood, the biological consequence and rationale for sexual behaviour. But the payoff is less for the individual than for his/her species. So it is a different kind of demand from the business of daily survival, though the process of reproduction may have vast influence on survival itself. This is the reason that the brain uses many of the mechanisms to regulate sex that we might otherwise think of in connection with more obvious physiological demands such as getting enough food and water. We have a brain that not only 'knows' how to make us focus on sex when it matters, but also ensures that we do, not at all for our sake but for the preservation of future generations. The brain is being altruistic, but in so doing, it enables Darwinian selection. If there was no sexual behaviour, no urge to procreate, no brain mechanisms for selecting a mate and for seeing off the competition, no care of the young so that enough survived, then there would be no genetic material on which selection could act. And sexual selection (who mates with whom), the second Darwinian mechanism, relies totally on the brain. That means we need a brain that not only makes us breed, but makes the 'right' choice about with whom we breed.

Sexual Selection and Competition

This form of selection (sexual selection) depends not on the struggle for existence in relation to other organic beings or external conditions, but on a struggle between the individuals of one sex, generally the males, for the possession of the other sex. The result is not death to the unsuccessful competitor, but few or no offspring. Sexual selection is, therefore, less rigorous than natural selection. Generally, the most vigorous males, those which are best fitted for their places in nature, will leave most progeny. But in many cases victory depends not so much on general vigour as on having special weapons confined to the male sex. A hornless stag or spurless cock would have a poor chance of leaving numerous offspring. Sexual selection, by always allowing the victor to breed, might surely give indomitable courage, length to the spur, and strength to the wing to strike with the spurred leg, in nearly the same manner as does the brutal cockfighter by the careful selection of his best cocks.

Charles Darwin. (1872) *The origin of species.* Sixth ed.
Ed. R E Leakey. (Hill and Wang, New York.)

. . . The success which really counts is reproductive success. Those animals that leave relatively more offspring than others are 'fitter' or more successful. The 'fittest' animals are not necessarily the biggest, strongest, fastest, or sexually most attractive; merely those that leave the most progeny.

D Pilbeam. (1970) *The evolution of man.*
(Thames and Hudson, London.)

Sex is an antisocial force in evolution. Bonds are formed between individuals in spite of sex and not because of it. . . . Societies that lack conflict. . . are most likely to evolve where all of the members are genetically identical. When sexual reproduction is introduced, members of the group become genetically dissimilar. . . . The inevitable result is a conflict of interest. The male will profit more if he can inseminate additional females. . . . Conversely, the female will profit if she can retain the full-time aid of the male. . . . The offspring may increase their personal genetic fitness by continuing to demand the services of the parents when raising a second brood would be more profitable for the parents. . . . The outcomes of these conflicts of interest are tension and strict limits on the extent of altruism and division of labor.

E O Wilson. (1975) The new synthesis. *Sociobiology.*
(The Belknap Press, Cambridge, Massachusetts.)

There is one major big difference between sex and the other survival tactics. Getting food and water, or staying warm and dry, presents much the same problems for all adult animals. Resources such as these come from the environment, the external world. But sex, to state the obvious, does not come from the environment, it comes from within the species. Moreover, species divide into two, each gender having somewhat different aims and objectives. So while we can justifiably point to similarities between the brain mechanisms for sex and other survival behaviours, there will be differences. Not just because animals need to distinguish sex from other survival processes, or know when to use it, but because there are elements in sex which simply do not exist in other realms of behaviour.

When we think of sex, we think of hormones and that is where we should start. Remove the ovaries from a female cat, rat or mouse, and she will never mate again. Within 24 hours, she has become a sexual neuter. She will only mate if we replace the hormones that have been removed along with her ovaries. What hormones do we need? The female cat needs only oestrogen. Inject her with a tiny amount — about 100 micrograms of oestradiol (an oestrogen) might be enough (a microgram is 1 millionth of a gram, or 1 thousandth of a milligram), and a few hours later she is eager for a mate. If she had met a passing randy tom cat before her hormone treatment, she would probably have tried to scratch his eyes out. Now she is quite different, rubbing herself against him and adopting a position which is unmistakably sexy. If there is food around, she might ignore it. A minuscule amount of this steroid hormone has produced a dramatic change in her behaviour, altering her reaction from hostility to sex, her preference from food to mating. What is oestrogen doing to the brain to produce these astonishing changes in behaviour?

Before we try and answer that, let us try the same experiment with our female rat. We are disappointed to find that oestrogen alone is not very effective, though if we give enough for long enough we may get some females to behave sexually. But add a small amount of progesterone, a second ovarian steroid hormone, a few hours after the oestrogen and the result is much more obvious: all our female rats are now as sexy as the female cat (though, of course, with male rats). These two experiments show that whilst ovarian hormones are required for both cats and rats (and many other species) the exact mixture varies.

She was very pretty — exceedingly pretty. With a dimpled, surprised-looking, capital face; a ripe little mouth, that seemed made to be kissed — as no doubt it was; all kinds of good little dots about her chin, that melted into one another when she laughed; and the sunniest pair of eyes you ever saw in any little creature's head. Altogether she was what you would have called provoking, you know; but satisfactory, too. Oh, perfectly satisfactory.
Charles Dickens. *A Christmas carol.*

The Greek, the Turk, the Chinese, the Copt, the Hottentot, said Stephen, all admire a different type of female beauty. That seems to be a maze out of which we cannot escape. I see, however, two ways out. One is this hypothesis: that every physical quality admired by men in women is in direct connexion with the manifold functions of women for the propagation of the species.
James Joyce. (1916) *A portrait of the artist as a young man.*

She had been very pretty when she was young. 'The Belle of Hornton', they had called her in her native village. . . . Another of her favourite stories was of the day she had danced with a real lord. . . before the evening was over he had whispered in her ear that she was the prettiest girl in the country, and she cherished the compliment all her life. There were no further developments. My Lord was My Lord, and Hannah Pollard was Hannah Pollard, a poor girl, but the daughter of decent parents. No further developments were possible in real life, though such affairs ended differently in novelettes. Perhaps that was why she enjoyed reading them.
Flora Thompson. (1939) *Lark Rise to Candleford.*
(Oxford University Press, Oxford.)

There was a boy in Alabama, I think, they raised never to see a girl till he was twenty-one — they was kind of 'xperimenting'. He was raised by men. So when he was twenty-one his daddy carried him to where the high school children would pass by. . . . And he seen them from the windows coming along so pretty, with their ribbons and long hair. . . , and smiling and playing. And he said, 'Daddy, Daddy, come here. Looky looky, what are those?' 'Those are ducks.' Give me one, Daddy.' 'Which one do you want?' 'It don't make no difference, Daddy, any one.'
So it's better to let them grow up with each other, so they can pick a little.
Angela Carter. (1991) *The boy who had never seen women. The Virago book of fairy tales.* (Virago, London.)

Every four or five days, a female rat becomes very sexy for a few hours, a process termed being on 'heat' or, more scientifically, in 'oestrous' (oestrous comes from a Greek word meaning a 'gadfly' or a 'sting', and is meant to suggest the frenzy of sexual appetite). This is because her ovaries secrete a surge of oestrogen every 4–5 days, followed, a few hours later, by a small amount of progesterone. Within an hour or so, she is oestrous. Then, a few hours after this, her ovaries expel a number of fertile eggs (ovulation). The eggs pass down her reproductive tract, where they meet the sperm deposited there by her male mate a few hours earlier. If she does not mate, or the mating proves infertile, then the whole process repeats itself. Ovulation and sexuality are locked together, so that fertility is maximal. She is highly likely to become pregnant every time she mates, and she will not waste time mating when she is not fertile. The ovaries are responsible for the whole process; because the release of eggs and hormones occurs at the right times, sex and fertility coincide. But the ovaries do not control the regular cycle of fertility-sexiness: the brain does.

In the female cat, it is slightly different. Her ovaries produce oestrogen, like the rat's, and this alone makes her sexually active. But her ovaries do not shed eggs. Instead, the ripe eggs wait in the ovary until she mates; only then does she ovulate. The female cat, unlike the rat, can be in heat for days, even weeks, and the stimulus of mating is needed for ovulation. This, of course, is another way of maximising fertility; the female cat only sheds eggs when there are sperm around to fertilise them. There are lots of variants in different species on these two themes; as in other areas of adaptation, we see that there are many possible answers to a single biological problem. The best one may depend on all sorts of other factors, for example, whether the species concerned is a prey or a predator (or both) or the kind of social or physical environment in which it lives.

Although we have not yet ventured very far into the complexities of reproduction, already we can see several roles for the brain. Although our female rat or cat may need the correct hormones from their ovaries to become sexually active, it is their brain that is actually responsible. The brain has a curious double-handed role. First, it makes sure the ovaries secrete the right hormone(s), then hormones act back on the brain itself to induce sexual behaviour. You can see why this oddly roundabout system

"Such an eye! — the true hazel eye — and so brilliant! regular features, open countenance, with a complexion! Oh! What a bloom of full health, and such a pretty height and size; such a firm and upright figure! There is health, not merely in her bloom, but in her air, her head, her glance. One hears sometimes of a child being 'the picture of health;' now, Emma always gives me the idea of being the complete picture of grown-up health. She is loveliness itself. Mr. Knightley, is not she?"

Jane Austen. *Emma.*

What stunned me was not the door opening, but what came through it. Viz., the loveliest girl I had ever seen in my life.

The thing about her that hit the spectator like a bullet first crack out of the box was her sort of sweet, tender, wistful gentleness. . . . And when I tell you that with this wistful gentleness went a pair of large blue eyes, a perfectly modelled chassis, and a soft smile which brought out a dimple on the right cheek, you will readily understand why it was that two seconds after she had slid into the picture I was clutching my pipe till my knuckles stood out white under the strain and breathing through my nose in short, quick pants. With my disengaged hand, I straightened my tie, and if my moustache had been long enough to twirl there is little question that I would have twirled it.

P G Wodehouse. (1936) *Laughing gas.*
(Penguin Books, Harmondsworth, UK.)

I like being a private eye, and even though once in a while I've had my gums massaged with an automobile jack, the sweet smell of greenbacks makes it all worth it. Not to mention the dames, which are a minor preoccupation of mine that I rank just ahead of breathing. That's why, when the door to my office swung open and a long-haired blonde named Heather Butkiss came striding in and told me she was a nudie model and needed my help, my salivary glands shifted into third. She wore a short skirt and a tight sweater and her figure described a set of parabolas that could cause cardiac arrest in a yak.

Woody Allen. (1992) Mr Big. In: *The complete prose of Woody Allen.* (Picador, London.)

works so well. No good being sexy unless you are fertile. Or vice-versa. How does the brain know that its command to the ovaries to produce eggs has been successful? Because the ovaries secrete hormones when they shed eggs (or, in the case of species like cats, when the eggs in the ovary are ripe and ready for shedding): it is the signal the brain has been waiting for. So as soon as hormone levels start to rise, the brain causes the rat or cat to feel and behave sexily. She looks for a mate.

Ovaries are controlled by the pituitary gland, which sends out command signals to the ovaries in the form of large peptide hormones (called gonadotrophins). The rhythmic secretion of gonadotrophins from the pituitary (28 days in women, 4–5 days in the rat) determine the length of the reproductive cycle. One way of treating infertile women is to give them the right mixture of gonadotrophins, so that their ovaries produce an egg, which can be fertilised either naturally or artificially. As discussed in Chapter 2, the pituitary gland lies just under the base of the brain, connected to it by a very special set of blood vessels. Down these blood vessels, come the chemical command signals from the limbic part of the brain (the hypothalamus, in fact). These signals are also peptides, though much smaller ones than those produced by the pituitary (which are several hundred long). Small they may be, but they are utterly vital for reproduction. The most important one is called GnRH (gonadotrphin-releasing harmone) and it is 10 amino-acids long. No brain signals, no fertility. It is the brain that determines the way that the pituitary secretes gonadotrophins, which in turn send secondary commands to the ovaries. Then the ovaries tell the brain that all is well. Rather like the company CEO sending a memo (GnRH) to his senior managers, who then pass on the information to those to will do the job (gonadotrophins), who then report back (hormones from the ovaries). Instead of paper memos or emails, the body uses a variety of chemical signals (little peptides from the brain, bigger ones from the pituitary, steroids from the ovary).

Now for the males. The first difference is that male rats or cats do not seem to have sexual cycles (though that does not mean they are always sexy, as we will see). A given male may show regular changes in sexual activity, but this is likely to be due to the females, rather than him. If we castrate a male rat or cat, his sexual behaviour decreases but only rather slowly. It may take weeks or more for him to reach the lowest level of

The Variety of Sexual Behaviour

We believe that a deep comprehensive understanding of human sexual behavior develops most surely from a correct view of our species' place in the animal kingdom. Acquiring this view requires comparative study. In addition, there is substantial intrinsic interest in the sexual behavior of nonhuman species and its determinants. . . . Sexual processes are virtually ubiquitous in the animal kingdom. Sexual and evolutionary processes are so closely linked as to almost inseparable. To understand evolution, one must understand sex, and vice versa.

No single physiological variable. . . is as important in determining the occurrence or level of sexual responsiveness as the amount of gonadal hormones in the blood. This kind of relationship is unusual if not unique in behavioral physiology. In no other area of behavior do hormones appear to occupy such a commanding role, and no hormones have nearly as important an influence on sex behavior as the gonadal hormones.

G Bermant and J M Davidson. (1974) *Biological bases of sexual behavior.* (Harper and Row, New York.)

We know that in the wild or in naturalistic conditions, females display a wide variety of behaviors to initiate and sustain sexual behavior. Each behavioral component ultimately influences production of offspring. These behaviors are therefore likely to be controlled by the nervous system in ways that are unique to the female of each species. The use of (laboratory measures) of sexual behavior have been useful in addressing many questions regarding the facilitation and persistence of sexual responsiveness; . . . As studies of brain and behavior become more sophisticated, it has become clear that our understanding of the neurobiological mechanisms controlling behavior will be significantly deepened if more naturalistic aspects of the behavior are incorporated in to our studies.

J D Blaustein and M S Erskine. (2002) Feminine sexual behavior: Cellular integration of hormonal and afferent information in the rodent forebrain. In: *Hormones, brain and behavior.* Eds. D W Pfaff, A P Arnold, A M Etgen, S E Farhbach, *et al.*, pp. 139–214. (Academic Press, Amsterdam.)

Sexual behaviour is *sexually dimorphic*, in the sense that certain activities are typical of one sex, rather than the other. . . . . However, use of the term *sexually dimorphic behaviour* does not imply that a pattern occurs exclusively in one sexual activity, and even then there may still be some left (though not very much). Females, we recall, lost all their sexual ability within about 24 hours after their ovaries were removed. We can restore the males to full potency by giving them testosterone, the major hormone secreted by the testis, so this is what is missing. But if we measure levels of testosterone in the blood of a male after castration, we find that it is all gone within 24 hours. Even so, the male still continues to be able to mate in the absence of testosterone, declining only slowly in the subsequent weeks. Similarly, though giving females their hormones rapidly restores their sexual behaviour, it is much slower for males and it may take several days or weeks. Our conclusion is that there is a much more immediate control system in females than males, though in both, hormones are very important. An intriguing difference. How does the brain of the male carry on supporting sexual behaviour, for a while at least, in the absence of testosterone, and what limits this ability? And why this sex difference in the way that hormones control sexual behaviour? These are questions we need to address later.

For now, however, we can begin to see how the hormonal system that is responsible for regulating sexual behaviour looks rather similar to those chemical signals concerned with more immediate demands, such as food, water, or salt intake. Let us remind ourselves about salt. If concentrations of salt in the blood decline below a tolerable limit, this invokes the classical homeostatic response (all this is considered in Chapter 6). An important part of this response is a sharp increase in the secretion of the steroid hormone aldosterone from the adrenal gland. This hormone has two major actions. One is a peripheral one: it acts on the kidney to retain salt, thus making the most of what stores there are, and limiting further loss of precious salt. The other is a central one on the brain: this increases salt appetite so that the individual concerned goes in search of sources of salt. Aldosterone thus not only acts as part of the adaptive response on the body (retaining salt) it also sends the brain a signal that salt is low, thus creating a 'demand' for increased salt intake.

Now consider the action of testosterone. Increased secretion acts on the periphery to facilitate sexual behaviour by, for example, increasing the formation of sperm, causing the penis and other parts of the reproductive tract to enlarge, and encouraging growth (in man) of the beard and other sex. . . . In monkeys and apes both sexes may employ hindquarter presentation and mounting postures as part of sociosexual communication. Such *heterotypical* behaviour has been described in many vertebrates. Sexual dimorphism in behaviour is a question of degree, therefore, rather than absolute differences between males and females.

Alan F Dixson. (1998) *Primate sexuality*.
(Oxford University Press, Oxford.)

In evolutionary terms, sexual reproduction must be extremely important, since many species devote so much energy to it. The advantage of sexual reproduction is obvious, since it enormously enhances variability. An asexual organism simply produces identical copies of itself and thus its potential for change is limited, occurring only via gene mutation. In this setting, the acquisition of two favourable mutations by a single individual requires two independent events, whereas in sexually reproducing species the chances of the genes coming together through genetic exchange are much greater.

R E Leakey. (1979) Introduction. In: *The illustrated origin of species*
(Charles Darwin). (Hill and Wang, New York)

Prediction in a complex world is a chancy business. Every decision that a the survival machine takes is a gamble, and it is the business of genes to program brains in advance so that on average they take decisions which pay off. . . . There are risks whichever way you turn, and you must take the decision which maximizes the long-term survival of your genes . . . Some form of weighing up of the odds has to be done. But of course we do not have to think of the animals as making decisions consciously. All we have to believe is that those individuals whose genes build brains in such a way that they tend to gamble correctly are as a direct result more likely to survive, and therefore propagate those same genes.

R Dawkins. (1976) *The selfish gene*. (Oxford University Press, Oxford).

signs of masculinity (to increase his sexual attractiveness). It also sends a message to the brain, generating a 'demand' (some would call it a 'drive') for sex. This is as essential in the context of successful reproduction, sexual selection and procreation, as 'wanting' salt is in the context of the homeostatic control of body fluid composition. No wonder, then, that the structure of the system underlying sexual behaviour looks so like that concerned with other, quite distinct, demands. In females, it is similar. The hormones from the ovaries prepare the womb (uterus) for the arrival of the fertilised egg. They also signal to the brain (the limbic system) that the female is fertile, and set up the 'demand' for a mate. Now we begin to understand why the limbic system is so closely involved in sex, and why some of the things we learn about the role of the limbic system in other 'demand' states might tell us interesting things about sex.

So far, we have been discussing males and females separately. Now, it is time to put them together. Let us watch a pair of sexy rats. The male rushes over to the female, and spends quite a while sniffing her rump, his nose tucked under her tail. Then he may wander off, returning to do it all over again. The female is, meanwhile, waggling her ears in a way we have not seen before. She also makes a series of little darting rushes forward. If we had a bat-detector handy (this is a machine that detects the ultrasonic cries of bats) we would hear that she is giving out very high pitched squeaks. This goes on for quite a while. What is happening?

What is happening is an exchange of sexual information. The hormones of the female are doing more than act on her brain to make her sexy, they are also changing her smell by activating glands in her genitalia, and the sensitivity of the skin over her flanks. The male finds her smell very attractive. At the same time, her brain recognises the presence of a male (using sight and smell; testosterone makes him look and smell different) and she responds to this by wiggling her ears, making little forward runs and sending out typical high-pitched squeaks. This, the male also finds very attractive, but it also tells him that the female is receptive, she wants to mate. Attraction and receptivity are not the same in the world of the rat any more than in our own. A pair of rats need both to mate successfully. Sight, smell and hearing all continue to signal to each rat that the other is both attractive and receptive. This is the 'courtship' phase. Finally, the male mounts the female. As she detects this by the feel of the

My body was overreacting to every stimulus, from inside or outside, my period came every three weeks in a heavy iron-smelling flood, along with backaches, headaches and cramps. Each time I'd swell, and then lose pounds in a couple of days off school, moping around the house, insulated with aspirin and groggy daydreams. The metabolic misery had its pleasurable side. I'd writhe in a chair and read, and wrap the bloody sanitary towels in brown paper and poke them into the back of the fire, where they smouldered slowly, like me.

Lorna Sage. (2000). *Bad blood*. (Fourth Estate, London.)

Three girls pile out of the train and clack down the icy stairs. Three waiting men greet them and they all pair off. It is biting cold. The girls have red lips and their legs whisper to each other through silk stockings. The red lips and the silk flash power. A power they will exchange for the right to be overcome, penetrated. The men at their side love it because, in the end, they will reach in, get back behind that power, grab it, and keep it still.

Toni Morrison. (1992) *Jazz*. (Chatto and Windus, London.)

And what am I supposed to do with these old thighs now, just walk up and down these rooms? What good are they, Jesus? They will never give me the peace I need to get from sunup to sundown, what good are they, are you trying to tell me that I am going to have to go all the way through these days all the way, O my God, to that box with four handles with never nobody settling down between my legs. . . . O Jesus I could be a mule or plow the furrows with my hands if need be or hold these rickety walls up with my back if need be if I knew that somewhere in this world in the pocket of some night I could open my legs to some cowboy lean hips but you are trying to tell me no and O my sweet Jesus what kind of cross is that?

Toni Morison. (1980) *Sula*. (Chatto and Windus, London.)

Linda was feeling, what she had never so far felt for any man, an overwhelming physical attraction. It made her quite giddy, it terrified her. She could see that Fabrice was perfectly certain of the outcome. So was she perfectly certain, and that was what frightened her. How could she, male on her sensitive flanks, her behaviour changes, she arches her back, and stands still, just the right position to allow the male's penis to enter. Scientists call this 'lordosis' (arching the back). After several mounts, the male ejaculates, and walks off to sit by himself rather quietly in a corner and does nothing much. That was the copulation phase. A few minutes later, the whole sequence may happen again. Finally, the male stops mounting, seemingly satiated. That is the post-copulation refractory phase. The male rat does not exactly roll over and go to sleep, but he looks as if he might like to.

It is important that we remember that two rats in a cage are not a model of the real (rat) world. But even in these simple conditions, we can see that the brain is doing a lot of work during the sequence of a successful mating. The male's brain has to recognise a female rat, interpret the signals given by her smell (these are called 'pheromones'), the sounds she makes and her behaviour as sexual. So his nose, ears and eyes are all transmitting sexually-important information. His brain then has to formulate the appropriate response (either more investigation or, ultimately copulation). After ejaculation, some mechanism results in (temporary) sexual satiation. The female's brain is doing similar, but not identical things: responding to the sensations emitted by the male, and making copulation possible by taking up the stereotyped 'lordosis' position at the right moment. But before we try to understand all this any more, particularly whether sex is really adaptive, and which parts of the brain does what, we should ask the obvious question: how much of what we have learned about hormones and sex in rats, cats and other non-primate species applies to humans?

The female rat's oestrous cycle is not, in some ways, a very good model for a women's menstrual cycle. This is because the rat has only half a cycle. The rat's cycle begins by her ovary secreting increasing amounts of oestrogen for a couple of days. Then her ovary sheds its eggs (ovulates). After ovulation, the rat's cycle starts all over again. In women, there is a phase of about 14 days when the ovaries produce increasing amounts of oestrogen, then the ovary ovulates. Then there is a phase (also about 14 days) in which progesterone levels are quite high (this is the part missing in the rat). When they fall, the woman menstruates. Hence the usual 28 day cycle. Despite all the folk-lore, mystique and even political

Linda, with the horror and contempt she had always felt for casual affairs, allow herself to be picked up by any stray foreigner, and, having seen him only for an hour, long and long and long to be in bed with him? He was not even good-looking, he was exactly like dozens of other dark men in Homburgs that can be seen in the streets of any French town. But there was something in the way he looked at her which seemed to be depriving her of all balance. She was profoundly shocked, and, at the same time, intensely excited.

Nancy Mitford. (1945) *The pursuit of love.*
(Hamish Hamilton, London.)

My dear boy, no woman is a genius. Women are a decorative sex. They never have anything to say, but they say it charmingly. Women represent the triumph of matter over mind, just as men represent the triumph of mind over morals.

Oscar Wilde. (1974) *The picture of Dorian Gray.*
(Oxford University Press, Oxford.)

auras surrounding menstruation, it is actually wholly insignificant from a reproductive point of view. Only humans, apes and Old-World monkeys menstruate, all the other species get on fine without it. The females of some species have more human-like hormonal patterns that rats, for example guinea pigs, sheep and, of course, monkeys. They secrete progesterone as well as oestrogen, and have longer reproductive cycles than the rat. But they still have a very restricted period of 'heat' at mid-cycle (the time of ovulation or egg-shedding).

Women do not. At one time, it was fashionable to say that not only women, but other non-human primates like monkeys and apes had become 'emancipated' from the effects of hormones. Their sexual behaviour, it was said, had become independent of the control exerted by hormones in so-called 'lower' animals, one consequence of their greatly developed brains. We primates, unlike other lesser mammals, were not slaves to our hormones. Recent information has tempered that view. Even in the 1930s and 1940s, studies on wild and captive monkeys and apes had shown clearly that a female primate's sexuality did vary reliably with her cycle, though the way this happened differed according to who she was and her standing in her social group. Whether women also show cyclic changes in sexuality has been a subject of considerable controversy for years. You might think that this suggests that, if it happens, it cannot be very important, otherwise it would be clear-cut. However, it is quite difficult (for obvious reasons) to measure the sexual activity of large numbers of women (we have to rely, for the most part, on what they say they do and feel), and there may be important individual differences. In other words, women are not all the same. You might think this is equally obvious, but it is striking how many researchers in this area lump all their subjects together, trying to find a consistent pattern and thereby missing another but equally interesting possibility: some women respond to their hormones in one way, some in another, some, perhaps, hardly at all. There do, indeed, seem to be three (heterosexual) patterns: increasing sex behaviour during the first half of the cycle peaking at mid-cycle, peaks just before and just after menstruation, and no peaks at all. One complication is whether the phases of the woman's cycle alter her attractiveness, whether she is equally attractive to her partner throughout her cycle; and/or her receptivity, whether her cycle affects how she responds to his advances, or how attractive she

A great wedding breakfast was prepared. Cupid reclined in the place of honour with Psyche's head resting on his breast. . . . Jupiter was served with nectar and ambrosia by apple-cheeked Ganymede, his personal cup-bearer; Bacchus attended to everyone else. Vulcan was the chef; the Hours decorated the palace with red roses and other bridal flowers; the Graces sprinkled balsam water; the Muses chanted the marriage-hymn to the accompaniment of flute and pipe-music. . . Venus came forward and performed a lively step-dance in time to it. Psyche was properly married to Cupid and in due time she bore him a child, a daughter whose name was Pleasure.

> Apuleius. (1967) *The golden ass. Translated by Robert Graves.*
> (Penguin Books, Melbourne.)

In the Arabian Nights, we have a series of stories, some of them very good ones, in which no sort of decorum is observed. The result is that they are infinitely more instructive and enjoyable than our romances, because love is treated in them as naturally as any other passion. There is. . . .no pretence that a man or a woman cannot be courageous and kind and friendly unless infatuatedly in love with somebody. . . ; rather indeed, an insistence on the blinding and narrowing power of lovesickness to make princely heroes unhappy and unfortunate.

> Bernard Shaw. (1901) *Three plays for puritans.*
> *Preface: Why for puritans?*

Very few people ever state properly the strong argument in favour of marrying for love or against marrying for money. The argument is not that all lovers are heroes or heroines, nor is it that all dukes are profligates or all millionaires cads. The argument is this, that the differences between a man and a woman are at best so obstinate and exasperating that they practically cannot be got over unless there is an atmosphere of exaggerated tenderness and mutual interest.

> G K Chesterton. (1958) Two stubborn pieces of iron. In: *Essays and poems.* Ed. W Sheed. (Penguin Books, Harmondsworth, UK.)

From the British point of view marriages between the British and the Anglo-Indian communities were deeply frowned upon — but not from the Anglo-Indian: an unwritten rule was for the girls to try and marry the finds him. Either or both will change sexual interaction, and this is what researchers usually measure ("how often and when") though there is more than one underlying mechanism. However, it is clear that women do not, in general, show the very restricted phases of sexual activity characteristic of most other species.

We also have a natural experiment: the menopause. At the menopause, the secretion of oestrogen and progesterone from the ovaries ceases. This has a prominent effect on the vagina, which becomes dry and perhaps uncomfortable during coitus; oestrogen acts on the genitals in humans as in rats. But there is no marked decrease in sexuality, though because of age and, perhaps, familiarity with a partner, sexual behaviour is often quite low around the menopause. Hormone replacement therapy (HRT), which usually includes some oestrogen, does wonders for the dry vagina, but has less effect on a post-menopausal woman's sexual feelings. Before we rush to the conclusion that this means that hormones do not matter too much for human female sexuality, we have to recall that the post-menopausal ovary goes on secreting appreciable amount of another set of hormones: those that resemble the 'androgens' more usually associated with men. More on these later.

The females of some species of monkeys and apes develop huge swellings round their genitals at mid-cycle (oestrogen causes it) which act as a none-too-subtle signal to the male that she is sexually active (and fertile). Mothers taking their children to the zoo have a hard time explaining what these great red swellings are all about. There is been a good deal of chat about the fact that women do not advertise their fertility state, unlike some non-human primates, though, in truth, not all monkey or ape species do this. It is very hard, for example, to tell whether a female gibbon is fertile, but very easy in the case of a female chimp. Some have suggested that concealing fertility is a sexual strategy developed by women (and other primate species with 'monogamous' relationships) so that their male partners cannot tell when they are not fertile, and will be less tempted to stray in the direction of other, possibly fertile, females. We discuss the ways that such sexual strategies determine different patterns of behaviour in males and females later. However, this is the place to mention that Solly Zuckerman, in a famous book published in 1932, suggested that the persistence of all primate societies was due to the equally persistent

British soldier. 'Not to propagate the species but to improve the strain, so our aim was to marry British soldiers, not to marry Anglo-Indian men.'

Charles Allen. (1975) *Plain tales from the raj.*

(Andre Deutsch, London.)

They had an unexpected visitor. . . . The Comte de Frontenac. . . when his wife, Mademoiselle's companion, who had eloped with him as a young girl but who had been avoiding him for years, greeted his arrival and his conjugal demands with screams of terror and revulsion, Mademoiselle. . . was confirmed in many of her feelings: 'I scolded Madame de Frontenac and told her she was bound in conscience to go to bed with her husband. . . As for me, I have always had a great aversion to love, even legitimate love, so unworthy of a noble soul has this passion always seemed to me. . . . I saw clearly that deeds done out of passion seldom breed rational consequences. I saw that passion dies quickly, that one is wretched for the rest of one's days if one's marriage is based on anything so short-lived, that one is better off to marry rationally: there may be aversion at first, but there will be all the more love later.'

Francis Steegmuller. (1955) *La grande mademoiselle.*

(Hamish Hamilton, London.)

Married Woman's (as it was known for short) was one of Savannah's most exclusive societies. . . . . . Husbands were as much a part of Married Woman's as their wives. They were, after all, the ones who footed the bill for the dinners and for refurbishing the house beforehand. And they were, of course, the major qualification for membership: A woman had to be married to belong. The rules stated that if a member obtained a divorce, she would be forced to resign and forfeit her dues. More than one marriage had been held together by that rule alone.

John Berendt. (1997) *Midnight in the garden of good and evil.* (Vintage, London.)

She was determined never again to be a party to the hideous transformation which overcomes the partners of a bad marriage, who grow fangs and horns and sprout black monstrous wolfish hair, who claw and cling and bite and suck.

Margaret Drabble. (1987) *The radiant way.*

(Weidenfeld and Nicolson, London.)

sexual attraction between its members. In other words, sex is the glue binding these animals together. It is a view that has not survived the succeeding years very well. Most people now think that social bonds are more complicated than this, and, anyway, some primates show prolonged periods of no sex, but stay together. But it was a remarkable attempt to relate physiology and social behaviour, in a way that had not really been done before. In humans (and maybe even in some other animals), something we call 'love' is a powerful sexual bond. We will have more to say about what neuroscience can tell us about love in Chapter 9.

By now you are half-way to the 'emancipation' camp for women. Here is something that may give you pause for thought. It turns out that testosterone, the steroid hormone we all associate with maleness and masculine sexuality, plays a considerable part in the sexuality of women. This was first suspected following some observations in the late 1950s to early 1960s. There were studies on women who had had both their ovaries and adrenals removed. Removal of the ovaries, by itself, was found to diminish sexuality a little, but this was much more marked after both ovaries and adrenals has been taken out. The adrenals and ovaries of women both produce testosterone (about equal amounts) and levels in the blood are about one tenth those of men. Giving women replacement testosterone after either removal of the ovaries or both operations markedly stimulated their sexual interest ('libido'). Similar results have been seen with other women, with intact ovaries and adrenals, given (small amounts of) testosterone. Experimental work on female monkeys confirms this: their attractiveness to the male is heavily dependent on oestrogen levels (their vaginas smell different, their rumps look redder), but their receptivity (whether they will mate with him) owes more to testosterone, which acts on their brain. Nowadays, some post-menopausal women (who can have low levels of androgens) are given androgen-like steroids as well as other hormones to spice up their sex lives. You will have noticed that none of this was deducible from working on non-primate species like rats, cats or guinea pigs. Perhaps there is something special about primate sexuality after all. It certainly seems there is no such thing as 'male' or 'female' hormones in primates. Neither, in fact, are there in rats. Though the male rat may secrete lots of testosterone, his brain converts much of it into oestrogen. So much (not all) of the things that

Sex Differences

The time-honored phrase *vive la difference* reflects the sentiments of most people about variations between the sexes. . . . The combination of events that lead to establishing these sexual dimorphisms is referred to as the process of *sexual differentiation*. The elucidation of this process is a fascinating problem, both for its intrinsic interest and because its study yields important insights into the physical basis of behavior. . . .Of course, there are many behavioral differences between the sexes other than those related to copulation. An obvious example is that of aggressive behavior. . . . Less obvious are various aspects of feeding behavior, spontaneous activity, and play and emotional behavior.

G Bermant and J M Davidson. (1974) *Biological bases of sexual behavior*. (Harper and Row, New York.)

Psycho-analysis has taught us that a boy's earliest choice of objects for his love is incestuous and that those objects are forbidden ones — his mother and his sister. We have learnt, too, the manner in which, as he grows up, he liberates himself from this incestuous attraction.

S Freud. (1950) *Totem and taboo*. (Routledge and Kegan Paul, London.)

A vast number of human males, whilst they may be only too anxious at times for female company, are equally keen for much of the time to get away from women and relax in the ease of male companionship. Chimpanzee males seem to feel rather the same. Of course they cluster round pink sexually attractive females when these are available. But more often they travel about and feed in all-male groups, and they are more likely to groom each other than they are to groom females or youngsters.

J van Lawick-Goodall. (1971) *In the shadow of man*. (Collins, London.)

There is a substantial body of evidence for the role(s) played by "biological" or "inborn" forces directing erotic interest to males or females and promoting the conviction that one is a man or a woman. Some writers, identified as social constructionists, ignore these "biological" influences and cite, to the exclusion of the biological, socialization experiences and massive cultural influences that impact on psychosexual development. Biological reductionists, in contrast, ignore socialization and cultural energy. People are not solely walking containers of DNA and sex steroid molecules. Nor are they solely cultural blotters. A balanced view must be seen.

R Green. (2002) Sexual identity and sexual orientation. In: *Hormones, brain and behavior* **4**, pp. 463–485. (Elsevier Science Press, New York.)

testosterone does for the male rat's sexuality is, in fact, the result of oestrogen acting on the cells of the male's brain. The startling conclusion is that maleness and femaleness is not defined by the hormones the adult secretes, but by how the brain of each sex responds to these hormones.

Sexuality in human males is also responsive to testosterone. Without the benefit of knowing any endocrinology (or even that hormones existed), our forefathers discovered that reliable custodians of harems had to be castrated before puberty. Choir masters keen to prolong the pure singing voice of a boy also knew that castration was effective. Castration after puberty (or, in more modern times, treatments that reduce the effects of testosterone) has less effect, though there is a gradual and partial loss of both sexual interest and, perhaps more prominently, the ability to achieve penile erection. This shows that sexual motivation in men is sensitive to testosterone, but also that peripheral effects on the genitals are also part of its action. In some species (such as some monkeys, but not man), the glans penis (the tip) grows arrays of little barbs, the penile spines, when testosterone levels rise. These spines are thought to increase the female's sensory information, encouraging ovulation in some species, but perhaps only pleasure in others. There is a current debate about whether, in some cases at least, the decreasing sexual vigour of ageing men is due to falling testosterone. Levels do go down in some older men, but whether this is functionally significant is not certain. Note that men are not emancipated either, but that the first exposure to testosterone (at puberty) seems to alter the precise way it controls sexuality. Something happens in the brain.

Now it is time to ask what steroid hormones like testosterone and oestrogen do in the brain. Steroids, like other hormones, act on cells that contain (express) the appropriate receptors for them. Brain cells can only respond to steroid hormones if they contain the right receptors. The hormone is the key, the receptor the lock. Unlike some other hormones, steroids dissolve in fat (are lipid-soluble), so they pass easily across the membrane of a nerve cell. The receptors lie inside the neuron; when a steroid binds to them, they travel within the cell and attach themselves to a special site in DNA. DNA, of course, makes up the genes, so steroids can directly alter the activity of any gene that has a steroid-binding site on it. A good way of detecting neurons that can bind steroids, and thus respond to them, is to map those that contain steroid receptors. Mapping

Sexual Strategies

Attitude surveys in a wide variety of human societies around the world have shown that men tend to be more interested than women in sexual variety, including casual sex and brief relationships. That attitude is readily understandable because it tends to maximize transmission of the genes of a man but not of a woman.

Jared Diamond. (1997) *Why is sex fun?*
(Weidenfeld and Nicolson, London.)

. . . We do not subscribe to the often expressed view — that animals, unlike humans, have sexual interactions only for reproduction, not for pleasure. On the contrary, in all likelihood humans are the only species that understand the reproductive consequences of sex. Animals can be presumed to engage in sex primarily for pleasure, although there is some evidence that social factors, such as dominance or access to resources such as food, contribute to sexual motivation in some species.

E M Hull, R L Meisel, B D Sachs. (2002) Male sexual behavior.
In: *Hormones, brain and behavior.* Eds. D W Pfaff, A P Arnold, A M Etgen,
S E Farhbach, R T Rubin, pp. 3–35. (Academic Press, Amsterdam.)

Although evolution. . . has tended to make females the exploited sex. . . females, through their *behavior*, can at least partially redress the balance. Because a few males can fertilize many females, a female has more of a choice about who she mates with than does a male. . . . Obviously, genes will be favored that cause her to make this choice in a way that benefits her reproductive success. Such behavior may consist of simply choosing the largest male, or the one who has proved himself the strongest by defeating in single combat every other male in the vicinity. But she can also choose in such a way as to increase the male's investment in their offspring. . . . The females of many species require the males to provide a large amount of food or to construct a nest as a condition for mating. If the male has made large investments of some kind prior to mating, he will be more likely to take an interest in the well-being of the young: it is just too expensive to abandon the family and start over.

S LeVay. (1993) *The sexual brain.* (MIT Press, Cambridge, Massachusetts).

The sexual drive is nothing but the motor memory of previously experienced pleasure. The concept of drives is thus reduced to the concept of pleasure.

Wilhelm Reich. (1942) *The function of the orgasm.*
(Farrar, Strauss and Giroux Inc., New York.)

receptors for either oestrogen or testosterone shows that most are in the neurons of the limbic system. The amygdala and hypothalamus are two areas that have large amounts. It looks as if our search for the 'sexual brain' ought to start here.

If we make a small area of damage (a lesion) in the front of the hypothalamus of a male rat, he stops copulating even though his testosterone levels are normal. If we take a castrated male rat, whose sexual behaviour has declined, and implant a tiny pellet of testosterone in the same area, he starts to try to mount the female. Pellets elsewhere in the hypothalamus do not work. This is beginning to look interesting: have we found the male's 'sex centre'? Then we do the same experiments in females. We find a similar result with their steroids, except that the sensitive part of the hypothalamus is not quite the same it lies just behind the 'male' area. We are getting positively excited: we have separate sex centres for males and females, just what you might expect.

Our fun is spoiled by an observant colleague who points out that our lesioned males seem still to be very interested in the females; it is simply that they cannot seem to mate. We suddenly remember that the penis and spinal cord also need testosterone for adequate sexual behaviour. Perhaps that is what is missing, but giving testosterone does not change things very much. When we do a more complicated experiment, we find that males with damage in the front of the hypothalamus will still do work (e.g. press a bar) to get at a sexually-attractive female, though when they do, they still do not mate. After a while, they stop pressing the bar. If the hypothalamus is the seat of sexual motivation, how can we explain this curious mixture of results? It looks as if sexual performance, rather than sexual motivation, is dependent on the hypothalamus. However, it does seem that the two are inter-linked: hence the males give up trying to get access to the females after failing to mate a few times. Not quite what we were expecting.

It seems to get more complicated. Females will also mount other females. Lesions in the front of their hypothalamus stops this, but not their ability to show the receptive lordosis position to a male. Light dawns: what we have really found is a part of the brain concerned with a given pattern of sex behaviour: 'masculine' (though observable in both sexes) and 'feminine' (ditto). But where then is the seat of sexual

It is customary in this age to attribute a comprehensive and quite unanalysed causality to the 'sexual urges'. These obscure forces, sometimes thought of as particular historical springs, sometimes as more general and universal destinies, are credited with the power to make of us delinquents, neurotics, lunatics, fanatics, martyrs, heroes, saints, or more exceptionally, integrated fathers, fulfilled mothers, placid human animals, and the like.

Iris Murdoch. (1973) *The black prince.*
(Chatto and Windus, London.)

. . . The wasting fires of lust sprang up again. The verses passed from his lips and the inarticulate cries and the unspoken brutal words rushed froth from his brain to force a passage. His blood was in revolt. . . . He moaned to himself like some kind of baffled prowling beast. He wanted to sin with another of his kind, to force another being to sin with him and to exult with her in sin.

James Joyce. (1916) *A portrait of the artist as a young man.*

What do you want me to do? He said.
I want you to be considerate of a young girl's reputation.
I never meant not to be.
She smiled. I believe you, she said. But you must understand. This is another country. Here a woman's reputation is all she has.
Yes mam.
There is no forgiveness, you see,
Mam?
There is no forgiveness. For women. A man may lose his honor and regain it again. But a woman cannot. She cannot.

Cormac McCarthy. (1993) *All the pretty horses.*
(Vintage, London.)

Of course Freud's immediate reception in America was not auspicious. A few professional alienists (psychiatrists) understood his importance, but to most of the public he appeared as some kind of German sexologist, an exponent of free love who used big words to talk about dirty things. At least a decade would pass before Freud would have his revenge and see his ideas begin to destroy sex in America forever.

E L Doctorow. (1976) *Ragtime.* (Pan Books, London.)

motivation (desire)? In females, damaging the part of the hypothalamus that responds to ovarian steroids does seem to prevent them being sexy in all ways. Surely the brain cannot have a 'sex centre' for females but not for males?

The picture gets a little more blurred. If you make small lesions of the hypothalamus of female rats, (in the same area that interferes with masculine sexual behaviour in males) they wreck the females' maternal behaviour; they neglect their new-born pups. How can the same bit of brain do both, rather distinct, behaviours? More to come: damage to the part of the brain that alters 'feminine' sexual behaviour also causes rats to put on masses of weight. It seems to be part of an appetite-regulating centre. Can it be both? Mapping biologically different behaviours in the hypothalamus is getting less convincing. If there is a sexual brain it does not seem very distinct. Yet rats (or people) can tell the difference between a sexual object and one that is edible.

Similar experiments on the amygdala show that it, too, plays a role in sexual behaviour, but one that is different from the hypothalamus. Damage to the amygdala interferes with the time male rats spend sniffing the genitalia of females, though eventually they mate much as normal. They also will not work (press a bar) to get access to a sexy female. Some people interpret these results as suggesting the amygdala is the seat of sexual 'motivation' but a different idea is more plausible. We know, from a variety of other studies, that the amygdala is concerned with 'labelling' sensory experiences as 'sexual' or 'edible' or whatever, and with certain forms of learning, for example, associating a neutral event (like a light) with a reward (like sex). So it is not surprising that amygdala damage prevents rats associating a 'neutral' stimulus like a light with sex and so they no longer press a bar to get access to one when the light comes on. In a more natural context, such lesions will reduce their exploration of females, since the sensory information they get may not have the same 'meaning' or 'reward value' as in rats with an intact amygdala. We have already seen that impairing sexual performance can reduce sexual motivation. So impairing the quality of sexual information may do the same. In females, there is rather less effect. It looks as if the amygdala is somehow concerned with gathering sexual information, but is not the seat of sexual motivation either. Neither is it exclusively concerned with

No other writer has managed to turn his failures and frustrations as a human being into such a success story, just as no other man. . . has made of impotence a source of so much strength. Self-doubt, insecurity, tentativeness modulate each and every one of his sentences, which explains, amongst other reasons, why they are so long. Proust made an art not just of introspection, but of irresolution. He courted the world as if he were an outsider looking in, but his vision. . . was essentially that of a confident contrarian who knows the twisted ways of the world because he knows them in himself so well. . . . He exposes love for self-interest, beauty for bad taste, purity for perversion.

A Aciman. (2002) Proust regained.
New York Review of Books **49**, pp. 55–64.

Of course, people had been taking mad risks for sex, lust, love, for as long as we'd been people. Wars had been fought for what you could , if you were being uncharitable, characterise as basically a bit of slap and tickle. Holy books had been rewritten, the laws of God changed to facilitate the having of some desperately yearned-for piece of ass. Desire was the backhanded compliment humanity had no choice but to pay itself. It was just the way we were, it was what we did. We couldn't help ourselves.

Iain Banks. (2002) *Dead air (Abacus, London).*

sex. Other sorts of information (e.g. about food) and different associations (eg. between a neutral stimulus and something unpleasant) are disturbed by damaging the amygdala. So another unanswered question is how the amygdala seems to be able to classify some stimuli as 'sexual' and others as 'fearful' or even 'eatable.' By now, you will have realised that we do not really understand the details of how hormones such as testosterone control sexuality, even in laboratory rats. But so far, we have been concerned about turning sex on; what about turning it off?

It may come as a surprise to learn that turning sexual behaviour and reproduction off is as important biologically as turning it on. This is because reproduction, as we have already mentioned, is so costly. Costly for the male, who has to fight off rivals, and may even have no time to eat. Costly for females, who have to nurture their young both through pregnancy and lactation, putting enormous strains on their bodies and their energy supply. Add to this the job of defending the young against would-be predators. In some species, the males may stay around to help; in others, it is the females alone that bear the burden. Both may expose themselves to increased risk of becoming prey during the distracting business of breeding. It is in the interest of both males and females that the young have the best chance of survival; that is, the risk of breeding pays off.

Go into the fields in the spring, and you will see lambs aplenty. None in autumn, though, if you are observant, you will notice the rams paying extra attention to the ewes. There is a season for mating and a season for births in most species living in the so-called temperate zones — those north or south of the Equator. The birth season is nearly always the spring — the time when food is getting plentiful, and the days warmer. At other times of the year, reproduction is turned off. There is much more about breeding seasons, an example of an annual rhythm, in Chapter 11. Another, quite different, set of circumstances also require reproduction to be shut off. The remarkable and important adaptations to social stress are discussed in Chapters 4 and 10. Here, we have only to note that all animals (we really mean mammals) live in a social group. This group is essential for survival: animals do much better living in groups than on their own in most cases. Groups have a structure, a hierarchy; some members are at the top of the pile (they are dominant), others are at the bottom — the subordinates. It is the latter we need to think about. Being subordinate is a potent social stress, and it is not a good life. Subordinate monkeys, for

Sex and Violence

. . . An important aspect of both civilian and martial rape is that it is an instrument of domestication: breaking for house service. It breaks the spirit, humiliates, tames, produces a docile, deferential, obedient soul. Its immediate message to women and girls is that we will have in our own bodies only the control that we are granted by men and thereby in general only that control in our environments that we are granted by men. . . .

If there is one set of fundamental functions of rape, civilian or martial, it is to display, communicate, and produce or maintain *dominance*, which is both enjoyed for its own sake and used for such ulterior ends as exploitation, expulsion, dispersion, murder.

Claudia Card. (2001) Hypatia Vol. 11, No. 4.

Understanding why men are more violent than women requires an understanding of the highly asymmetrical gender roles. . . assigned at birth on our patriarchal culture. . . and powerfully conditioned to conform throughout the rest of their lives. . . . The differences in those gender roles makes it possible for men to ward off or undo feelings of shame, disgrace or dishonor by means of violence, whereas that is significantly less for women.

J Gilligan. (2001) Preventing violence. (Thames and Hudson, New York.)

The enlarged brain that accompanied the transformation of the simple forest-dweller into a co-operative hunter began to busy itself with technological improvements. The simple tribal dwelling places became great towns and cities. The axe age blossomed into the space age. But what effect did the acquisition of all this gloss and glitter have on the sexual system of the species? Very little, seems to be the answer.

Desmond Morris. (1967) The naked ape. (Jonathan Cape, London.)

Perhaps the characteristic of human sexuality which sets it most clearly apart from that of most animals is its relative separation from reproduction. Sex has obviously come to play a much wider sociobiological function than the production of offspring. . . . If human sexuality has a wider function than in most other species, it is because there are fewer biological constraints. Hence the need for social constraints.

J Bancroft. (1989) Human sexuality and its problems.
(Churchill Livingstone, Edinburgh.)

example, lose out on competition for food, water, shelter, and (of course) for mates. They also have to keep a constant eye out for attacks on them from stronger, more dominant animals. They struggle to survive (Chapter 4).

Even if they had the chance, reproduction would be wholly unwise for them. To add an extra burden onto their already overburdened, subordinate lives would, surely, be the last straw. So their brains take them out of the competition, by both turning off their reproductive hormones, and making them behaviourally unresponsive to them even should they reach reasonable levels. A subordinate female monkey does not ovulate; a subordinate male does not even try to mate (though, just to make sure, his testosterone levels are low as well). In many non-primate species, a similar picture can be seen. Better to wait: perhaps one day their status will change, and they will have a better chance. The right time for them to breed is when they are no longer so stressed. And how is reproduction suppressed when social conditions are inauspicious? Why, by using the chemical signal β-endorphin, the same peptide that turned off reproduction in the very different context of the non-breeding season. Let's take a closer look at β-endorphin.

B-endorphin, like other peptides, is formed in the brain by breaking up a much bigger precursor, parent peptide called POMC (pro-opiomelanocortin). POMC is split by several enzymes into a whole family of daughter peptides, many of them with strong behavioural and physiological actions. One is ACTH, a peptide that has already appeared in the story about stress (Chapter 4). It activates the adrenal glands to secrete the major stress steroid cortisol (corticosterone in rats). Another is the peptide MSH which stands for melanocyte stimulating hormone, a name which does not reflect its true function in man. It is concerned with food intake (Chapter 5), and it is also sensitive to stress. The third is β-endorphin. If you infuse β-endorphin into the brain, it reduces gonadotrophin secreted from the pituitary (thus shutting off the testes or ovaries) and it inhibits sexual behaviour. Even if you fill them up to their ears with testosterone, male rats will not mate if you inject β-endorphin into their brains. If you were to measure β-endorphin in the fluid surrounding the brain (the cerebrospinal fluid), you would find it much higher in subordinate monkeys than top-ranking ones. It is higher because the brain is making more of it. So this may be why these unfortunate animals do not mate (or ovulate) very often, though how social stress increases β-endorphin is another matter.

Actually, it is not necessarily true that β-endorphin is increased in lower-ranking males only as part of their adaptation. The dominant males (we are focussing on males) need to be very sure that all the babies in the group are theirs. Constant vigilance is therefore their lot, since other, less top-ranking, males may try and sneak a tryst. If subordinate males do not want to mate, or if subordinate females do not ovulate even though they mate, then this helps the bosses. So the changed β-endorphin in the subordinates' brains may be a clever scheme whereby the boss males make sure the competition is reduced, and it is their genes that are passed on into the offspring. It is also important, in many species, to turn off sexual behaviour during pregnancy, both to protect the developing foetus (the female's point of view) and to ensure that the male does not compete with other males only to mate with a female who is no longer fertile (the male's point of view). β-endorphin is increased in the brains of females during pregnancy, and may play an important role in reducing sexuality during this critical time in a female's reproductive life.

So β-endorphin is a peptide that turns off sexuality. There may well be many others, since to inhibit reproduction is desirable under many different conditions. One that we know about is CRF (corticotropin-releasing factor), a peptide we discuss in other parts of this book (Chapter 4), and closely concerned with an individual's ability to respond to stressors. Though the most obvious actions of CRF behaviourally are to increase anxiety and fear (necessary if one is to cope with some sorts of threat), it also inhibits sexual behaviour. This may be because sexuality is biologically inappropriate under conditions of threat. Peptides like CRF may also alter the priority of response. The latter means that, if there is a choice of possible responses (drink, sex, run away) the peptides coding the currently predominant behavioural state (hopefully the most appropriate one) will also determine that priority is given to the most imperative stimulus or demand. You can see this if you deprive a rat of food, and then allow him access to a bowl of food or an oestrous female. Depending on the balance between the chemical state in the brain, the rat will choose first the female (usually) or the food. But make conditions rather more severe, you may get the opposite. A peptide called NPY (discussed in Chapter 5) has a now familiar dual role: it encourages feeding but inhibits sex. Another example of a peptide signal in the limbic system determining the priority of response.

Incidentally, if you change the features of the female (e.g. make her less attractive) then you will, of course, alter the priority of response even though you keep the brain chemistry the same. This shows how external events and current chemical state of the limbic system interact with each other.

But, what you and every pharmaceutical company in the land wants to know is whether here are peptides that increase sexuality: a biological aphrodisiac. There is one obvious candidate: GnRH, a rather small (10 amino-acids) peptide, and we have already met it. It is a major controlling peptide for the reproductive function of the pituitary. Like other such peptides, it is produced by the neurons of the hypothalamus. There is no doubt that GnRH is a major 'breeding' signal from the brain to the pituitary. Without it, animals and humans remain infertile.

The obvious question is: does GnRH have a behavioural role as well? After all, it would make sense. No good having the gonads all ready for a fertile mating if there is no sexual behaviour to go with it. So is GnRH a sexual stimulant? About 30 years ago, several groups reported experiments that seemed to suggest just this. They gave female rats, whose own ovaries had been removed, a small amount of oestrogen. This was not enough to make them sexually receptive. Then they were given GnRH directly into the ventricles of the brain. They rapidly became very sexy indeed. A clear indication, you may think, that GnRH fulfils its suspected role as a sexual activator. This, indeed, was the conclusion of those in the field at the time, encouraged no doubt by the thought that this behavioural role of GnRH fitted well with its physiological function. Sadly, the succeeding years have not really borne this out. The problem is that all sorts of different chemicals can activate sexuality in oestrogen-treated rats, so the effect of GnRH was not very specific. Furthermore, it did not do much for males, and when it was tried in man it was also not very effective (though a few people claimed to show some beneficial effects on sexual performance). Though peptides related to GnRH have been developed for the clinical treatment of fertility, and are very valuable, there is no established behavioural role for GnRH, which is a pity, since the original logic is still strong. One wonders if one day someone might have a new idea about GnRH and its possible function in behaviour.

Before we leave GnRH, we should mention some other rather fascinating things about it. The neurons that make it begin life in the part of the brain concerned with smell, and this is where you will find neurons containing GnRH in the foetus. These neurons track their way into the hypothalamus, where they arrive in time for birth, and remain there during the rest of life. There is only a very small number in the adult brain, but some of the nerve fibres containing GnRH wander off into the brain in directions away from the pituitary, further hinting at a wider role. Recall the important role of smell in sexual behaviour (watch that male rat or dog sniff the genitals of a passing female; and which of us does not wear either perfume or deodorant?) and you will see why the relation between GnRH, smell and sex is an intriguing one.

Before we give up the search for a neurochemical sexual code, we had better take a look at the monoamines. Recall that the monoamines are a general name given to a group of chemicals the brain uses as transmitters: serotonin, dopamine and noradrenaline are the best known (see Chapters 3, 4 and 5). They have a strong family resemblance to each other, not only chemically, but in the way they are arranged in the brain (see Chapter 3). As it happens, there are many rather effective drugs that can act on each of these systems, which allows researchers to test their role in sexuality. And a role they certainly have. In general, drugs that increase serotonin dampen sexual behaviour. This can be a troubling side effect when they are used, for example, to treat depression in humans, though helpful in treating socially unacceptable forms of sexuality (e.g. fetishism, paedophilia). Increasing the action of dopamine, on the other hand, generally stimulates sexual behaviour, that is, it becomes easier to induce sex in sluggish animals. Decreasing dopamine makes rats very uninterested in sex. There are stories of people getting dopamine active drugs, for example for Parkinson's disease, who begin to show inappropriate and unusual sexual behaviour, though this may simply be because they have regained their ability to move. Noradrenaline has rather mixed effects, though a drug called yohimbine, which increases noradrenaline activity in the brain, is a traditional aphrodisiac. So all the monoamines can alter sexuality. But their candidacy as 'sexual' chemicals in the brain is seriously undermined by realising that they do similar things to other behaviours, such as eating, aggression, drinking and so on. This has not deterred attempts by certain drug companies to try and develop drugs that act on dopamine as sexual stimulants.

Of course, such drugs might very well increase sexual responsiveness, but only as a more general action, and whether this is worth the candle remains to be seen. Since all these chemicals interact with a considerable number of different receptor molecules in the brain (serotonin, for e.g. has about 14, see Chapter 3), there is always the chance that one might be particularly concerned with sexual behaviour. If this is the case, then one might imagine a drug targeted to that receptor being used to regulate sexuality. So far, this has not happened. At the moment, it does not look as if the monoamines are more concerned with sexuality that any other adaptive behaviour.

So is there a 'sexual brain'? That is, a defined part of the brain given over to sexual behaviour and, one assumes, the associated hormones and other features of reproduction? And does all the experimental evidence, gained mostly from years of patient research on rats (and a few other species) actually apply to humans?

The answer to the sexual brain question seems to be an unsatisfactory 'yes and no'. Yes, because, as we have repeatedly pointed out in this book, an animal (or a human) knows when to respond sexually, or when it experiences a sexual demand (the motivation to find sex). Sexual behaviour is quite distinct from other adaptive behaviours, so the brain must have mechanisms for recognising sexual stimuli, generating a sexual response to them, and initiating sexual activity when hormonal conditions are optimal. And hormones such as testosterone seem to pick out those parts of the brain that contain receptors to this steroid, and this may 'mark' the sexual brain. However, testosterone has other behavioural actions, for example, it can increase aggression, though this might justifiably be seen as a part of an overall sexual strategy devised by the limbic system to ensure successful sex. So we can see which parts of the brain have testosterone (or, in the female, oestrogen) receptors and use this as a marker for the 'sexual brain'. Little patches of hypothalamus, amygdala, brainstem and other parts of the limbic system fit. But after this, the trail goes cold. Even in the limbic system, there is another problem. All the areas that contain receptors for testosterone etc. also do other things. They control other adaptive behaviours, other hormone systems. So how does a pulse of testosterone (for e.g.) set up a special 'brain state' that allows the male rat to respond, say, to those ultrasonic cries from the female? Or her special smell? The visual, smell and sensory parts of the brain are busy with many other things (food, drink, avoiding danger and so on): somehow, they channel sexual information to the 'sexual' limbic system, where it only becomes effective if hormonal (and other) conditions are right. How all this happens is still a big, big mystery. We still cannot point to an area of the brain, or a bunch of nerve cells in the limbic system, and say (truthfully) that this is the sexual brain (as distinct from other categories). But there must be one. Perhaps the secret lies in a level of analysis which has hardly begun for sex: the chemical content of certain nerve cells. Those steroid receptors may be a good signpost, but are they a necessary feature of everything in the brain that is 'sexual'? Surely not. And is everything in the brain that has a testosterone receptor part of the 'sexual brain'? I doubt it. The most intriguing question (not limited to sexuality) is how a relatively simple molecule like a steroid hormone can induce powerful, but temporary, motivational and emotional changes in brain function, and how these come to be part of the animal's priority in life.

Sexuality in humans is much more than responding to hormones, but we need to ask whether, deep in the human brain, there lies a limbic system not too unlike that of rats and rabbits, or, more likely, monkeys and apes. If there is, it may be functioning not too differently from all those other limbic systems. After all, they have been pretty successful in making sure that the best genes are transmitted to succeeding generations. This is hardly a new concept: much of the older morality (and some religions) was based on the idea that man has an 'animal' brain which needs to be corralled by uniquely human ethical, religious and social controls (a supposed function of the 'higher' brain). The obvious power of the sexual limbic system in other species suggests that, if we humans have one too, it is going to need some equally powerful moderating influences. What does neuroscience have to say?

Not a lot. If we examine the human brain anatomically, we see all the limbic components of other animals. The hypothalamus looks rather like theirs, the amygdala likewise, particularly if we compare ourselves to other, non-human, primates. There is (rather limited) evidence that the human limbic system has nerve cells that contain steroid receptors, just like rats. The limbic system of monkeys certainly does. Hormone secretion is important in humans, though, as we have seen, there may be detailed differences (in females at least) between primates and others, and a partial shift from internal (hormonal) controls to external (social and psychological) ones. Damage to the human hypothalamus can interfere with sexuality (we have to distinguish between direct effects on sexual behaviour and indirect ones via changes in hormone secretion). Rare cases of amygdala damage in man have been reported to result in unrestrained sexuality. As we have seen, drugs that alter monoamines can influence human sexuality, suggesting common features between man and rat. But the great mass of experimental data available for rats is simply not there for humans. It is even rather sparse for non-human primates, who are expensive to maintain in labs, difficult to get, and raise ethical questions about whether they should be used at all. So we have to make a best guess. Mine is that the human brain indeed contains most of the limbic elements we see in monkeys, and many we see in rats. But, once again, there is one big difference. Surrounding this elemental but powerful limbic system is a huge neocortex. Monkeys and apes have quite a large neocortex as well, but not as big as ours. Rats have very much less. If we want to look for distinguishing aspects of human sexuality, it is here we need to look, not in the limbic system. Like many other adaptive behaviours, the abilities of the human neocortex add enormous versatility to an otherwise basic process. This is what Sigmund Freud thought.

So far, we have been thinking about sex as if there were only two great divisions in the biological world of the mammal, the male and the female, and thus a 'male' and a 'female' brain. But whilst there is merit in this approach when we try to understand the general principles by which the brain controls sexual behaviour, it omits two enormously important facts: whilst males and females of any species have a common interest in maximising reproductive success, the way they go about this may not be the same; and neither are males or females all the same, as everyone knows.

The idea that the sexual strategies of male and females may be different is an old one. It comes from assuming the basic premise that both sexes have a common biological objective in trying to pass their genes on to as many offspring as possible, with the caveat that those offspring must survive to breed in their turn. But the facts of physiology show that the two sexes ought to adopt different ways of achieving this. The reproductive capacity (the number of young they can bear) is limited for females by the duration of pregnancy (some species, such as rats, reduce this so that the young are born very immature but they have to have large litters, because so many die), the period of lactation (when the females of many, but not all, species are infertile) and the demands of rearing the young. This means that it is a good biological principle that females choose their breeding conditions (when, how and with whom) very carefully, because they have only so many opportunities. They need to make each attempt as successful as possible. Each one is a major investment. They should choose also their mate with great care, to make sure they get the 'best' genes. Males, on the other hand, have no such restraint. Their strategy might seem to be to mate with as many females as possible, since this might be the best way of maximising the number of offspring (hence genes). Now, of course, there are species in which the male takes some (or even all) of the rearing duty, and others in which he will spend much energy getting food for the young. There is a clear difference in overall sexual strategy, and we cannot avoid thinking about how the brain might go about implementing it.

Let us pay a visit to cloud nine, on which sits the Director-General. He/she/it has decided that animals will have a limited life span and that sex is the way that all the mammals will procreate, and issues the corresponding order. Down on cloud twenty-one, the Chief of the design team scratches his/her/its celestial head. After a moment's inspired (divinely-inspired, perhaps?) thought, he (etc.) has the answer. He will make sex very nice (so we will all want to do it) and he will so arrange how we do it to increase the chances of each gender being reproductively successful. We will adopt the best tactics, but be unaware of the overall strategy. Natural selection will operate on the outcome of the strategy. If the tactics are no good, then there will not be any individuals left to continue using them. The tactics are what the brain does, in the service of the overall, sublime, strategy. If, therefore, we were to understand how the brain controls sexuality, we need to talk tactics. Darwin said it all, when he put forward his ideas on natural and sexual selection, though he wasn't so very interested in the role of the brain.

Now, I have to tell you that even exceedingly eminent biologists, who understand this distinction very well, sometimes let themselves lapse into writing about males 'choosing' a promiscuous strategy, or females 'opting' for a selective sexual strategy. They do nothing of the sort. Assume, for the moment, that the male's brain has in it the mechanisms that result in promiscuity, or in females those that cause her to look for particular features in her mate. The fact that they do so (the tactics) results in the strategy being achieved (maximum reproductive efficiency). The tactics represent the 'choice' not the strategy. The fact that we are almost certainly the only species that understands the link between sex and reproduction enables us to manipulate the tactics.

There are no animal societies in which sexual behaviour is unregulated, though the form of regulation differs considerably. Social control is the first, and in many ways, the most potent reason why sex is always unevenly distributed. If we look at the apes, our nearest biological cousins, we see this. Gibbons, for example, form monogamous pairs, and this limits who will mate with whom. Gorillas, however, have a 'harem' system, in which a large, dominant male gathers a number of females around him. He defends access to them. Although there may be other adult males in the group, he does all, or nearly, all the mating. Chimpanzees, on the other hand, live in large heterosexual bands, and a male will mate with many females, a female with many males. But not randomly. Even in this type of society, sex is not haphazard. It is the latter type of group that shows the second mechanism most clearly: sexual selection. If we want a simple rule about what determines the distribution of sex in a multi-sexual group it would be: the males compete with each other, and the females then choose the males. But females also compete, and males do not find all females equally attractive. And vice-versa. As we all know.

It is a biological fact that aggression and sex go together. Were you to hack your way through the thick forest that lines many of the rivers in West Africa, you might see a small, greenish monkey called a talapoin. These tiny monkeys (they weigh about 1 kilogram, less than your cat) live in quite large groups (30 or more) and quite peaceably for most of the year. But come the breeding season, and two things happen. The males (who otherwise keep their distance from the females) move into the female groups, and fights break out everywhere. It is the same in other monkeys who live in multimale groups, for example, in the more familiar rhesus monkey, found throughout Northern India. Many males get injured during the annual breeding frenzy. If you were to inject out-of-season males with testosterone and the females with oestrogen, you would replicate this behaviour. So testosterone acts on the brain in at least two ways: to increase sexual motivation, but also to supply a tactic whereby a male can improve his access to a sexually-attractive female by fighting for her. Notice that you have to treat the females as well, otherwise there is no incentive for the males (though simply giving them testosterone may increase aggressiveness to some degree on its own). Outbreaks of aggression during the breeding season are not limited to monkeys; witness those stags locking antlers during their rutting season, the general hostility of breeding bulls, and, most dramatically, the 'musth' shown by male elephants. Musth is an annual period of uncontrollable aggression, accompanied by increased secretion of glands on the head, and urine dribbling down their legs. The latter are probably transmitting smell signals to other males and females. Many zoos cannot cope with male elephants in musth. The 'laddish' behaviour so common in young human males may be a similar phenomenon; certainly, folklore attributes this to 'too much testosterone' — not a bad guess. But not all non-human primates are aggressive during the breeding season; for example, those that live in monogamous groups. So the brain (probably the limbic system) has a flexible set of testosterone-dependent tactics, depending on the type of mating system the species uses. The same parts of the brain may also determine whether or not the species in question adopts a monogamous or polygamous mating system, though testosterone does not determine which system, only its implementation. Perhaps this is the moment to mention that the distinction between these tactics in non-human primates at least is not an absolute one. Some species can modify their mating systems according to habitat and circumstances. So, of course, can we.

In species of monkeys that live in multi-male groups, little pre-pubertal males, like little females, are tolerated by the adult males. They romp around, climbing over these formidable, canine-armed, monsters, pulling their tails, eating their food. But as soon as a little male begins to secrete testosterone at puberty, everything changes. Their licence come to an end. No longer do they dare get anywhere near adult males, who are now very aggressive towards them. In fact, it is highly likely that they will be driven from the troop, to live a lonely life with other vagabond males, at least for a while. Eventually, they may manage to join another troop, working their way circumspectly up the social hierarchy until, one very fine day, they can mate with a female of their own, first surreptitiously, then more openly. This process, quite widespread amongst non-human primates, serves two purposes. It reduces the competition faced by the resident male, but perhaps more importantly, it ensures that inbreeding is limited, and males mate with females who are unlikely to be related to them. Note the distinction between why something happens (genetic dilution) and how. There are brain mechanisms that allow adult males to detect when a young male becomes a potential rival (involuntary testosterone-dependent signals) and ensure that this is not tolerated.

What do we know of the way that testosterone links aggression and sex in the male's brain? Rather little, as it happens. This is because the scientists that study sexual behaviour in the lab are usually not so interested in studying aggression (and vice versa), and because the inbred rat, the species they mostly use, is rather docile. Put several of these male rats into a big new cage with a sexy female, and they will politely take turns to mate with her. But put a smallish male rat into the resident cage of a larger one (that is, his territory), and you are likely to end up with a badly bitten intruder, particularly if the resident male lives with a sexy female. So aggression depends on the context of other behaviours, a point we emphasise in the chapter that discusses the role of the brain in aggressive behaviour (Chapter 10).

Damage to the amygdala reduces aggression as well as sexual behaviour in male rats, even if they are given lots of testosterone. And the amygdala has plenty of testosterone receptors. As we discuss elsewhere in this book, the amygdala lies in a strategic position between the neocortex, which processes complex information from the visual, hearing and bodily sensation systems; and the limbic system, which adds emotional and motivational value to these sensory experiences. The cortex provides the sort of information that allows a male, for example, to recognise a female of the same species, or a male. But it is the amygdala that assigns that information its value. For example, that the current image is a sexy female, or a rival (aggressive) male. It also receives direct information from the smell (olfactory) system, which plays such a prominent part in sexual activity. This does rather suggest that the inbuilt tactic linking aggression and sex may reside in this part of the limbic system, though exactly how this comes about is unknown. Is it only in males? Does testosterone alter the level of certain neurochemicals in the male amygdala that encourage both a sexual response to attractive females, and an aggressive one to other males? If so, what are they? And where is the 'decision' to attack (a male) or approach (a female) taken (the frontal cortex is a distinct possibility, in primates at least)? So we can break down a complex series of behavioural events of great biological and social importance into different components, each of which may depend upon different parts of the brain, or upon different chemical codes in a particular part of the limbic system. You might now be thinking that more information on this would come in very useful for understanding (and even, perhaps, controlling) the problems associated with violent behaviour of young human males in our society.

But is success in defeating rival males actually reflected in reproductive success? In most cases in wild animals, the answer is 'yes' but not inevitably so. Some very dominant male monkeys actually sire fewer offspring than their immediate second-in-commands, perhaps because they are too busy maintaining their status, or the stress of being a chief is hampering reproduction. And lower ranking males can adopt a number of strategies, for example, surreptitious matings, to increase their reproductive ability despite their lesser social rank. Using guile and deception, a very neocortical brain activity, males can improve their 'fitness' by assuaging the imperative demands of their limbic system.

And now, what about the female? Female monkeys and apes can also regulate the breeding potential of their rivals. How they do it depends to some extent on their social structure. For example, whether they live in large, multi-male groups, or monogamous family ones. Females monkeys also form dominance hierarchies, though these are less obvious than for males. Top-of-the pile females tend to mate more, and have more babies, than subordinates. Females may compete for the males, and the more dominant ones (or those who form alliances with other dominant females) are likely to be more successful. But females employ more subtle means. A good example occurs in the tiny marmoset, a monkey that lives in family groups. No matter that a daughter has grown up, and seems fully adult — she is not fertile. Her mother (involuntarily) ensures this is so, and she will only be able to ovulate when she leaves the family group and sets up on her own. This is quite common in many mammals. How does this come about? One way, of course, is for lower ranking females to be denied access to scarce food, as we have seen, under-nutrition can reduce fertility. But more direct signals, smell signals perhaps, may play a part. Within the brain, as we have seen, peptides such as β-endorphin may play a role.

But an important factor, recognised by Darwin, is the way females choose their mates. The gaudy display by males of many species during the breeding season may warn off other males, but its principal function is to attract females. This, together with a male's social standing (many females prefer socially dominant males) is the driving force behind sexual selection. Does all this ring a bell or two? How many Western men wear shoulder pads to increase the 'maleness', or grow beards, or moustaches to emphasise 'male' hairiness? And how often do we see younger, attractive women draped over the arms of rather elderly but very rich or famous men?

This human behaviour shows rather beautifully the respective roles of the 'cognitive' and 'limbic' parts of the brain in sexual selection. The woman's limbic brain, honed by millions of years of successful evolution, is making sure she mates with the best male around. Best in the sense that he has genes that maximise his survival, and hence that of future children, and qualities that ensure he provides for those young. In the forests of yesteryear, this might have been the man with the broadest shoulders, the strongest arm, the most prowess at hunting. Fast forward several millennia. The strategy remains the same, but the tactics have altered. The qualities that served so well in the forest do little in the more recent world of high finance. Yet there are still men who offer better genes or better provision, only the attributes have altered. So she shifts her selection criteria. Her neocortex informs her about the subtleties of modern 'fitness' (it is the only part of the brain that can) but her limbic system plays the same old tune. She thinks she is making a deliberate choice, and, to some extent, she is but what she now finds attractive is dictated by current circumstances driven by ancient needs. If you are now outraged by this interpretation of the mechanisms behind womens' sexual selection, be reassured that similar (but not identical) processes are operating in human males. Now, I am not for a moment suggesting that the changed tactics of human females is necessarily a 'conscious' decision (though, of course, it can be). What I am saying is that there is an ancient link between the limbic system and those parts of the brain that evaluate the social environment. The limbic system, as part of its role in maximising reproductive fitness, somehow taps into the information about the qualities of potential mates represented in the higher cortical areas. This cortical information alters as social and technological evolution proceeds.

We have spent some time thinking about the sexual behaviour of monkeys and apes because of what this may tell us about the basic neurobiology of sexuality, particularly in large-brained animals like us. One of the things monkeys and apes do is to use sexually-derived behaviours for other purposes. At the local zoo is a large compound housing about 30 or so macaque monkeys. Let us watch them for a while. We notice that as a smallish male walks past a much larger, evidently dominant one, the latter mounts the younger male, quite briefly. Homosexuality in a monkey troop? Paedophilia, even? Not at all. The less dominant male reaffirms his lower rank by 'presenting' his behind to the more dominant, just as a female might do when she wanted to mate. But this is not sex. It is submission. Whilst such behaviour is not unknown in other species, its most noticeable in primates. Humans export sexually-derived activities to all corners of their lives. Look at your local advertising bill-board. You can think of a thousand other examples. This is the cortex, knowingly using an ancient part of the brain for its own purposes.

So far, we have discussed human sex as a consensual and socially-regulated activity between males and females. It is not always so. Across history, across cultures, across continents: wars mean rape. Now, of course, rape occurs without war, whatever your definition of rape might be. But it is striking that conquering armies nearly always rape the women of the conquered, despite all the social and military attempts to control the behaviour of soldiers. There are plenty of ancient examples, not necessarily associated with war. Zeus famously raped Leda. The army of Alexander raped the women of Babylon. The practice continues in our time. Russian soldiers raped the women of Berlin in 1945, rape was commonplace during the recent wars in Bosnia, Sierra Leone and Vietnam.

Why do soldiers rape? The curious fact is that even well-brought up young men, from societies in which rape is not tolerated and practically unthinkable (even though it may occur), and who would never contemplate rape in their home towns, can and do commit rape in times of war. Is there anything we can say about the role of the brain in rape?

The features of what we can call 'military' rape are: the soldiers have often been in considerable danger, and extreme fear; their adversaries may have been demonized, either because of supposed or actual atrocities committed earlier, or because of effective propaganda by their officers or political leaders; and there is often some distinct racial or religious difference between the two sets of combatants. What has broken down is the normal social control on unbridled sexual behaviour, but there may also be a 'positive' erotic effect of victory itself. Together with an unusually long period of sexual abstinence, since women are usually unavailable during a war, this somehow leads to the socially abnormal behaviour of rape. We should be quite clear about this: rape in war is not a throwback to some earlier, primeval, form of sexual behaviour (as some believe). Everything we know about human society, let alone that of non-human primates or even the rest of the mammals, shows clearly that sexual behaviour is never uncontrolled by social forces. In particular, it is never without some degree of selection (usually very considerable) by the females of the species. Yet military rape is random, uncontrolled and has absolutely no element of choice by the female. Of course, drunkenness may play a part in some, perhaps many, instances of military rape. But this does not explain why rape is so common as part of military victory, yet comparatively rare even in the most raucous societies.

Most of what we understand about the social control of sexual behaviour comes from the study of stable, established societies, ones in which the members have lived together for a long time. Whereas there may be various degrees of aggressive interaction, the overall structure of the social group is evident to all. In human terms, elaborate social controls, using complex signals and established learned patterns of behaviour, regulate sexuality. These controls represent, if you like, the moderating influence of the 'higher' brain, such as the frontal cortex, on the motivation for sex generated by the limbic system. Let us assume, for the moment, that the evolutionarily most advantageous strategy for the human male's limbic system is, indeed, as some have suggested, to impregnate as many females as possible. The whole complexity of social control is to limit that propensity within the rules of the man's social group, which may differ not only between groups, but within groups, (i.e. according to social class) and change with time. They are essentially learned controls, and an individual male learns to navigate through them to achieve the objective of successful sex. This includes rules governing their behaviour both with other males and with females, who exercise, as we have seen, considerable power over mate selection. In some cases, the society delegates this power to others: for example, the female's father or other family members.

Imagine a long and bloody battle, filled with death, the expectation of death, and increasing hate towards a defined, stereotyped, foe as friends and colleagues become casualties. During the battle, few soldiers (I am assuming this is a war between male armies) think of sex. Indeed, their brains are careful to switch them from sex to survival. As in many other situations of extreme demand to do what they can to avoid being killed. And were you to measure their levels of testosterone in the blood (and thus in the brain), they would be very low indeed. In contrast, levels of peptides in the brain such as β-endorphin and CRF would be very high, and both would further decrease the appetite for sex. The brain of a soldier in battle is in a non-sexual survival mode, though not necessarily in aggressive mode. The predominant emotion is fear.

Now imagine the battle won, the town taken. Victory itself will tend to cause a surge of testosterone in the victorious soldiers, just as it does in those winning a tennis match (they may also get a short-lived surge). But amplified in war, perhaps, because a battle is so much more significant than most games of tennis. Since the number of testosterone receptors in the brain will have increased during the period of low testosterone, the limbic brain is all that more sensitive to increased amounts. Within the limbic system, the emergency alerting peptides, CRF, β-endorphin and an array of others, will decrease restoring the sexual responsiveness of the brain to testosterone. So all is set for a resumption of sexuality, perhaps even enhanced sexuality. The gun is primed, but the trigger is pulled by the social context in which the soldiers now find themselves. For all the social controls are absent. In the brain, this is not a limbic event, but a cortical one. The town's population is 'alien,' that is, not part of their social structure, and not, therefore, bound by the rules. All the learned social inhibitions are absent; so the resultant sexuality is not 'primeval' it is 'abnormal' in the sense that it would be very unlikely in the soldiers' home social group. But it may be 'normal' for war, just as some species of male monkeys kill the young of groups they invade and take over, or unborn foetuses are resorbed under similar situations in other species. Men with damage to their frontal lobes may behave sexually in an unrestrained and socially inappropriate way. Soldiers entering a defeated, alienated, town, whose inhabitants have been assigned to inferior and non-group status, can no longer rely on their frontal lobes regulating their sexuality according to learned social rules. Of course, there may be other factors, such as a desire to humiliate the defeated population. Now, I understand that this interpretation may sound like an apologia for rape in war: it is not. My job, as a neuroscientist, is to try to understand behaviour which is common, context-dependent, and, just maybe, biologically sensible however repugnant. But we choose, as a species with our big brains, to modify what may be one biologically optimum strategy because there are others (social as well as biological) that take precedence. In fact, you could say that much of what our big brain does is limit and channel the indiscriminate behaviour that our limbic system might otherwise encourage. In the case of the defeated town, it does make biological sense for the victors to impregnate as many of the newly subjugated women as possible, whether or not their stay is a long one, or they are gone by next week. In Berlin, about 100,000 women were said to have been raped following capture of the city by the Russians in 1945. Many will have become pregnant, and these babies would carry the genes of the captors. Even in 1945, however, many women underwent abortions, thus neutralising the rampant limbic systems of their molesters by using their 'cognitive' or cortical brains, and those of their doctors. Increasing reproductive 'fitness' is part of victory, in the absence of human technology (cortically-driven), though, of course, some societies do not permit abortion, even after rape. However, the fact that the big cortical human brain understands the link between (forced) sex and reproduction, and moreover can alter the natural outcome (birth), determines, to a degree, how we handle rape at a 'clinical' level. No other species can do this, even those in which rape can be said to occur.

The reactions of German women to the experience of rape varied greatly. For many victims, especially protected young girls who had little idea of what was being done to them, the psychological effects could be devastating. Relationships with men became extremely difficult, often for the rest of their lives. . . . Other women, both young and adult, simply tried to blank out the experience. "I must repress a lot in order, to some extent, to be able to live," one woman acknowledged, when refusing to talk about the subject. Those who did not resist and managed to detach themselves from what was happening appear to have suffered much less. Some described it in terms of an 'out-of-body' experience. "That feeling." one wrote, "has kept the experience from dominating the rest of my life." . . . .

Men who returned home, having evaded capture or been released early from prison camps, seem to have frozen emotionally on hearing that their wife or fiancee had been raped in their absence. . . . They found the idea of the violation of their women very hard to accept. . . an anonymous diarist recounted to her former lover. . . the experiences which the inhabitants of the building had survived. "You've turned into shameless bitches," he burst out. "Every one of you. I can't bear to listen to these stories. . ." She then gave him her diary to read. . . when he found that she had written about being raped. . . . He left a couple of days later, saying he was off to search for food. She never saw him again. . . .

Rape has often been defined by writers on the subject as an act of violence which has little to do with sex. But this is a definition from the victim's perspective. To understand the crime, however, one needs to see things from the perpetrator's point of view. . . . The soldiers concerned appear to have felt that they were satisfying a sexual need after all their time at the front. In this, most soldier rapists did not demonstrate gratuitous violence, provided the woman did not resist. . . . The basic point is that, in war, undisciplined soldiers without fear of retribution can rapidly revert to a primitive male sexuality, perhaps even the sort which biologists ascribe to a compulsion on the part of the male of the species to spread his seed as widely as possible.

Antony Beevor. (2002) *Berlin. The downfall 1945.*
(Viking Books, London.)

This neural and endocrine view of rape is a biological one, not an ethical one. There is no reason why biology should take precedence over ethics or moral values in this situation as in any other. It is just that the biology (or, rather, the neurobiology) may be driving the tendency to rape after victory, and analysing this will lead us not to condone it, but to understand why it happens. Understanding a behavioural phenomenon like war rape is the surest way to being able to do something about it. I have chosen to discuss rape in war because, in some ways, it is the best example of uncontrolled sexual conduct within a context of little or no social control. That is not to say that all examples of rape are necessarily the result of similar factors to those operating in war. Rape, like all behaviour, can occur for several reasons and in different contexts.

The response to rape is also an interesting one. If a woman has been raped, then she may be carrying a baby with the genes of her assailant, rather than her 'legitimate' partner. Men in modern society, scientifically educated, will know this; primitive men, with no understanding of reproductive biology, may not. We know that even in our current, Western, society, so tolerant of sexual behaviour, most rape is unreported. Why? Because women find it shameful, and are fearful of the consequences of admitting that they have been raped. Fearful, that is, of damaging their ability to sustain a current relationship, or even be successful in a future one. Now, please understand that I do not mean to imply that rape has no adverse consequences for the woman herself. Quite the contrary: rape is a well-known harbinger of post-traumatic stress disorder, for one thing (Chapter 12). But the odd thing is how difficult it is for men. The partner of a raped women 'knows' that it is, by definition, an unwilling act, 'knows' that she might have had to yield to avoid serious injury or death, 'knows' that consequences, such as sexually-transmitted diseases or a pregnancy, can be dealt with in many cases, 'knows' that it is not her fault. Yet, it seems that men find acceptance of a raped partner difficult. Despite all this 'cognitive' information, something is tending to make her distasteful, at least for a time. There is an analogy. Recall the case of eating a piece of fish (Chapter 5), after which you became ill. You avoid the fish in future, even though you 'know' perfectly well it was not the fish, but something else that was responsible. No amount of logic, no amount of telling yourself not to be so stupid helps. You do not like that

This is not rape out of control. It is rape under control. It is also rape unto death, rape as massacre, rape to kill and to make the victims wish they were dead. It is rape as an instrument of forced exile, rape to make you leave your home and never want to go back. It is rape to be seen and heard and watched and told to others: rape as spectacle. It is rape to drive a wedge through a community, to shatter a society, to destroy a people. It is rape as genocide.

Quoted by Dahlia Gilboa. (2001) *Mass rape: War on women.*
Internet document.

In war, rape is an assault on both the individual woman and her family and community. Many hundreds of thousands of women have been raped in wars in this century alone, as reported in areas as diverse as Korea, Bangladesh, Liberia, Southeast Asia, and Uganda. Bosnian refugees have described how, in the former Yugoslavia, military forces publicly raped women to systematically force families to flee their villages, contributing to the goal of 'ethnic cleansing.' Assaults are often gang-related and sadistic, including other forms of physical torture. These women may also experience loss of home and community, dislocation, injury, and untreated illness, and these women may witness the murder, injury, or rape of loved ones. The effects of these types of trauma are immeasurable, long lasting, and shattering to both inner and outer worlds.

National Center for PTSD Fact Sheet.
U.S. Department of Veterans Affairs.

The rape was in his bloodstream and he would never get it out. The odor of it was in his blood stream, the look of it, the legs and the arms and the hair and the clothing. There were the sounds — the thud, her cries, the careening in a tiny enclosure. The horrible bark of a man coming. . . . All unsuspectingly, she had stepped out of her doorway and they had grabbed her from behind and thrown her down and there was her body for them to do with as they wished. . . . These men. They were speaking a foreign language. Laughing. Whatever they felt the urge to do, they did. One waited behind the other. She saw him waiting. There was nothing she could do. And nothing he could do. The man grows crazier and crazier to do something just when there is nothing left for him to do.

Philip Roth. (1997) *American pastoral.* (Vintage Books, New York.)

sort of fish any more. It is one example of a biologically-relevant behaviour. It is obviously useful to avoid eating things that make you ill, even if the process sometimes gets a bit scrambled.

A man whose sexual partner has been violated is in a similar position. The biologically sensible thing to do is to go off and find another, since he can no longer be sure that the genes in the future baby will be his. This is not a conscious, 'cognitive' decision. It is programmed into his limbic system. Just like avoiding a fish associated with illness, the male partner of a raped woman finds it very hard to override this unconscious, basic process, put into his brain to help his reproductive fitness, even though the more recent 'cognitive' part of the brain tells him that this is not so. Humanity versus biology. Some men may, of course, succeed: that does not alter the argument. Some people eventually eat the fish again but they are aware of a period when they illogically did not like it. Now, in the case of rape, there may be all sorts of other apparent reasons for men to discard their raped wives: disgrace, dishonour, the attitude of the family and so on. But I wonder whether this is not, to some degree, a surrogate for a more primal, biological, aversion, similar to the conditioned taste aversion so well known for food.

In no other sphere of human activity is the interplay, and conflict, between the ancient limbic structures and the newer cortical brain more apparent. Sex is a struggle, not only socially, but inside the brain itself.

Chapter 9

Bonding, Motherhood and Love

We are sitting comfortably in a little hide, like the ones bird watchers use. It is spring, and the early sun is warm. But outside the hide are not woods or even a tree, but a field. Rather an odd field, for it is rectangular, and divided up into six smaller squares by white lines, like those you might see on a grass tennis court. Pencils, paper, a tape recorder and an event recorder lie to hand. In one of the corner squares of the field is a pile of hay. In the opposite one, tethered to a pole, is a small lamb, making not very strenuous efforts to get free but bleating in that plaintive and persistent way so typical of lambs that have been separated for a short time from their mother. The other squares are empty. Outside the gate that leads to the field is a ewe, and we are here to see how she behaves when she enters the field. There are two things you should know about this ewe. She has never had a lamb of her own (and she is not pregnant), and she has a tiny tube passing from a valve in her neck into the fluid-filled spaces (the ventricles) of her brain. Ten minutes earlier, she has had a small volume of saline (a control procedure) injected into her brain ventricles.

She enters the field. Now, ewes are greedy creatures, and so she makes a beeline for the hay, and begins to eat. Every so often she wanders into some of the other (empty) squares. She even goes to see the lamb, but does not spend too long there, giving it a cursory sniff or two, but otherwise not paying it very much attention. It continues to bleat piteously. However, she does spend more time with the lamb than in any of the empty squares. Most of her time is spent in the square containing the food, which she continues to eat between exploring the rest of the field. After 30 minutes, the ewe is taken out, and another similar ewe is tested. This one, however, has had half a microgram (1 microgram = 1 millionth of a gram) of a peptide called oxytocin injected into her brain ventricles 10 minutes beforehand. After she enters the field, she gives the food a quick examination, taking a mouthful, but quickly goes over to the bleating lamb. She stays with the lamb for most of her 30 minutes, licking it, even trying to suckle it and looking just like all the mother-ewes you have ever seen in flocks of sheep. Just to make sure this experiment is reliable, we repeat it, this time giving the first ewe the oxytocin, and the second the saline. And we do it on several other ewes. The result is always the same: when they get oxytocin, they look like concerned mothers, but after saline they largely ignore the lamb and feed themselves.

Oxytocin has been known for years, but not as a brain peptide. Let us leave the ewe to nuzzle her lamb, and visit the nearby milking shed. Here we see them milking cows the old-fashioned way. Each squeeze of a teat is followed, a few seconds later, by a squirt of milk. Oxytocin does that. A squeeze (or a suckle) is sensed by the hypothalamus, which sends a pulse of oxytocin down to the pituitary and into the blood. This acts on the udder (or breast, in humans) which squirts out the milk. If you watch a gaggle of tiny rat pups suckling their mother, every few minutes you see them wriggle mightily. They have just received a shot of milk, the result of a pulse of oxytocin in their mother's blood. Some lactating women have been known to squirt milk across the room! Next door, there is a ewe giving birth. Her womb (uterus) contracts hard in waves to expel the newborn lamb. Oxytocin again. Women near term can be induced to give birth by being infused with oxytocin (more usually, with an artificial peptide closely resembling it). As the baby, or little lamb, snuggles up to its mother, more oxytocin ensures a good supply of milk. Oxytocin is clearly an essential part of the process of giving birth (rats lacking it cannot give birth properly) and of the delivery system for feeding the baby.

How extraordinary, then, that it took so long for its role in the brain to be discovered — a role that fits so well with its other actions. For good mothering needs not only a successful birth, and an efficient supply of milk, it also needs the mother to be 'maternal'. That is, to be motivated to care for her young (provide food, warmth, protection, a shelter) and to make sure the baby stays close, and to look for it if it strays. To do that,

Parental Care

When considering the many different forms by which parental care is expressed in mammals and the variety of control mechanisms involved, it becomes quite evident that no general model can be proposed to explain this complex behavior. . . .

. . . Maternal behavior may be stimulated by a variety of means that include simultaneous selective activation and inactivation of different subpopulations of neurons within the same structure. A better knowledge of the chemical identity of such neurons and of their interconnections is crucial to understanding the mechanisms of action of hormones and neurotransmitters for the stimulation of parental behavior. . . .

The overwhelming majority of studies on parental care have been concerned with the neurobiological mechanisms underlying its immediate activation. In contrast, the factors controlling the ongoing expression of maternal behavior, the maintenance of maternal responsiveness across lactation, and the processes leading to the dissolution of the maternal bond remain largely unexplored.

> G Gonzalez-Mariscal and P Poindron. (2002) Parental care in mammals: Immediate internal and sensory factors of control. In: *Hormones, brain and behavior.* Eds. D Pfaff *et al.*, pp. 215–298. (Academic Press, Amsterdam.)

The daily energy budget of a nursing mother exceeds that of most men with even a moderately active lifestyle and is topped among women only by marathon runners in training.

> Jared Diamond. (1997) *Why is sex fun?* (Weidenfeld and Nicolson, London.)

Many parents express a preference for sons, especially as first-born. Some actually try to achieve them. The recipes vary from the heroic to the hopeful. In ancient Greece, tying of the left testicle was said to do the job, while medieval husbands drank wine and lion's blood before copulating under a full moon. Less drastic — but equally ineffective — methods included mating only in a north wind or hanging one's underpants on the right side of the bed.

> Steve Jones. (1993) *The language of the genes.* (Harper Collins, London.)

A mother animal with young will behave aggressively toward a large number of intruders. It has been suggested that this strong tendency to aggression is characteristic of all vertebrate mothers. . . . A few days after giving birth, a the limbic system cleverly makes the baby a prized object, something the mother does not want to lose. It is called 'attachment' or 'bonding' or 'motherly love' and oxytocin, a little peptide of only eight amino-acids, may be one essential chemical signal responsible for it. Take a kitten from its mother, and watch the mother's frantic attempts to find it, and listen to her calling for it. The kitten does the same, so it has a survival machine in its brain as well. Take a rat pup from the nest, and place it a few feet away. After a minute or two, the mother leaves her litter, picks up the pup, and takes it back to the warmth and security of the nest. Oxytocin is yet another example of a chemical signal in the limbic system that is responsible for a number of concerted actions in the brain and in the body — birth, maternal behaviour and milk ejection. All these optimises the survival of that new bundle of genes, the baby. The brain makes the mother invest in her offspring.

But oxytocin is not the only chemical signal responsible for a female becoming maternal. The body makes sure the brain has multiple ways to become aware that there is a foetus growing in the womb, and that it needs post-partum care. The precise signals may vary according to species, and one important difference between them is how mature the young are at birth. Peer into a rat's nest after a recent birth, and you see a crowd of little pink, blind, almost foetal-like objects struggling to find a nipple. Each pregnancy may produce 8 or more pups, very immature (it's called 'altricial' birth); many will die. If they did not, the world would have been packed with rats long ago. The strategy of the rat (sometimes called the 'R' strategy) is to produce many pups, thus improving the chances that one or two will survive. She does this by having short pregnancies, giving birth to immature pups, and getting pregnant again rather soon. Now come with me to a nearby field, and watch a lamb being born. A few minutes after birth it is on its feet, and looking for a teat. It has got a woollen coat and is, essentially, a little ewe or ram. This is precocial birth; there is only one (sometimes two) young, and the duration of pregnancy is much longer than the rat's. A rat may have more young at one go than an ewe during the whole of the latter's life. Not only is pregnancy short in the rat, but the duration of maternal behaviour is short too, whereas the ewe stays looking after its (more mature) youngster for longer (not quite what you would expect). The ewe's approach to reproduction is sometimes called female mouse may be so aggressive that it will kill any males unable to escape from her ferocious and unrelenting attack.

> K E Moyer. (1974) Sex differences in aggression. In: *Sex differences in behavior*. Eds. R C Friedman, R M Richart, and R L Vande Wiele.
> (John Wiley, New York.)

It is now demonstrated that maternal care in infancy and early childhood is essential for mental health. This is a discovery of which the importance may be compared to that of the role of vitamins in physical health, and is of far-reaching significance for the prevention of mental ill-health.

> J Bowlby. (1953) *Child care and the growth of love*.
> (Pelican Books, London.)

What do studies of infant, maternal; and adult attachment have in common? . . . .First, approach the parent, infant or partner; second, learn the identity of this individual; and third, invest in this individual while rejecting all other individuals. . . . A working hypothesis is that not only the tasks but the neural mechanisms of attachment behaviour have been largely conserved. In a general sense, neuropeptides. . . seem especially suited as mediators of attachment. . . . Oxytocin has emerged as one candidate from studies in rats, sheep and monogamous voles. . . . Oxytocin is, at most, one element in a cascade. . . . In the very near future, we can hope that discoveries of the molecular and cellular mechanisms of addiction might be applied to the neurobiology of attachment, providing a new understanding of one of our most complex and intriguing emotions.

> T R Insel and L J Young. (2001) The neurobiology of attachment.
> *Nature Reviews Neuroscience*, pp. 129–136.

the 'K' strategy. It is typical of species that have to move around (that is, do not live in nests or shelters). Animals do not always divide up into these two strategies neatly (kangaroos have very immature babies indeed, but only one at a time usually), but the difference between them at the extremes is clear enough, and will require somewhat different brain mechanisms. Humans have a mixture of strategies. A long pregnancy, but a rather immature baby (it cannot walk etc. though it is not blind). And, of course, parenting in humans goes on for years — some would say a lifetime.

During pregnancy, the ovaries and the placenta produce huge amounts of steroid hormones, particularly oestrogen and progesterone. These play an essential role in the pregnancy itself; low oestrogen, for example, is incompatible with pregnancy in humans. But they also signal the brain that the female is pregnant. The pattern varies in different species, but in general, oestrogen rises to very high levels just before birth, and progesterone may drop just before it, or just after. Experiments show that, whilst mimicking these hormonal patterns does not always induce a virgin female (eg. a rat) to become maternal, they certainly make it more likely. Interestingly, oestrogen can increase the number of oxytocin receptors (the molecules that detect and respond to oxytocin) in the brain, one way that these two chemical signals interact in the limbic system.

Then there is prolactin (already mentioned in Chapter 6). Prolactin is a large peptide hormone released from the pituitary. As its name implies, it is essential for milk production (as opposed to milk ejection which is the role of oxytocin) and is very high in lactating women. But for years, people have wondered if it has other roles. In particular, whether it plays a part in maternal behaviour. The evidence is rather mixed, though the suspicion persists that it contributes in some way. For example, giving prolactin can persuade female rats to begin to build a nest. Male marmosets form persisting pair-bonds (more about that later) with a single female. When that female gives birth, the male takes an active role in parenting. There are reports that his prolactin levels go up, just like the female's, but not everyone agrees about this. Prolactin is sometimes raised abnormally in people by a pituitary tumour. This results in infertility and lowered sex drive, one of the natural (and adaptive) features of a lactating female. Prolactin does the same in males (including

Alfred and I are happy, as happy as married people can be. We are in love, we are intellectually and physically suited in every possible way, we rejoice in each other's company, we have no money troubles and three delightful children. And yet, when I consider my life, day by day, hour by hour, it seems to be composed of a series of pinpricks. Nannies, cooks, the endless drudgery of housekeeping, the nerve-wracking noise and boring repetitive conversation of small children (boring in the sense that is bores into one's brain), their absolute incapacity to amuse themselves, their sudden and terrifying illnesses, Alfred's not infrequent bouts of moodiness, his invariable complaints at meals about the pudding, the way he will always use my tooth-paste and will always squeeze the tube in the middle. These are the components of marriage, the wholemeal bread of life, rough, ordinary, but sustaining. . . .

Nancy Mitford. (1945) *The pursuit of love.*
(Hamish Hamilton, London.)

But fathers and their ways are enigmatic. I know without being told, for instance, that Mr Smeath lives a secret life of trains and escapes in his head. Cordelia's father is charming to us on the rare occasions when he is seen, he makes wry jokes, his smile is like a billboard, but why is she afraid of him? Because she is. All fathers except mine are invisible in daytime; daytime is ruled by mothers. But fathers come out at night. Darkness brings home the fathers, with their real, unspeakable power.

Margaret Atwood. (1990) *Cat's eye.* (Virago, London.)

He went on looking at his hands for a moment. Then he said slowly:
"I hope I've been a good father to you."
I laughed a little and said: "I'm so glad you're feeling better now."
"I'm proud of you. A good son. I hope I've been a good father to you. I suppose I haven't."
"I'm afraid we are extremely busy now, but we can talk again in the morning."
My father was still looking at his hands as though he was faintly irritated by them.
"I'm so glad you're feeling better now," I said again and took my leave.

K Ishiguro. (1989) *The remains of the day.*
(Faber and Faber, London.)

impotence), adaptive, perhaps, in species that form pair-bonds, but not in those that do not.

Time to pay another visit to the farm, and a field full of ewes with their lambs. Each ewe has her lamb beside her. If the lamb wanders, the ewe will pick it out of the flock, and shepherd it back. Experiments confirm what every farmer knows: a ewe not only recognises her lamb, but is bonded specifically to it. Other lambs are either ignored or even rebuffed. Although ewes (and women) may have a propensity to respond positively to all babies, they much prefer their own. If a mother is to ensure that it's her genes that survive, this is clearly a prerequisite. How does this come about?

It's a fascinating story. It turns out that it all depends on birth itself. As the lamb passes down the vaginal canal, it stimulates a nervous pathway. This does many things: it increases oxytocin release both in the blood (to enhance delivery) and in the brain (to enhance maternal behaviour). But it also alters the state of the mother's smell system. For a short while after birth, she is extremely sensitive to the smell of a lamb — her lamb, since that is the one that is around. Her lamb's smell becomes imprinted in her brain, a kind of memory, so that not only can she recognise her youngster, but she can respond in a special way to it. Lots of clever experiments, mostly on sheep or rodents, have shown this, and that it is dependent on activation of noradrenaline in the brain. This sensitises the female's brain to the smell of her newborn (recall the role of noradrenaline in improving the strength of a sensory signal, described in Chapter 4). High levels of oestrogen help this to occur. We begin to see how an interlocking series of chemical and neural messages are responsible for the amazing phenomenon of being a good mother ewe. Does it happen in humans?

There is an obvious prediction. Mothers who have their babies by Caesarian section should have problems in forming the maternal bond, since nothing passes down their vagina during birth. In fact, there is rather little evidence for this (though it is true for rats). Does this mean that humans are different? In a way, yes: but we must also remember that other animals have fail-safe means of making sure that important behaviours like mothering occur when they should; we should also remember that the long period of human parenting must mean that there

Mrs Arbuthnot: Men don't understand what mothers are. I am no different from other women except in the wrong done me and the wrong I did, and my very heavy punishments and great disgrace. And yet, to bear you, I had to look on death. To nurture you I had to wrestle with it. Death fought with me for you. All women have to fight with death to keep their children. Death, being childless, wants our children from us. Gerald, when you were naked, I clothed you, when you were hungry I gave you food. Night and day all that long winter I tended you. No office is too mean, no care too lowly, for the thing we women love. . . . . And you needed love, for you were weakly and only love could have kept you alive. Only love can keep anyone alive.

Oscar Wilde. *A woman of no importance. Oxford Drama Library.* (Clarendon Press, Oxford.)

Parental feeling, as I have experienced it, is very complex. There is, first and foremost, sheer animal affection, and delight in watching what is charming in the ways of the young. Next, there is the sense of inescapable responsibility, providing a purpose for daily activities which scepticism does not easily question. Then there is an egoistic element, which is very dangerous: the hope that one's children may succeed where one has failed, that they may carry on one's work when death or senility puts an end to one's own efforts, and, in my case, that they will supply a biological escape from death, making one's life part of the whole stream, and not a mere stagnant puddle without any overflow into the future. All this I experienced, and for some years it filled my life with happiness and peace.

Bertrand Russell. (1968) *The autobiography of Bertrand Russell.* Vol II. (George Allen and Unwin, London.)

. . . For a brief moment she remembered that awful afternoon in Mochudi, when the nurse had come up to her, straitening her uniform, and she saw that the nurse was crying. To lose a child, like that, was something that could end one's world. One could never get back to how it was before. The stars went out. The moon disappeared. The birds became silent. . . .

are other mechanisms for making the bond persist (smell etc. like other memories, has a finite lifespan). However, mothers who suckle their babies (more oxytocin) interact with them more than those who bottle-feed (less oxytocin).

We know curiously little about what happens in the brain of any species to make a female behave maternally. We do know that there has to be some way of ensuring that sensory information from the pups (their smell, the sounds they make, their movements) are decoded and register with that part of the brain that is 'maternal'. Where is this part? Many scientists in the field now think of a 'maternal circuit'. This is a collection of interconnected parts of the brain that, together, represent what we describe as maternal behaviour. Not surprisingly, the hypothalamus figures large in this circuit. Damage to the front of the hypothalamus disturbs maternal behaviour. Interestingly, it is the same area that, in males, plays an important part in sexual behaviour (Chapter 8). But infusing oxytocin into this area of the hypothalamus has not reliably induced maternal behaviour, which leaves the question of exactly how oxytocin acts unanswered. The amygdala is an obvious part of the limbic system that might be involved in maternal behaviour. After all, this is the part of the brain that adds 'value' or 'emotional meaning' to sensation. The evidence is not strong. It may be that several parts of the limbic system (including both hypothalamus and amygdala) need extra oxytocin. Receptors for oxytocin in the limbic system are increased by the hormones of pregnancy. We need to know more about this. Not only is parental behaviour an essential element of reproduction, and thus survival of the species, but it can go wrong. Even in humans, there are those mothers who remain indifferent to their babies; what is different about their brains? Why do not they bond?

It was the psychologist John Bowlby who emphasised the significance of early attachment (bonding) in humans. The quality of this experience so early in life, he thought, laid the foundation for all meaningful adult relationships. This carries two suppositions: that a child (or young animal) passes through a special 'sensitive' period, during which events can have long-lasting results, in a way that later events do not; and that there is something similar about maternal-infant bonding and other sorts of affiliation. Subsequent work has supported him.

. . . And she thought of the moment when. . . she had laid the tiny body of their premature baby, so fragile, so light, into the earth and had looked up at the sky and wanted to say something to God, but couldn't because her throat was blocked with sobs and no words, nothing, would come.

Alexander McCall Smith. (2003) The no. 1 ladies
detective agency. (Abacus, London.)

When the sun slipped below the horizon, it was not only the day that died. . . but my family as well. With that second sunset, disbelief gave way to pain and grief. They were dead; I could no longer deny it. What a thing to acknowledge in your heart! To lose a brother is to lose someone with whom you can share the experience of growing old, who is supposed to bring you a sister-in-law and nieces and nephews, creatures to people the tree of your life and give it new branches. To lose your father is to lose the one whose guidance and help you seek, who supports you like a tree trunk supports its branches. To lose your mother, well, that is like losing the sun above you.

Yann Martel. (2002) Life of Pi.
(Canongate Books Ltd., Edinburgh.)

"But" said Sam, and tears started in his eyes, "I thought you were going to enjoy the Shire, too, for years and years, after all you have done."
"So I thought too, once [Frodo says]. But I have been too deeply hurt, Sam. I tried to save the Shire, and it has been saved, but not for me It must often be so, Sam when things are in danger; some one has to give them up, lose them, so that others may keep them. . . ."

J R R Tolkien. (1954) The lord of the rings.
(George Unwin and Allen, London.)

A human mother is attached to her little child; she also bonds with her mate (partner) and both feel strong affiliations to their parents. In each case, there is a strong attachment to a particular person (which may exclude others). Three words: bonding, attachment, affiliation, with essentially the same meaning. There is a fourth, which you will not find mentioned much in the neuroscientific literature, because neuroscientists find it troubling. It is called love, and poets have no problems with it.

I am not so concerned here with the psychological aspects of love, on which there is a literature, as with the biological functions of love and its neural basis. Love or attachment, whatever you call it, implies that a particular person becomes special, in that social interaction (and usually proximity) is rewarding, that loss (temporary or permanent) is both feared, avoided and, if it happens, is treated as a serious adversity, and great efforts are made to rectify this loss or deficit. You may recognise this description as one that could apply to more mundane requirements, like food, water, adequate heat and so on. Just as there are two levels of understanding for, say, hunger (what is its function? how does it happen?) so there are for love. The biological function of love (its role in survival) lies in the fact that attachment implies an individually-distinct interaction. One person invests time, resources and attention in another because the outcome will be biologically beneficial: increased success at reproduction is the most prominent. Of course, there will be costs. A mother protecting an infant may herself be in danger; one individual providing food for his/her partner may risk having less to eat him/herself, and so on. But only if there is investment in particular others can survival be maximised. So it is important to choose your investment wisely, which is why so much scientific effort is put into trying to understand how sexual pairings come about, or how different strategies of parental behaviour succeed. The same general ideas apply to 'friends', those whom with one is more likely to act altruistically. A concept developed from game theory, called the evolutionary stable strategy, describes the various ways in which one individual can act in a seemingly selfless, or selfish, way, and what this may mean for subsequent benefit and survival. Relatedness is an important consideration: the closer a relation, the more likely you are to share genes with him/her. So being seemingly altruistic is actually an advantage, since you are giving your genes a helping hand. But social

Love

Sitting awkwardly (in sociological accounts of marriage) is the concept of love. Whilst those in the artistic world have grappled persistently and often effectively with this topic, scientists have been somewhat half-hearted, perhaps revealing an ambivalence. Falling in love therefore remains an enigma, possibly the last defended stronghold against the analytic prying of scientific man.

> J Bancroft. (1989) *Human sexuality and its problems.*
> (Churchill Livingstone, Edinburgh.)

. . . The distinction between 'liking' and 'loving' has been mentioned. Liking appeared to involve primarily perceived attributes of the other participants, while the criteria of loving involved the relationship itself. (Love) appears to be a poorly articulated emotion, and adolescents have only vague notions as to how it should be identified. Whether or not they label their feelings as 'love' — and furthermore, one may add, whether they act out the role of romantic lovers — will depend on the cultural climate. The more the culture idealizes the lover, the more will they be rewarded for labelling their feelings as love and for acting as lovers are supposed to act.

> R A Hinde. (1979) *Towards understanding relationships.*
> (Academic Press, London.)

The cure of psychic disturbances requires in the first place the establishment of the natural capacity for love. It depends as much upon social as upon psychic conditions. . . . The fact that man is the only species which does not fulfil the natural laws of sexuality is the immediate cause of a series of devastating disasters. . . (which) results in mass death, in the form of wars, as well as in psychic and somatic disturbances of vital functioning.

> Wilhelm Reich. (1942) *The function of the orgasm.*
> (Farrar, Strauss and Giroux Inc., New York.)

. . . Even in societies that recognize monogamy by law or custom there is much extramarital and premarital sex, and much sex that is not part of a long-term relationship. Humans do engage in one-night stands. On the other hand, most humans also engage in many-year or many-decade stands, whereas tigers and orangutans engage in nothing but one-night stands.

> Jared Diamond. (1997) *Why is sex fun?*
> (Weidenfeld and Nicolson, London.)

relations are also significant. Like lending your friend a hundred pounds today, so that in the future you have a resource which is likely to help you should you need it. Reproduction in all its forms is heavily dependent upon bonding (love in humans), since breeding is a highly uneven activity, but one that is essential to genetic survival. It is the 'ultimate' function, that is, the cause of attachment.

We should also recall that different species have markedly different solutions to the problem of successful reproduction. Why this happens is an intriguing question. Is it because there is no one optimal solution? Or that no species has the optimal solution, and all are making compromises? Or, more likely in my view, is it because reproduction has to fit other aspects of a species' life style, its habitat, its size, whether it is a predator or a prey, what it eats, and so on. In other words, adaptation is a 'joined-up' activity, and adaptive mechanisms in one domain have to take account of the properties of the others. The varied pattern of reproductive strategies means that bonding patterns, an essential feature of them all, will also differ equally markedly between species.

Nevertheless, a different question to that of the function of bonding is how it comes about. What actually happens in the brain? What is the 'proximate' cause of bonding (attachment, affiliation, affection)? Let us summarise what we are looking for. Bonding implies that a particular individual has a special value for another. So we have to consider how sensory information (sight, smell, sound) signals the particular attributes of this individual. Then we have to know how this is translated into a 'value' such that interaction is rewarding, and separation is aversive. Finally, we have to see whether all bonding (maternal, sexual, social) has essentially the same mechanism, though it occurs in different contexts.

Many of the brain mechanisms that might be involved have already been discussed in this book in other contexts. We have seen how sensory information goes both to the cortex (for analysis) and to the limbic system (particularly the amygdala) for emotional evaluation. We have seen how this information can, somehow, be transmitted to the 'reward' system, which, it is currently thought, is a single system but capable of being linked to a variety of sensory (or, indeed, motor) experiences. What we know of the parts of the brain involved in bonding suggests that, indeed, they contribute to this more general mechanism. For example, the dopamine

Monozygotic twins share most of their properties. Apart from physical resemblance, they think alike, feel alike, and act alike. . . . Whatever attracts you to one twin — the way he walks, the way he talks, the way he looks, and so on — should attract you to the other. And this should cast identical twins in tales of jealousy and betrayal of truly gothic proportions. In fact, nothing happens. The spouse of one identical twin feels no romantic attraction toward the other twin. Love locks our feelings in to another person *as that person,* not as a *kind* of person, no matter how narrow the kind.

> S Pinker. (1997) *How the mind works.* (Allen Lane, London.)

(Nature says) "You are my child. Do not expect me to love you. How can I love — I who am blind necessity? I cannot love, neither can I hate. But now I have brought forth you and your kind, remember you are a new world unto yourselves, a world which contains in virtue of you, love and hate, and reason and madness, the moral and immoral, and good and evil. It is for you to love where love can be felt. That is, to love one another".

> C S Sherrrington. (1941) *Man on his nature.*
> (Penguin Books, London.)

Love brings us a good measure of pain. Artists struggling to decide whether this commingling of pleasure and discomfort is absolutely inescapable or merely commonplace might be surprised to learn that some scientists ask the same question. To what extent must an animal preparing to mate also prepare for the possibility of pain? For many species, such pain is not just psychological, but can be quite physical as well. Pain and sex are big, important topics and their confluence during mating is clearly more important than a happenstance or the perverse confabulation of artists. . . discussion of [these] issues should help any future scientists who might tackle why love hurts so good.

> S M Breedlove. (2003) Love and pain meet in the brain.
> Book review of 'Central states relating sex and pain'.
> *Nature Neuroscience*, p. 785.

system is currently thought to play a central role in reward (Chapter 5); disruption of this system interferes with bonding. The opioids, peptides such as β-endorphin, are also known to be associated with reward, or 'pleasure' and blocking their action experimentally reduces maternal attachment to an infant. Interestingly, doing the same to the infant increases its attachment behaviour, perhaps because it needs to repair the deficit by behavioural means. Some researchers think that opioid peptides are the chemical 'glue' that is responsible for all forms of social adhesion. Oxytocin, as we have seen, plays a part in maternal bonding. It may also do so in other contexts, including monogamy. The point has already been made that behavioural strategies for successful reproduction differ. One prominent difference is between species that characteristically form monogamous, long-lasting, mating pairs, and those that show a more promiscuous pattern. Oxytocin receptors have been found to be more prominent in the brains of the former (e.g. prairie voles) than in related species that are more promiscuous (montane voles).

But it is unlikely that all human affiliative behaviour can be described solely in this way, though mechanisms may exist in the human limbic system as in those of other animals. The great human cortex will have its say. This may be one reason why human attachment can last so long. It is not only dependent on the hormonal and chemical systems that feature so large in rats and sheep, but it has, in part, become emancipated from them. So there is a progression from 'hormonal' to 'cortical' bonding, and this applies to maternal behaviour, partner bonding and the affection you feel for your parents, relatives and friends. But remember, the basic evolutionary objective remains the same which is to maximise the spread of your genes in your society. All you need is love.

Bonding is part of what all social animals, including our species, does as part of its interaction with the rest of society. We have a particularly complex system of assessing those to whom we should behave in a particular way; either because we would lose something if we did not, or because we feel 'affection' for them or 'obligation' towards them. We are bound by social rules that we learn as we grow up. These processes require some of the most complicated activities of the human brain, way beyond the capacity of the limbic system. In particular, they rely upon a region of the cortex called the prefrontal lobe.

Love etc. The proposition is simple. The world divides into two categories: those who believe that the purpose, the function, the bass pedal and principal melody of life is love, and that everything else — everything else — is merely an etc.; and those, those unhappy many, who believe primarily in the etc of life, for whom love, however agreeable, is but a passing flurry of youth, the pattering prelude to nappy-duty, but not something as solid, steadfast and reliable as, say, home decoration. This is the only division between people that counts.

Julian Barnes. (1991) *Talking it over.*
(Jonathan Cape, London.)

Love is not blind; that is the last thing it is. Love is bound; and the more bound the less it is blind. A man's friend likes him but leaves him as he is: his wife loves him and is always trying to turn him into somebody else.

G K Chesterton. (1958) The flag of the world. In: *Essays and poems.*
Ed. W Sheed. (Penguin Books, Harmondsworth, UK.)

Why. . . it happens every day. It's the old story. Boys and girls fall in love, that is, they are driven mad and go blind and deaf and see each other not as human animals with comic noses and bandy legs and voices like frogs, but as angels so full of shining goodness that like hollow turnips with candles put into them, they seem miracles of beauty.

Joyce Cary. (1944) *The horse's mouth.*
(Michael Joseph, London.)

There is a love that equals in its power the love of man for woman and reaches inwards as deeply. It is the love of a man or a woman for their world. For the world of their centre where their lives burn genuinely and with a free flame.
The love of a diver for his world of wavering light. His world of pearls and tendrils and his breath at his breast. Born as a plunger into the deeps he is at one with every swarm of lime-green fish. . . . Pulse, power and universe sway in his body. He is in love.
The love of a painter standing alone and staring, staring at the great coloured surface he is making. . . . The white light in a northern sky is

The prefrontal cortex is so-called because it forms the very front of the brain, and is part of the frontal lobes. It lies immediately behind your forehead. The high forehead typical of humans reflects the considerable size of this part of the brain. Interestingly, folklore associates cleverness with high, domed foreheads and low cunning and criminality with a shallow brow. Comparison of human brains with apes such as the chimpanzee, and even more markedly with monkeys, shows that human brains really do have a bigger prefrontal cortex, even allowing for absolute differences in brain size. It is involved in a range of extremely complex functions, though these are part of everyday life. They have a direct and powerful role in adaptation — to help you plot the route through life that is most beneficial for you, and enabling you to make decisions that are in your own best interest. Particularly those that involve other people.

Every medical student learns about Phineas Gage. His name sounds like the hero of a Victorian novel, but he was real enough. He was in charge of a railway construction gang in the US in 1848, and one of his jobs was to lay the explosive charges that were used to clear the ground for new lines. He did this by drilling a hole, inserting the charge and then 'tamping' it: that is, pushing the charge to the bottom of the hole using a 'tamping iron', a long steel bar. On this particular day, the bar must have struck a spark from the rock, because the charge exploded as he tamped, turning the tamping iron into a projectile. The bar passed through the front of his head, and landed some distance away. Over the next few months, after he had (rather miraculously) recovered from the immediate effects of this appalling injury, Phineas Gage began to behave very strangely. Whereas previously he had been a reliable, dependable, sociable man, a natural leader, he became extravagant, foul-mouthed, unreliable, deceitful and anti-social. He lost his job, and wandered round the country exhibiting himself and the tamping iron, abandoned by family and friends. In short, his personality had changed dramatically, and he was unable either to plan his future, see that his behaviour was detrimental to it, or to understand that others found his behaviour objectionable. However, all his other abilities, including both sensation and movement, were unaffected. He could still recognise things and people, and retained all his old manual skills.

silent. The window gapes as he inhales his world. His world: a rented room, and turpentine. He moves towards his half-born. He is in love.
Mervyn Peake. (1946) *Titus Groan.* Eyre and Spottiswoode, London.

The baby, Nicholas, was born in April. Alix fell helplessly, hopelessly, recklessly in love with the baby. He was all the world to her. She no longer knew if she was happy or unhappy, cheerful or depressed, as she gazed at the infant lying in his pram, asleep in his cot, kicking on a rug before the fire. She was obsessed, in love. Sebastian [her husband] spent more time out of the house. Alix did not care.
Margaret Drabble. (1987) *The radiant way.*
(Weidenfeld and Nicolson, London.)

And he knew finally the meaning of all the small footprints on all the deserted beaches he had ever walked, of all the secret cargoes carried by ships that had never sailed, of all the curtained faces that had watched him pass down winding street of twilight cities. And, like a great hunter of old who has traveled distant miles and now sees the light of his home campfires, his loneliness dissolved. At last. At last. He had come so far. . . so far. And he lay upon her, perfectly formed and unalterably complete in his love for her. At last.
Robert J Waller. (1992) *The bridges of Madison county.*
(Warner Books Inc., New York.)

It was so simple, as she watched him, as his regular breathing calmed her, that she did not even see it happening at first. She began to think of the rooms in our house and the hours that she had worked so hard to forget spent inside of them. Like fruit put up in jars and forgotten about, the sweetness seemed even more distilled as she returned. There on that shelf were all the dates and silliness of their early love, the braid that began to form of their dreams, the solid root of a burgeoning family. . . .
Alice Sebold. (2002) *The lovely bones.* (Picador, London.)

Mme Gherardi maintained that love, like most other blessings of civilisation, was a chimera which we desire the more, the further removed we are from Nature. Insofar as we seek Nature solely in another body, we

You will have guessed by now that Phineas Gage had damaged his prefrontal cortex. In fact, his brain was never examined, but a recent computer-aided reconstruction (using his skull) shows what must have happened, and confirms the drawing his doctor made at the time. The tamping iron destroyed much of his prefrontal cortex, particularly on the left side. The important point is that there is part of the brain which is concerned not with sensation or movement, but with how we use complex, processed sensory information to survive: a part of the brain that is our social command centre. Without it, our fate would resemble that of Phineas Gage.

Since the prefrontal cortex is so much bigger in primates than others, it is not surprising that most of what we know about it comes from either experimental studies on non-human primates (monkeys and apes) or on humans. Until recently, studying humans was limited to assessing the effects of prefrontal damage, usually (but not always) the result of accidents or war. Damage to the human brain is a haphazard business, different people will have different amounts destroyed, and some will have multiple injuries of other parts of the brain as well. It has often been quite difficult to know exactly what had been damaged, though the recent development of imaging techniques has made this easier. Experimental methods have greater precision, but the tests that can be used to assess the effects are necessarily different from those we can use on humans. Most of these studies have been done by experimental psychologists, who are often not very interested in real-life social behaviour, but more concerned with the kind of learning, motivation and emotion one can study in the rather formal conditions of the laboratory.

Damage to the prefrontal cortex results in severe deficits in what is called 'executive function'. This is a term for the process by which you assess, evaluate and decide things. It is how you formulate your behavioural strategy. Such a strategy may be concerned with what is best to do in the next few minutes, or how to react to the current situation, but it also involves much longer-term planning: how you work out the best way to achieve an objective, be that a physical one (to get a meal, for example, or, more generally, to ensure a regular supply of food) or a social one (for e.g.: reacting to someone else's behaviour towards you or, more generally, set up and maintain a relationship, or prepare yourself for a particular *become cut off from Her; for love, she declared, is a passion that pays its debts in a coin of its own minting, and thus a purely notional transaction which one no more needs for one's fulfilment than one needs the instrument for trimming goose-quills that he, Beyle, had bought in Modena. Or do you imagine (thus according to Beyle, she continued) that Petrarch was unhappy merely because he never knew the taste of coffee?*

W G Sebald. (1999) *Vertigo.* (The Harvill Press, London.)

kind of job). Attention, planning, ambition, insight, empathy, social awareness are all terms that include much of what the prefrontal lobes do. If you have to take a decision about what to do, this requires that you have enough information about the events going on in your environment. So it is not surprising that what psychologists call 'working memory' is also impaired by frontal lobe damage. Working memory is a sort of neural video clip of what is currently going on around you. Imagine a machine that records everything that is happening, without any selectivity. Like such an information processor, the brain has limited storage capacity. There is a great deal of information at any one time in your environment, so the brain can only hold it for a short time. Psychologists argue about how long 'working memory' lasts, but its probably only a few minutes at best. It may be what you think of as 'now.' After that, it is short-term memory, and this is much more selective. By then, you may have made your decision.

fMRI is a relatively recent technique that measures changes in blood flow in local areas of the brain. Blood flow depends on function: essentially, the harder the area of brain is working, the greater its blood flow. So fMRI is an indirect index of neural activity. The prefrontal lobes are activated by tests that require planning or strategic decisions, as you would expect. Gambling is a good example. Do you go for a bet with high odds (bigger winnings) but with less chance of success, or one that promises a more reliable, but lesser, payoff? Telling lies also activates this part of the brain, suggesting that the 'social' part of the brain has a special mechanism for dealing with deception. The prefrontal lobes may also be concerned with other sorts of memory processes such as actively retrieving a visual memory. They may change as we get older. Children have less social control over their behaviour than adults; they also show less prefrontal activation in situations when they are asked to inhibit a response. This may represent the brain growing up.

Damaging the prefrontal cortex also results in changes in emotionality. fMRI studies show that it is activated by rewards or punishment. Not far from the frontal area that responds to rewards (e.g. being given money) is one also activated by jokes, which is perhaps why we like hearing them. Near the prefrontal cortex, and sometimes included

There's nothing you can do that can't be done.
Nothing you can sing that can't be sung.
Nothing you can say but you can learn how to play the game.
It's easy.

Nothing you can make that can't be made.
No one you can save that can't be saved.
Nothing you can do but you can learn how to be you in time.
It's easy.
All you need is love.

Beatles. *All you need is love.*

He felt the hot tears wet his neck and the hollows of his neck, and he remained motionless, suspended through one of man's eternities. Only now it had become indispensable to him to have her face pressed close to him; he could never let her go again. He could never let her head go away from the close clutch of his arm. He wanted to remain like that for ever, with his heart hurting him in a pain that was also life to him.

D H Lawrence. (1972) *The horse dealer's daughter.* In:
The second Penguin book of English short stories
Ed. C Dolley. (Penguin Books, Harmondsworth, UK.)

Emma continued to entertain no doubt of her being in love. Her ideas only varied as to the how much. At first, she thought it was a good deal; and afterwards, but little. She had great pleasure in hearing Frank Churchill talked of; and, for his sake, greater pleasure than ever in seeing Mr. and Mrs. Weston; she was very often thinking of him, and quite impatient for a letter, that she might know how he was, how were his spirits, how was his aunt, and what was the chance of his coming to Randalls again this spring. But, on the other hand, she could not admit herself to be unhappy, nor, after the first morning, to be less disposed for employment than usual; she was still busy and cheerful; and, pleasing as he was, she could yet imagine him to have faults; and farther, though thinking of him so much, and, as she sat drawing or working, forming a thousand amusing schemes for the progress and close of their attachment, within it, is an area called the anterior cingulate. It is part of the inside of the prefrontal cortex. Showing people photos of their loved partners (but not their friends) activates the cingulate cortex. The anterior cingulate of cocaine addicts react when they watch a video tape of cocaine use; this does not happen in controls who are not addicted. Those with damaged prefrontal lobes react much less angrily to things which might otherwise annoy them. Electrically stimulating this part of the brain results in the opposite effect: blood pressure rises, the pupils dilate, and the gut stops contracting. These are all signs that the body has gone on alert. The so-called tranquillising result of damaging the frontal lobe gave rise to one of the most striking, and perturbing, episodes in recent medicine.

In 1935, two American physiologists were describing the results of an experiment to a scientific meeting in London. They had trained two chimpanzees to watch whilst they put food under one of two cups. Then an opaque screen was lowered for a few seconds. When it was raised, the watching chimpanzee could reach for the cup that had been baited. One of the chimpanzees became highly agitated whenever she got it wrong, throwing what amounted to a temper tantrum, and eventually refusing to do the test any more. Then the prefrontal lobes on both sides were removed. The chimpanzee continued to do the test, but now she was calm and did not react angrily when she made a mistake. A remarkable transformation in her emotionality, and one that fascinated one member of the audience, a neurosurgeon called Egas Moniz.

It occurred to Moniz that the prefrontal lobes might be involved in abnormal states, such a persistent anxiety or other mental illnesses. After he had returned home to Portugal, Moniz had the idea of isolating the prefrontal lobes in such patients. He did this by cutting the connections between the frontal lobes and the rest of the cortex. In the ensuing years, this operation was perfected, so that it could be done by inserting a special knife up the nose and into the front of the brain. No one knows how many prefrontal lobotomies, more properly called leucotomies (cutting the white matter), were carried out in the enthusiasm which swept the neuropsychiatric world over the next 20 years or so. 40,000–50,000 in the US alone is a common estimate. They *fancying interesting dialogues, and inventing elegant letters; the conclusion of every imaginary declaration on his side was that she refused him. Their affection was always to subside into friendship. Every thing tender and charming was to mark their parting; but still they were to part. When she became sensible of this, it struck her that she could not be very much in love; for in spite of her previous and fixed determination never to quit her father, never to marry, a strong attachment certainly must produce more of a struggle than she could foresee in her own feelings.*

Jane Austen. *Emma.*

Of course, the fervid passion of the first few weeks cannot last eternally; but to that love there sometimes succeeds another and a better love. When that has come about, husband and wife are twin souls who have everything in common. Not a secret is there between them, and if children should result of the union, even the most difficult moments of life will have a sweetness of their own.

Fyodor Dostoevsky. (1931) *Letters from the underground.*
Translated by C J Hogarth. (J M Dent, London.)

Some people hold the opinion that a schoolgirl, simply on account of her age, should not consider herself properly in love. Rather she has a 'crush' or some other such derogatory expression. But surely the love of the fifteen-year-old girl is as pure and definite as love can be: she becomes as vulnerable as a beetle on its back — what reasonable woman in her twenties or thirties could give as much as that? Where is the older woman who hasn't learnt to put herself first? Who doesn't offer morsels of herself to her lover, one at a time, cautiously, ready for their rejection? The fifteen-year-old has not yet learnt the skill of self-division: she gives everything. This is surely the love of the poets.

Olivia Fane. (1994) *Landing on clouds.* (Mandarin, London.)

In that spring, my life was in his hands. Love fastened to our hearts and never going thence, each day I pushed back the limits of my soul to hold more l love of him, renouncing possession to receive love afresh, a new and everlasting wonder.

I found him in everything I touched and saw and knew, till all was reflection and shadow, rooted in knowledge and love of Mark. And so I were carried out for a variety of psychiatric complaints, some quite minor, in the belief that the procedure relieved many conditions that were difficult or impossible to treat by other methods at the time. Reading the scientific rationale for prefrontal leucotomy written during these years, so eloquently described by Elliot Valenstein, one is struck by one consistent fact: they are utter fantasy. Reverberating circuits, persistent cortical electrical patterns, circulating memories, fixed arrangement of cellular connections, crowding of the brain...they are all there, and characterised by a common feature — an absolute lack of any experimental or clinical evidence for any of them.

What Moniz had evidently not noticed was that the American chimpanzee had become rather bad at the memory task after removal of the prefrontal cortex. The astonishing fact is that it took so long for the side-effects of leucotomy to become an overwhelming reason why the operation, apart from a few very rare cases, is no longer done. All or some of the features observed in Phineas Gage became only too apparent after the operation, an irreversible one, had been carried out. Partly this was because those carrying out the procedure seldom made a serious attempt to assess its consequences. Another reason was that many patients were seriously and apparently incurably mentally ill, and prefrontal leucotomy offered the only chance of some sort of improvement. Indeed, in some cases there was benefit. Dangerously aggressive patients became calmer, those imprisoned by their obsessions were sometimes relieved, people incarcerated in mental hospitals for decades might rejoin the community. But they were not the same people. They were socially inept, and those close to them no longer received the same affection and regard.

The prefrontal lobes play a very special role in survival and adaptation. But not in the sense that damage to other parts of the brain — say the amygdala or hypothalamus — imperil survival. Prefrontal leucotomy, or even lobectomy (removal of the lobes) does not prevent an animal (or person) from eating when hungry, being thirsty and drinking, sleeping or even having sex. So why is the prefrontal cortex so essential for survival? The answer lies in the nature of the disturbance that follows prefrontal damage. To survive in the complex world of human society requires equally complex assessment of individual roles in that society. 'Frontal' *clutched with fervour the shining momentary now, made it Eternity, and thought myself both honest and clever, squaring accounts with Heaven.*

Han Suyin. (1952) *A many-splendoured thing.*
(Johnathan Cape, London.)

Eileen, who used to be pretty and still could be of she didn't look so moithered all the time, lying neatly, back turned, eyes closed, dead set against new fangled colours in her kitchen. Eileen Glover, nee Barlow, virgin bride of Ronald Glover, at St Andrews the Less, 1 December 1946, four weeks after he got demobbed. . . . Eileen, who loves Ronnie in the quiet, dutiful way Barlow women love their men. . . . Eileen, who is happy, but doesn't hold with silly talk.

Laurie Graham. (1996) *The ten o'clock horses.*
(Bantam Press, London.)

I watched him reach up and take a strand of my mother's hair and loop it around her ear. "I fell in love with you again while you were away," he said.
I realized how much I wished I could be where my mother was. His love for my mother wasn't about looking back and loving something that would never change. It was about loving my mother for everything — for her brokenness and her fleeing, for her being right there then in that moment before the sun rose and the hospital staff came in. It was about touching that hair with the side of his fingertip, and knowing yet plumbing fearlessly the depths of her ocean eyes.

Alice Sebold. (2002) *The lovely bones.*
(Picador, London.)

Abou Ben Adhem (may his tribe increase!)
Awoke one night from a deep dream of peace,
And saw, within the moonlight in his room,
Making it rich, and like a lily in bloom,
An angel writing in a book of gold:-
Exceeding peace had made Ben Adhem bold,
And to the presence in the room he said,
'What writest thou?' — The vision raised its head,

patients not only lack the ability to plan ahead or make executive decisions, but their behaviour may become rigid, another name for being maladaptive. They find it very difficult to alter their behaviour even though circumstances alter — an essential part of successful adaptation to constantly changing demands. This is called 'perseveration'. Add to this, their evident defect in recognising emotions and social nuances in others, as well as deficits in their own behaviour, and you have a being totally unsuited to life in human (or even primate) society. The prefrontal cortex thus enables adaptation and survival at the level of the social group, an essential requirement for a successful life as a human being. In a society less tolerant than even 19th century America, Phineas Gage would have lived for only a very short time after his accident — either driven out to die of starvation, or killed for transgressing the tolerable norms of the social group. Remarkably, intelligence tests usually show no change after prefrontal damage; but we should recall that these tests are designed to probe verbal, numerical or reasoning abilities. What is lacking is 'social intelligence', the ability to adapt to life with other people, understand the function and requirements of a social group, and form the relationships (attachments) that determine success or failure. Another way of thinking about the prefrontal lobes is that they allow you to choose between a set of tentative plans or strategies and select that best adapted to the current environment or demand state. Some call this 'Social Darwinism'.

You will have noticed, by now, little mention of chemical coding in the prefrontal cortex, though this is the main subject of this book. The nerve cells of the prefrontal cortex, like everywhere else in the brain, are electrochemical devices. The cortex itself is probably mainly dependent on glutamate and GABA, those mainstay transmitters that act as 'on-off' switches in many areas of the brain (recall that they are really not that simple — Chapter 2). But it is likely that the complexity of function of the prefrontal cortex lies mainly in the networks of neurons that are continually being set up and revised. Neuroscientists call these 'neural assemblies.' When we come to understand how this part of the brain really works, it will probably be by being able to describe how these assemblies change with time and circumstance.

Join me, for a few moments, on this comfortable verandah, overlooking an African game reserve. There is a television in the corner,

And with a look made of all sweet accord,
Answered, 'The names of those who love the Lord.'
'And is mine one?' said Abou. 'Nay not so,'
Replied the angel. Abou spoke more low,
But cheerly still; and said, 'I pray thee then,
Write me as one that loves his fellow-men'.

James Henry Leigh Hunt. (1784–1859) *Abou Ben Adhem.*

a mobile phone nearby, and across the room a fridge with cold beer. The obligatory Land Rover, in suitable safari-colours, is parked nearby. The chimpanzees sit in companionable groups, about half a mile away, grooming each other. We raise our binoculars. One pulls a nearby plant towards him, and slowly chews him way along the stem. A second chimp seems to be fishing for ants in a anthill, using a short stick for the purpose. Periodically, he (or she, it is hard to see) pulls the stick through his mouth, eating up the ants clinging to the twig. As it is getting late, we can see another making a night-nest in a nearby tree. Within a surprisingly short period of time, expertly pulling on the surrounding branches, he makes a comfortable-looking nest, and lies down. He will do it all over again the next evening, and on every evening after. I forgot to tell you that on the verandah of the bungalow is a rather strange-looking machine. It is vaguely familiar (perhaps from a film?) with its seats, but no wheels, and a large circular disc on the back. In front of the seats is a handle and some sort of gauge. Of course! It is a Wellsian time machine. . . . We climb into the seats (this must be a newer two-seater model) and set the gauge to 5000 years ago. And pull the lever.

There is the expected stomach-churning vertiginous rocking, the blurring of the scenery. . . and then we are in the same place, but 50 centuries earlier. No verandah, no fridge, no television, no phone and most definitely no Land Rover. And no chairs: we are sitting on the ground and nearby is the opening to a cave. We spy someone wearing skins (they smell awful), a fire, and a few pots nearby. We look across to where the chimps had been and. . . they (or, rather, their ancestors) are still there. Moreover, they are doing exactly what their descendants will be doing 5000 years later. Despite the fact that we share about 98% of the chimps genes, we, as species, have changed what we do and how we do it dramatically, whereas they have not. What then, is the critical factor (for it must be in the brain) that determines that chimps stay much as they were 10 000 years ago, whereas we change (most call this progress)? Were we to look at their brains, they would look a lot like ours, but the most obvious difference is the prefrontal lobes. Humans have distinctly larger frontal lobes than chimps, though chimps have larger ones than monkeys, and much larger ones than felines or rodents. I do not think one can confidently put all the credit for human progress on one part of the brain,

Social Interaction and Altruism

I have a hunch that we may come to look back on the invention of the Evolutionary Stable Strategy (ESS) as one of the most important advances in evolutionary theory since Darwin. It is applicable whenever we find conflict of interest, and that means almost everywhere. Students of animal behaviour have got into the habit of talking about something called 'social organization'. Too often the social organisation of an individual is treated as an entity in its own right, with its own biological 'advantage'. An example I have already given is that of the 'dominance hierarchy'. . . . Maynard Smith's concept of the ESS will enable us. . . to see clearly how a collection of independent selfish entities can come to resemble a single organized whole.

R Dawkins. (1976) *The selfish gene.* (Oxford University Press, Oxford.)

The fundamental idea [of kin selection] is simple. Although there is a baseline of genes that are shared by most or all members of a population, there are also a large number of genes that vary between individuals. Identical twins will of course have all their genes in common. Nonidentical twins and regular siblings have (on average) half of these genes in common. A parent and a child also share half their genes. Half-siblings share (on average) a quarter of their genes, cousins one-eighth, and so on. According to the theory of kin selection, an individual will help a sibling if the benefit to that sibling is more than twice the cost to him- or herself. Similarly, an individual will help a cousin if the benefit to to the cousin is more than eight times the costs to him- or herself. In other words, genes for altruistic behavior toward relatives are selected in evolution to the extent that the benefit to the recipient, *devalued by the degree of relatedness*, outweighs the cost to the individual who performs the altruistic act.

S LeVay. (1993) *The sexual brain.* (MIT Press, Cambridge, Massachusetts.)

Social behaviors involve two or more individuals and require the willingness of animals to aggregate and remain together. Social behaviors are typically identified as positive, including affiliations and social bonds, or negative, including aggression. . . .

It is likely that biological systems responsible for many types of positive interactions are based on shared biological processes. For example, the neural and endocrine mechanisms involved in adult social bonding and pair bonding have much in common with mother-infant bonding and maternal behavior. . . .

Social bonds may form between a parent and infant, between two adults, and among other members of a social group. These apparently very different bonding relationships have a common function — namely, to enhance reproduction and ensure reproductive success.

> C S Carter and E B Keverne. (2002) The neurobiology of social affiliation and pair bonding. In: *Hormones, brain and behavior.* Eds. D Pfaff *et al.*, pp. 299–337. (Academic Press, Amsterdam.)

It is a basic feature of human experience to feel soothed in the presence of others and to feel distressed when left behind. Many languages reflect this experience in the assignment of physical pain words ("hurt feelings") to describe experiences of social separation. . . . We conducted a functional magnetic resonance imaging (fMRI) study of social exclusion to determine whether the regions activated by social pain are similar to those found in studies of physical pain. . . . A pattern of activation very similar to those found in studies of physical pain emerged during social exclusion, providing evidence that the experience and regulation of social and physical pain share a common neuroanatomical basis.

> N I Eisenberger, M D Lieberman, and K D Williams. (2003) Does rejection hurt? An fMRI study of social exclusion. *Science* **302**, pp. 290–292.

There are three conditions which often look alike
Yet differ completely, flourish in the same hedgerow:
Attachment to self and to things and to persons, detachment
From self and from things and from persons; and, growing between them,
indifference
Which resembles the others as death resembles life,
Being between two lives — unflowering, between
The live and the dead nettle. This is the use of memory:
For liberation — not less of love but expanding
Of love beyond desire, and so liberation
From the future as well as the past.

T S Eliot. (1944) *Little Gidding.* (Faber and Faber, London.)

Oh, my lovely love, thought Madeline, my own sweet husband whom I love with all my heart. How beautiful, how beautiful he looks in the dim lamplight, his dark brows, his grey eyes, his good jaw slightly bearded at the end of the day, his delicate light fingers that have brought me so much pleasure lying curled up and easy on the arm of his chair as if begging me to put my hand in them. And how good he is. No, it doesn't matter how good he is; how good he tries to be, human good, not Sunday-school good. That's what matters. My sweet, dear husband. My darling, show-offy, gentle husband. My love.

Stanley Kauffmann. (1953) *The philanderer.*
(Secker and Warburg, London.)

. . . She was filled with a strange, wild, unfamiliar happiness, and knew that this was love. Twice in her life she had mistaken something else for it; it was like seeing somebody in the street who you think is a friend, you whistle and wave and run after him, and he is not only not the friend, but not even very like him. . . . Linda was now looking upon the authentic face of love, and she knew it, but it frightened her. . . . She tried to remember how she felt when she had first loved her two husbands. . . she could not recall it. Only she knew that never before, not even in dreams, and she was a great dreamer of love, had she felt anything remotely like this.

Nancy Mitford. (1945) *The pursuit of love.*
(Hamish Hamilton, London.)

She wondered whether there would ever come an hour in her life when she didn't think of him; didn't speak to him in her head, didn't relive every moment they'd been together, didn't long for his voice and his hands and his love. She had never dreamed of what it would feel like to love someone so much; of all the things that had astonished her in her adventures, that was what astonished her the most. She thought the tenderness it left in her heart was like a bruise that would never go away, but she would cherish it for ever.

Philip Pullman. (2000) *The amber spyglass,*
third part of His Dark Materials.

This state of exaltation was heightened, or even brought about, by the fact that I was in love then for the first time: I had identified love at once. The truth is that never since has any passion I have felt remained so hopelessly unexpressed within me or appeared so grotesquely altered in the outside world. It is strange that sometimes, even now, I remember unadulteratedly a certain morning when I touched my friend's wrist (as if by accident, and he pretended not to notice) as we passed on the stairs at school. I must add, and this is not so strange, that the child was not actually my friend. We had never exchanged a word or even a nod of recognition; but it was possible during that entire year for me to think endlessly on this minute and brief encounter which we endured on the stairs, until it would swell with a sudden and overwhelming beauty, like a rose forced into premature bloom for a great occasion.

Eudora Welty. (1998) A memory. In: *The collected stories of Eudora, Welty.* (Virago, London.)

Her life with others no longer interests him. He wants only her stalking beauty, her theatre of expressions. He wants the minute and secret reflections between them, the depth of field minimal, their foreignness intimate like two pages of a closed book.

Michael Ondaatje. (1992) *The English patient.* (Bloomsbury Publishing Co., London.)

Pasha suspected her of all the seven deadly sins, disbelieved every word she said and was ready to curse and hate her, but he loved her to distraction and was jealous of her very thoughts, and of the mug she drank from and of the pillow on which she lay.

Boris Pasternak. (1958) *Doctor Zhivago.* Translated by Max Hayward and Manya Harari, Wm. (Collins and Co. Ltd., London.)

Who then devised the torment? Love.
Love is the unfamiliar Name
Behind the hands that wove
The intolerable shirt of flame
Which human power cannot remove.
    We only love, only suspire
    Consumed by either fire or fire.

T S Eliot. (1944) *Little Gidding.* (Faber and Faber, London.)

but if I were asked to pick one, it would undoubtedly be the prefrontal cortex. If that is true, then the prefrontal cortex, and the genes that make it (there may be only a few), have had a remarkable impact on the activities of the limbic system, on human social behaviour and on the biology of this planet.

The Frontal Lobes and Decision-Making

The frontal lobe disorder is characterized foremost by a derangement of behavior programming. One of the essential functional deficits of the frontal-lobe patient appears to lie in an inability to maintain in his behavior a normal stability-in-time: his action programs, once started, are likely to fade out, to stagnate in reiteration or to become deflected away from the intended goal.

Part at least of the behavioural effects of frontal-lobe destruction could be seen as the consequence of an 'interoceptive agnosia', i.e. an impairment of the subject's ability to integrate certain information from his internal milieu with the environmental reports provided by his neocortical processing mechanisms.

W J H Nauta. (1971) The problem of the frontal lobe: A reinterpretation. *Journal of Psychological Research*, pp. 167–187.

One of the brain's great mysteries is cognitive control. How does the brain produce behaviour that seems organized and wilful? . . . cognitive control stems from patterns of activity in the prefrontal cortex that represent goals and the means to achieve them. . . .Virtually all complex behaviour involves constructing relationships between diverse, arbitrary pieces of information that have no intrinsic connection. Insight into the role of the prefrontal cortex in cognition can surely be gained from a better understanding of this process.

E K Miller. (2000) The prefrontal cortex and cognitive control. *Nature Reviews Neuroscience*, pp. 59–65.

If we ask whether we are free, the kind of answer we want may not be possible. A better question to ask is: do we make choices? The answer is certainly yes. Do our choices have any influence on our relationship to our peers and the environment? Again, yes. Are our choices constrained? Yes, because of natural law and historical circumstances, but not entirely because of random chance and deterministic chaos. Consider a game of cards. . . once the hands are dealt your freedom to play a certain card is limited by the rules of the game, the hand you are dealt, and your knowledge of strategy and tactics. But within these limitations you have many choices. . . . The moment of deliberation about which card to play seems to embody all of the freedom one could hope for. The fact that such deliberation is accomplished by your brain takes away none of the joy of the game.

J D Schall. (2001) Neural coding of deciding, choosing and acting. *Nature Reviews Neuroscience*, pp. 33–42.

Although of unquestioned importance, prefrontal functions are particularly difficult to characterize and understand. On the one hand, accounts based on highly specific deficits — such as impairment of 'delayed response' after frontal lesions in the monkey — seem too restricted to apply convincingly to the broad problem of disorganization in many different forms of behaviour. On the other hand, more general accounts — including concepts such as executive function, temporal structuring of behaviour, control by cognitive context or goal-subgoal selection — can be hard to apply in detail to any specific problem.

J Duncan. (2001) An adaptive coding model of neural function in prefrontal cortex. *Nature Reviews Neuroscience*, pp. 820–829.

Chapter 10

The Brain Goes to War

Let's sit on this little hill and watch the baboons as they walk across the veldt. There are about 30 of them in the troop, all sizes, some large adult males, some much smaller females, and plenty of juveniles of various ages. To us, they look like a random bunch of monkeys, but the primatologist sitting with us has more experienced eyes. She points out that there is an organisation, though it is not easy to see. The large males walk at the head near the middle of the group; several females surround them. On the edge of the group are other males, though they look less well-fed and in not so good condition as the glossy males in the centre. Very young baboons run around all over the place, no social barrier seems to exist for them. The troop comes across a clump of bushes bearing fruit, and stops to eat. The primatologist tells us to watch carefully. The larger males take their pick, as do some of the females with them. When they have finished, other baboons take their place. Last of all, the younger, smaller, peripheral males help themselves to whatever remains. Now it is time to drink, so the troop finds a small pool, all that is left after days of baking African sun. Again, we see the larger males take their fill, followed by the others though we also notice that size is not the only criterion that seems to matter. Occasionally, we hear the characteristic screech of an aggressive baboon, and see one or other animal running away, but mostly, all is quiet and seemingly peaceful. We borrow binoculars off our primatologist friend, and take a closer look.

The troop, now mostly replete, has moved into the shade of some nearby rocks. The big males lie down, and are immediately surrounded by attendant females who begin to groom them. We watch them; the males stretch out, closing their eyes in seeming rapture and lifting their arms so that the grooming females have better access. Some of the males have obvious penile erections whilst they are being groomed. The females seem totally absorbed, picking through the male's fur and appearing to eat whatever they find. The primatologist tells us that the popular idea that they are catching and eating fleas is utterly wrong. Healthy baboons are rather clean, and a flea would stand no chance; grooming keeps them parasite-free. What are they eating? We ask. Probably bits of skin, she says. We notice that some females groom other females; our primatologist tells us that the same females are often to be seen grooming each other, as if they were special friends. Other females groom infants. Infants seem to attract the females; several may sit round one. Occasionally, males groom each other, but there is not much grooming amongst the outer group of males, who continue to keep their distance. A brief fight breaks out, we cannot see why, but one smallish male runs off, screaming and baring his clenched teeth in what looks like a terrified smile. Another, much bigger, male is glowering at him, teeth also bared, but mouth wide open. We notice some extremely large canine teeth, like a pair of daggers. Though there is not much obvious fighting, the group does seem rather tense.

As the day grows cooler, some of the males begin to mate. Prompted by the primatologist, we notice that sexual behaviour is not random. Females mate with the males at the centre of the group. The primatologist tells us that that the females' interactions with the males are regulated by at least two interlocking factors: one hormonal (their cycle), the other social (their rank). We recall Chapter 8. Occasionally, a more peripheral male may try to sneak a liaison, and sometimes he is successful, but often his attempts are detected by the central males, and he is chased off. More screeching.

The quality and quantity of resources (particularly food and water) available to a group of animals, such as baboons, depends on their defending their territory against others who would otherwise take them. So there is another level of aggression, between as well as within groups. We watch our baboon troop as they near the boundary of their territory and come within sight of another group. Instantly, intra-group rivalry is forgotten. The males line up, barking furiously, showing their teeth and making little dashes towards the opposing group, who have similarly gone

Aggression

What is aggression? In ordinary English usage, it means an abridgement of the rights of another, forcing him to surrender something he owns or might otherwise have attained, either by a physical act or by the threat of action. Biologists cannot improve on this definition. . . except to specify that in the long term a loss to the victim is a real loss only to the extent that it lowers genetic fitness. . . . The essential fact to bear in mind about aggression is that it is a mixture of very different behavior patterns, serving very different functions.

E O Wilson. (1975) *Sociobiology. The new synthesis.*
(The Belknap Press, Cambridge, Massachusetts.)

Individual aggression is often categorised into a number of types. For instance, one system distinguishes 'instrumental aggression', deliberate and concerned primarily with obtaining an object of position or access to a desirable activity; 'emotional aggression', hot-headed and angry; 'felonious aggression', occurring in the course of a crime: and 'dissocial aggression', regarded as appropriate by the reference group or gang, but not so regarded by outsiders. Such categories, though useful for some purposes, usually turn out to be less clear-cut than they might appear for an obvious reason: a variety of motivations may contribute to a single act, and they may be present in various strengths and combinations. The very fact that such categorization systems can only be partially satisfactory is in itself an indication of the motivational complexity of even apparently simple aggressive acts.

R A Hinde. (1998) The psychological bases of war.
American Diplomacy, 3rd electronic ed.

Aggression is a significant problem in our society, with social, psychological and financial impacts that may be impossible to assess fully. Data. . . suggest that 3.7% of the population commit one or more acts of violence each year, and the lifetime prevalence of aggressive behavior may be about 24%.

R Kavoussi, P Armstead, and E Coccaro. (1997) The neurobiology of impulsive aggression. *The Psychiatric Clinics of North America* **20**, pp. 395–403.

into battle formation. The bolder females may join in. Often, all this ends with one group retreating after a while without much actual fighting; occasionally there is a considerable war.

We have been watching the role of social structure in adaptive behaviour. Access to essential resources for survival, like food, water and sex, are all regulated by the social structure in which the individual lives. This is as true for humans as baboons. In our baboon group, there is little overt aggression, because the animals have formed a social group with a hierarchy; that is, a system of social ranking. The position of each animal in this rank has been determined by previous interactions, most of them aggressive. Those at the top of the pile, the dominant baboons, have priority of access to sought-after resources like food, or mates or shelter. Each animal has learned its position, so there is no need for a fight every time two or more baboons go for the same object; they know who would win. Each animal 'knows its place', as our Victorian forebears would have said about each other. The hierarchy may not be simple: for example, several males may form a coalition which, together, could defeat a bigger male. Together, they are dominant; divided, they would lose rank. Females who are sexually attractive may temporarily increase their rank if they associate with a dominant male; but should the liaison break, the female returns to her original status. The social hierarchy is designed, it seems, to minimise overt aggression so that valuable energy is not wasted, or health put at risk unnecessarily, every time there is competition. Social stability is the result, but it is an uneasy stability. The hierarchy is constantly being challenged. Should a dominant male grow ill or old, he will be displaced. Should an alliance break, its members may be demoted. The social structure of the troop is continually reinforced and tested by signals and interaction between its members. Relationships between individuals wax and wane.

All this may sound rather familiar. Dominance hierarchies are not limited to baboons, or even to primates. They are certainly a feature of our own social structure, complex as it is. Being a member of a social group may confer all sorts of benefits, but it can also be a source of considerable stress. Being a subordinate is not good for a baboon's health; they tend to die earlier, as well as have less offspring, than more dominant animals. Can what we learn from studying the social lives of other animals inform

About 4400 people die every day because of intentional acts of self-directed, interpersonal, or collective violence. Many thousands more are injured or suffer other non-fatal health consequences as a result of being the victim or witness to acts of violence.

E G Krug, J A Mercy, L L Dahlberg, and A B Zwi. (2002)
The world report on violence and health.
Lancet **360**, pp. 1083–10.

While the general principles derived from studies of animals can be applied to understanding aggression in man, this must be done in a sophisticated manner. To cite some examples, in the human case the manner an individual perceives himself is a crucial issue; observational learning is more likely to affect him if it involves an individual he respects; the norms of the groups with which he identified are likely to have a profound effect on his behaviour; the extent to which he feels himself to be frustrated will be influenced by the extent to which he had acquired self-esteem and security; and the extent to which he avoids violence will be affected by the guide-lines for behaviour that he has acquired and by his future goals.

R A Hinde. (1974) *The biological bases of human behaviour.*
(McGraw-Hill Book Company, New York.)

us about our own society and the effects it has on each of us? Aggression and violence, some of it considered inappropriate, is a pervasive feature of contemporary human society, as well as in those of baboons and other non-human primates. Clinicians, social workers, policemen and school-teachers all know that understanding, preventing and treating socially unacceptable or inappropriate aggression is often incomplete and unsatisfactory. This helplessness reflects our basic ignorance of the causes of either 'normal' or 'abnormal' aggression (and fear). Part of the problem is that sociologists, psychologists and neuroscientists do not talk to each other much.

Our primary aim is to understand what part the brain plays in all this. How does it detects and determines the social hierarchy? How does it allows an individual to survive in a competitive environment? How does complex information about the social milieu of an individual regulate those parts of the brain that are responsible for meeting basic demands? Is an individual's physiology related to his/her rank? If so, how does the brain arrange this? We cannot hope to understand the role of the brain in general, and the limbic system in particular, in adaptation and homeostasis unless we can relate its function to the society in which all animals, including humans, live. The social group is as much part of an individual's biological environment as sun, rain, sources of food and pools of water. To begin, we need to think about the role of the brain in aggression.

Aggression is different from other behaviours that are concerned with survival. Unlike these other behaviours, it makes no biological sense on its own. Nothing is gained simply by winning a fight. This does not mean that winning a fight is not rewarding in itself, or that aggression cannot be pleasurable for its own sake. But no individual increases his/her 'fitness' simply by defeating another. The payoff is the increased access to some desirable resource that overcoming another can bring. So aggression mostly occurs in the context, and as part of, some other behaviour. The process of getting food in competition with all the other mouths around, drinking the scarce supply of water, mating with that most desirable partner or defending a territory that contains any or all of these coveted items may only be accomplished by using aggression. So whilst the appearance of aggression may look rather similar in different circumstances, its function may be very distinct. This will alter the brain's

The surprise at first was far worse than the pain. . . every man had his razor out. . . . and the obscure struggle reached its climax out of his sight. He had other things to watch: the long cut-throat razors which the sun caught slanting low down over the downs from Shoreham. He put his hand to his pocket to get his blade, and the man immediately facing him leant across and slashed his knuckles. Pain happened to him: and he was filled with horror and astonishment as if one of the bullied brats at school had stabbed first with the dividers.

Graham Greene. (1938) *Brighton rock.*
(Penguin Books, London.)

Mundt's appearance was fully consistent with his temperament. He looked an athlete. His fair hair was cut short. It lay mat and neat. His young face had a hard, clean line, and a frightening directness; it was barren of humour of fantasy. He looked young but was not youthful; older men would take him seriously. . . . There was a coldness about him, a rigorous self-sufficiency which perfectly equipped him for the business of murder.

John le Carre. (1963) *The spy who came in from the cold.*
(Victor Gollancz, London.)

Swelter's eyes meet those of his enemy, and never was there held between four globes of gristle so sinister a hell of hatred. Had the flesh, the fibres, and the bones of the chef and those of Mr Flay been conjured away and away down that dark corridor leaving only their four eyes suspended in mid-air outside the Earl's door, then, surely, they must have reddened to the hue of Mars, reddened and smouldered, and at last broken into flame, so intense was their hatred — broken into flame and circled about one another in ever-narrowing gyres and in swifter and yet swifter flight until, merged into one sizzling globe of fire they must surely have fled, the four in one, leaving a trail of blood behind them in the cold grey air of the corridor, until screaming as they fly down the endless passage ways of Gormenghast, they found their eyeless bodies once again, and re-entrenched themselves in startled sockets. . . .
He concentrated his entire sentience on the killing. He banished all irrelevancies from his canalized mind. His great ham of a face was

role. As we have seen, aggression may not accompany each act or series of competitive acts. It may have been used to predetermine the outcome.

The special tactical nature of aggression complicates scientific efforts to study it. Compared with aggression, studying other behaviours such as eating, drinking and sex seems easy (though it is not). To study eating, deprive a rat of food for a while; put it into an cage empty except for food and see what happens. If you want to study drinking, remove the rat's water supply for a few hours, and replace the food with water in the test cage. For sex, it is even easier: put the male (or female) rat into the cage, again empty, and introduce a sexy member of the opposite (or even the same) sex. The rationale for this approach is that such behaviours have definable characteristics, and equally distinct biological or motivational boundaries. Manipulations of the brain can be made to see what effect this has on these distinct behaviours, with the reasonable assumption this will yield information relevant to the neural mechanisms responsible for each. We cannot make such an assumption for aggression. Even if we were to be successful in inducing aggression in a cage all by itself, this would be irrelevant. It does not exist by itself. If we induce it as part of another behaviour (e.g. sex), we are really studying aggression in the context of sex, and the parts of the brain concerned may be very different from those controlling aggression under other circumstances (say, competition for food). As an example, we know there are very different hormones responsible for aggression between male rats (a sexual or territorial context) and those that cause a mother rat to defend her young by attacking an intruder (part of maternal behaviour).

Scientists have an understandable passion for classifying things. They do this to help them understand what they are studying. To classify satisfactorily means one has defined categories, and this is the first stage to knowing what there is to explain. So the concept of the 'species' helped enormously to define the biological world. Given its peculiar status, it is perhaps no surprise that attempts to classify aggression have been very messy indeed. A relatively straightforward one is to separate attack and defence. After that, it gets tricky. Some people have tried to classify aggression on the basis of the context or stimuli eliciting this behaviour; hence inter-male (or inter-female), maternal, self-defence and infanticide. A curious mixture of who, what and when. Predation (which is not

tickling as though aswarm with insects, but there was no room left in his
brain to receive the messages which his nerve endings were presumably
delivering — his brain was full. It was full of death.

Mervyn Peake. (1946) *Titus Groan.*
(Eyre and Spottiswoode, London.)

Freddie pushes me and everything turns dark in my head and I run at him
with fists and knees and feet till he yells, Hey, stop, stop, and I won't
because I can't, I don't know how, and if I stop, Malachy will go on taking
my story from me.

Frank McCourt. (1996) *Angela's ashes.*

Growltiger was a Bravo Cat, who travelled on a barge:
In fact he was the roughest cat that ever roamed at large.
From Gravesend up to Oxford he pursued his evil aims,
Rejoicing in his title of 'The Terror of the Thames'.
His manners and appearance did not calculate to please;
His coat was torn and seedy, he was baggy at the knees;
One ear was somewhat missing, no need to tell you why,
And he scowled upon a hostile world from one forbidding eye.

T S Eliot. (1939) *Growltiger's last stand. From: Old Possum's*
book of practical cats. (Faber and Faber, London.)

(A chimp fight)
Then they charged him. Darius, twice Mr Jeb's size, felled him easily and
sat on his chest, holding down his arms. Gaspar clutched his feet and
Pulul and Americo jumped on his head repeatedly. Then Gaspar leant
forward and sank his teeth into Mr Jeb's scrotum, producing a horrifying
scream of pain from the old chimp. But the battering he was receiving
from the others stunned him, and his body slumped. One by one the
others let him go.

William Boyd. (1990) *Brazzaville beach.*
(Sinclair-Stevenson, London.)

A boy of about ten came running along the pavement. He was very pale,
and so scared that he forgot to take his cap off to a German policemen

aggression) is included.   Human aggression has been separated into 'emotional' (i.e. aggression carried out with the main intention to harm someone) and 'instrumental' (aggression carried out with some other objective that is more important than their victim's injury). Are they really so different?   Do two categories reflect the complexity of human aggression? Aggression occurs over time and place in the real world; this means that there is a constant process of social adaptation to aggression or its consequences.   Animals and people learn whether or not aggression pays off, and the contexts in which to use it or how best to respond to it. The brain does all this.

Fear is a natural response to aggression and inextricably linked with it. Without fear, the subordinate male baboon threatened by the larger, more dominant one would neither run away nor display the characteristic behavioural traits of fearfulness.   The latter may placate the aggressor; submission is a common way to resolve a conflict without coming to blows in humans as well as baboons.   Without submitting, our little baboon is in acute danger from those stiletto-like canines.   So we also need to know whether there are special areas of the brain that recognise aggression in others and formulate an appropriate and biologically sensible response. The function of fear is not limited to social interactions and the maintenance of the social hierarchy.   Fear of unknown places, strangers, and possible predators are all just as important. Most studies of fear in the laboratory have little interest in the biological use of fear and how it may differ.

In 1939, a psychologist (Heinrich Kluver) who was interested in perception, teamed up with a neurosurgeon (Paul Bucy) and they removed both temporal lobes from rhesus monkeys. The result was an extraordinary collection of abnormal behaviours now always called the Kluver-Bucy syndrome. (I have always rather unkindly thought that Bucy's immortality came rather easily.) They included what Kluver called 'psychic blindness' which is an apparent inability to recognise common objects or understand their meaning. The lesioned monkeys tended to put anything and everything into their mouths ('oral tendencies'), and there was a remarkable increase in indiscriminate sexual behaviour (hypersexuality, they tried to mate with anything that moved; see Chapter 8). All this was interesting enough, but they also showed something else: there was a striking decrease in fear.

coming towards him. The German stopped, drew his revolver without a word, put it to the boy's temple and shot. The child fell to the ground, his arms flailing and died. The policeman calmly put the revolver back in its holster and went on his way. I looked at him; he did not even have particularly brutal features, nor did he appear angry. He was a normal, placid man who had carried out one of his many minor daily duties and put it out of his mind again at once, for other and more important business awaited him.

Wladyslaw Szpilman. (2000) *The pianist.*
(Orion Books Ltd., London.)

Normally they would attempt to bite any human hand that came near them, now they allowed themselves to be stroked. They were exceedingly placid and unemotional, even towards each other. They did not fight. A similar syndrome has been observed in humans after damage to the temporal lobe.

You can see that this syndrome is rather a mixture. Many behaviours are disturbed, and there is not a very clear relation, at first sight, between some of them. The parts of brain that Bucy removed were quite large and contained at least three separate parts of the brain: the temporal cortex (part of the neocortex), at least part of the hippocampus (traditionally part of the limbic system) and the amygdala. The amygdala is the almond-shaped chunk of grey matter that lies deep in the temporal lobes. It is a fully-accredited member of the limbic system. So it seems possible that the mixture of results was one consequence of several parts of the brain having been removed or damaged. A great deal of effort was put into trying to decide which part of brain was responsible for which altered behaviour. Psychic blindness seems mostly attributable to the temporal neocortex. Reduced aggressiveness and fear is mostly the result of removing the amygdala.

Note, however, the first problem: is the amygdala an 'aggression' part of the brain or one that is really concerned with fear? If you corner a wild cat, it will show all the classical signs of fear and try to escape; if it cannot get away, it may attack you. Remove the fear, and you remove the tendency to attack. But other experiments also implicated the amygdala, for example, stimulating it electrically increases the likelihood of aggression, but not randomly. Interestingly, these animals tended to go for things that they might normally attack — another member of their species, a potential prey, even a human experimenter — rather than an inanimate object. Localized seizures in the temporal lobe and sometimes specifically in the amygdala are associated with aggressive outbursts in human beings. These violent episodes occur during episodes of abnormal electrical activity. Patients with temporal lobe tumours may exhibit assaultive rages. Many years ago, a man climbed a tower in Texas and shot 44 people at random, before being himself shot by police. He had a temporal lobe tumour.

Damaging the amygdala (it has to be on both sides), reliably decreases aggression in a number of different species and they become very tame.

From this, it follows that I must now consider myself as existing in a different way and must, as it were, appropriate goodness of another sort, suitable for this new existence. Because my life, my security, my liberty, and my happiness today depend on the cooperation of others like myself, it is clear that I must look upon myself no longer as an isolated individual but as part of a larger whole, as a member of a larger body on whose preservation mine depends absolutely, and any disorder in which I would necessarily feel.

Jean-Jacques Rousseau. (1861) *A letter from Jean-Jacques Rousseau*. Trans. Arthur Goldhammer, *New York Review of Books* **50**, pp. 31–32.

You take a straight tip from the stable, Cokey: if you must hate, hate the government or the people or the sea or men, but don't hate an individual person. Who's done you a real injury. Next thing you know he'll be getting into your beer like prussic acid; and blotting out your eyes like a cataract and screaming in your ears like a brain tumour and boiling round your heart like melted lead and ramping through your guts like cancer.

Joyce Cary. (1944) *The horse's mouth*. (Michael Joseph, London.)

A pavilion had been erected for the King on one side, and another for the Constable on the other. The barricades and the pavilions were decorated with cloth. There was a curtained gateway at each end, like the dramatic hole through which the circus people ride into their arena. In one corner of the corral, visible for all to see, was a great bundle of faggots with an iron stake in the middle, which would not burn or melt. This was for the Queen if the law went against her. Before Arthur had started his life's work, a man accusing the Queen of anything would have been executed out of hand. Now, because of his own work, he must be ready to burn his wife.

For a new idea had begun to form in the King's mind. The efforts to dig a channel for Might had failed, even when it was turned to the spirit, and now he was feeling his way towards abolishing it. He had decided not to truckle with Might any more — to cut it out, root and branch, by establishing another standard altogether. He was groping towards Right

During the 1970s, neurosurgeons in India and Japan (both rather conformist societies at that time) destroyed the amygdala in children who were destructive, aggressive and uncontrollable (nowadays we would probably diagnose these children as 'conduct disorders'). The results were never properly recorded, and this operation, not surprisingly, is no longer done. But it remains a good example of the uncritical application of experimental data to clinical situations.

So it all begins to look as if the amygdala is central to aggression. But wait. At the same time, as one set of neuroscientists were studying the role of the amygdala in aggression, another was establishing that it was important in fear. Particularly, in conditioned fear. In 1965, the psychologist Larry Weiskrantz opened up a new idea about what the amygdala might do, one that has intrigued a generation of neuroscientists. You will recall Pavlov's famous experiment with the bell and the dog. Ring the bell just before you feed the dog, and after a while the sound of the bell alone will cause the dog to salivate. It has learned to associate the sound of the bell with subsequent food. You can also set up an association between a tone (or a light, or most stimuli) and something unpleasant, like a mild electric shock. Rats will learn to avoid the shock when the tone (or whatever) appears. But not if their amygdalae are removed. A bombshell! The amygdala is necessary for Pavlovian conditioning. This, of course, is one sort of learning. Imagine yourself transported into World War 2, and sitting in your living room. Suddenly, the characteristic wail of an air-raid siren breaks out. Now, nobody under the age of about 70 today, even if transported back in time, would flinch. The older ones might dive for the nearest shelter. The siren, simply a tone, had come to be associated with something fearful, and therefore had become fearful itself, but only in those who had experienced the war. That is conditioned fear, and it is this that is abolished in rats by damaging the amygdala. But in humans, damage to the amygdala of both sides impairs the recognition of fear in others and this is not quite the same.

Transported safely back from the 1940s, now you have to imagine yourself sitting companionably drinking a cup of coffee with a couple of friends. Suddenly, the door bursts open and a man enters carrying a gun. Did I forget to mention that you are hooked up to a machine that measures your physiological response? And that you are in Belfast or Beirut in the *as a criterion of its own — towards Justice as an abstract thing which did not lean upon Power. In a few years, he would be inventing Civil Law.*

T H White. (1958) *The once and future king.*
(Fontana/Collins, London.)

The peasant wife was destined for a life of suffering — so much so, indeed, that her life became a symbol of the peasant's misery, used by nineteenth-century writers to highlight the worst aspects of Russian life. The traditional peasant household was much larger than its European counterpart. . . . The young bride who arrived in this household was likely to be burdened with the meanest chores, the fetching and the cooking, the washing and the childcare, and generally treated like a serf. She would have to put up with the sexual advances of not just her husband, but his father too. . . . Then there were the wife-beatings. For centuries, peasants had claimed the right to beat their wives. Russian proverbs were full of advice on the wisdom of such violence. . . .

Orlando Figes. (2003) *Natasha's dance.* (Penguin Books, London.)

1970s or Baghdad in 2007? Your heart rate doubles, your blood pressure rises, levels of adrenaline in your blood increase, your face becomes pale, you feel the emotion of extreme fear, and even let out a half-smothered shriek. You fear for your life. Now suppose all this happens exactly as before, but this time you are actually taking part in a play, and the man with the gun is supposed to enter at that moment. No fear this time, though you, a rather good actor, may feign it convincingly. Let us try to analyse what has happened in the brain during each scenario.

I would bet a large amount that, if your amygdala was disabled in some way, not a muscle would you flinch in the first scenario, even though your friends are diving under the table, or even drawing guns of their own. They are adapting to the current demand, you are not. But nobody is born knowing about guns, what they look like, what they are for, and that they can be dangerous. We learn from being told, seeing films, even experiencing gun fights. So when the man bursts through the door, you recognise that he is carrying a small piece of metal that is a gun. Now here is the interesting point. The information carried by your eyes is processed, not by your amygdala, but by your cortex. A good deal of research shows that the part of the brain that actually recognises an object (e.g. a gun) for what it is lies in the cortex of the temporal lobe. In other words, this part of the brain, which is not limbic, performs high-level processing of visual information. You need to know what a gun is to be afraid of it. We recall Kluver's 'psychic blindness' after temporal lobe lesions. So there is a necessary connection between cognition (recognising the gun) and emotion (being afraid), and separating the two, though convenient perhaps for those studying either, is not sensible or realistic. Both are part of an effective adaptive response.

It gets more interesting. Neuro-anatomists spend their professional lives unravelling the unbelievably complex wiring diagram of the brain. This is not random; certain areas, as we have seen, connect preferentially with certain other areas, and this strongly suggests a shared function. It turns out that the temporal cortex has a huge projection to the amygdala; no other cortical area comes close. Suddenly, we see that the components of the Kluver-Bucy syndrome are not as separate as we thought. The cortex analyses the information (a gun), passes this to the amygdala, which labels it (danger). The limbic system, as we suspected all along,

Aggression in Males

The animal world is rife with sexual rivalry between males. Even the sweet-sounding song of the male nightingale is an example of this bitter struggle. His song warns other males to keep out of his territory and attracts females. The formation of territories is one way of demarcating procreational rights; the formation of a hierarchy is another. There is a definite link between power and sex; no social organization can be properly understood without knowledge of the sexual rules and the way the progeny are cared for.

F de Waal. (1998) *Chimpanzee politics*. Revised ed.
(Johns Hopkins University Press, Baltimore.)

King Benjamin, like many a royal master, found life full and demanding. He had to satisfy the sex requirements of his queen, and at the same time make sure no other male on his lands took liberties with his train of wife and concubines, at least not while he was in sight or knowledge of their actions. Clandestine flirtations between the sexes were many above ground, for rabbits obviously enjoy company, male with female; and that enjoyment is heightened or lowered by the degree of readiness of the female in her seven-day cycle to accept. . . copulation. As for male enjoying company with male, and female with female, this was sometimes apparent, especially in the neutral season, but usually they kept a little apart, a few feet — there was a minimum safety or 'individual' distance. Rabbits are essentially gregarious but not always sociable — their social structure is like that of a primitive community, which has advantages in times of danger.

R M Lockley. (1964) *The private life of the rabbit*.
(Andre Deutsch, London.)

In all mammalian species, from mouse to man, the male is the more aggressive sex. . . . The most frequent target of male hostility is a male conspecific to which the attacker has not become habituated. . . . There are several lines of evidence to indicate that the opportunity to engage in intermale aggression may be positively reinforcing to the participants. . . .

There can be no doubt that there is a relationship between sexual and aggressive behavior. . . . Freud has suggested that aggression is an essential and integral part of sexual feelings in the male.

K E Moyer. (1974) Sex differences in aggression In:
Sex differences in behavior. Eds. R C Friedman,
R M Richart, and R L Vande Wiele. (John Wiley, New York.)

cannot get along alone (it does not know what a gun is), and the cortex would not be very good at ensuring our survival without the recognition of threat supplied by the limbic system. Where is the memory, the learning process, that connects 'gun' with 'danger'? Most people suspect this lies in the amygdala itself, though how this is stored, and whether it is limited to the amygdala, are still unanswered questions.

At this point, we ought to recall that we have yet to account for the physiological accompaniments of fear (heart rate, hormone changes etc.). No problem here; there are extensive connections (in both ways) between the amygdala and the hypothalamus. These are plentiful enough to ensure that signals from the amygdala can reach the hypothalamus directly. The hypothalamus, as we know, is principally concerned with organising the hormonal and autonomic responses that accompany demand states. It is not the emotion that is the demand. It is the situation that results in the emotion. The emotional reaction is part, but only part, of the adaptive response (see Chapter 1). The response as a whole includes physiological adjustments, as important and necessary as emotion for survival in peril. But the amygdala, if it fulfils the role we think it has, not only must signal a demand state to the hypothalamus, but also some indication of what that state is. There must, it seems, be a coded message.

Or is the amygdala concerned with a range of emotional states, and with learning about situations that can predict rewards as well as danger? With pleasure as well as pain? If so, the important questions about the amygdala take on a very different hue. We need to know how different sorts of complex or even simple stimuli (e.g. smell) that signal or predict different categories of reward (e.g. food, drink, sex) or danger (social, physical, uncertainty) are encoded in the amygdala — and is this where it occurs? How are these very different sorts of information passed onto the other parts of the limbic system that will be responsible for composing and co-ordinating the most appropriate responses? Is there some sort of 'code' in the amygdala that represents these separate emotional states? And can we limit the role of the amygdala to 'emotion'?

You might think that we have wandered some way from aggression, but not so. Since fear is part of the response to aggression, as well as a cause for it, we need to consider both if we are to understand the role of the brain. 'Fear' is limited, for the moment, to the fear of being physically

Fear

. . . The evidence suggests that the concept of a single, or core, fear state should be replaced with a set of related but distinct states, each with its own class of incentives, neurophysiological profiles, and behavioral reactions. . . .

Psychologists and psychiatrists must work out the psychological principles for each of the fear states while neuroscientists, biochemists, and molecular biologists work out the physiological principles. As both corpora of knowledge are enriched, the obstacle to theory created by the assumption of a single fear state will be removed and our understanding of the complex relations between the two domains should become clearer.

> J Kagan and J Schulkin. (1995) On the concepts of fear.
> *Harvard Review of Psychiatry* **3**, pp. 231–234.

The great evolutionary biologist Charles Darwin. . . once described a visit to the reptile house in London Zoo, where he put his face close up to the glass in front of a puff adder, determined that he would not flinch if it struck at him. When the snake did strike at him behind the glass, however, he leapt backwards, propelled by ancient and automatic brain circuits. No amount of reason and rationality could stop this primitive reaction, which had helped Darwin's genetic predecessors survive in the snake-infested forests hundreds of thousands of years ago.

> Ian Robertson. (1999) *Mind sculpture.*
> (Bantam Books, London.)

The existence of mutually co-operative behaviour in moments of attack contrasts strongly with most social relations prevailing within the group. . . . In their behaviour at feeding times, monkeys and apes display the most conspicuous selfishness. With few exceptions, every monkey or ape living in captivity tries to obtain as much for itself and to take as much as it can from its fellows. . . . The dominant animal as a rule obtains all of a limited food supply. . . .

The selfishness and cruelty engendered by a system of dominance stand in striking contrast to the support offered one another by sub-human primates when they are attacked. . . . The support of a dominant individual is evoked either by a squeal of terror, or by a 'fear-threatening' gesture unassociated with injured; other fears, for example of losing one's job or one's partner, or making a fool of oneself in public may have different social and biological roles, and thus involve distinct parts of the brain. There is no doubt that the amygdala is concerned with fear. Those who work exclusively on experimental models of fear tend to limit this to conditioned fear, and even think this is all the amygdala does. If they are right, then where in the brain is the basis for unconditioned fear (e.g. heights, strange places, the dark and so on)? And is the sensation of fear elicited by a learned stimulus different from the unlearned variety? If not, then why are there different parts of brain responsible for the two sorts? Or is fear located in only one area of brain, somewhere other than the amygdala, which is concerned with the learning process but not fear itself?

The amygdala, as we have seen, is also concerned in other emotionally-related situations: for example, eating and sex. The amygdala is a complex structure. As we said earlier, a more comprehensive way to describe what it does is to say that it may have the general function of labelling an experience or external event with emotional or reward-related properties. This process is critically important if a biologically and socially appropriate decision about how to respond is to be made. If this is so, we need to understand how different labels are applied to events in the amygdala. But is the recognition of such responses in others also an important function of the amygdala? The growing literature on the role of the amygdala in humans in recognising fear (and, maybe, other emotions) in others is something else to take into account. Since social interaction depends on this ability, the brain has to do it somehow.

Let us leave the amygdala for the moment, remembering that, like any other part of the brain, it is part of a system (in this case, the limbic system) and cannot do anything effectively on its own. The hypothalamus has already made an appearance in this story. Some classical experiments by Philip Bard in 1928 implicated the hypothalamus in aggression. He found that removal of the brain above the hypothalamus led to a condition in cats called 'sham rage'. They showed extreme anger and the associated physiological responses to stimuli they would ordinarily have ignored. If the hypothalamus was also removed the animals no longer exhibited 'sham rage', so this part of the brain was critical. The hypothalamus, like the amygdala, is not a simple structure. It is composed of a number of any event existing outside the group. . . . the giving of such support is in the nature of a reflex. . . the form it takes will depend upon the scale of dominant relationships within the group of animals concerned. As such it has, perhaps, no right to be called 'mutual aid', in the sense in which this term is used in describing human behaviour. . . . the 'mutual support' afforded in situations of this kind is stimulated by the same factors that produce the effects of selfishness and cruelty.

S Zuckerman. (1932) *The social life of monkeys and apes.*

(Kegan Paul, London.)

anatomically separate elements ('nuclei') and their associated nerve bundles. In 1954, WR Hess did the opposite experiment. He stimulated the hypothalamus electrically and also observed aggression in cats, but most often if the electrodes were placed in a distinct region. An aggression-centre? But lesions in another part of the hypothalamus also induced aggression. The type of aggression produced by electrical stimulation of the hypothalamus seemed to differ depending on exactly where the electrodes were positioned. In some areas, it was 'offensive', it resembled an attack. In others, it was more 'defensive'. In yet others, it looked like predation. In some parts of the hypothalamus where one lab was getting aggressive responses, others were equally confidently getting changes in sexual or maternal behaviour. Despite the temptation, nobody has been able to assign a given hypothalamic nucleus specifically to aggression. This is not, it seems, how the hypothalamus is organised. Yet, its role in aggression is intriguing. Humans with tumours or other damage in the hypothalamus can become highly aggressive. They rage at stimuli they would have previously considered only annoying (rather like those 'sham rage' cats). There have even been attempts to make lesions in certain areas of the hypothalamus as 'sedatives' in the surgical treatment of highly aggressive patients. There is no doubt that the hypothalamus is important in aggression (and fear) but if you are having trouble getting a clear picture of what exactly it does, you are not alone. Let us remind ourselves that aggression can be part of very different behaviours; this may be part of the confusion. One thing seems likely, the classical anatomical arrangement of the hypothalamus into its constituent nuclei is not a map of separable behaviours like aggression.

The story does not stop at the hypothalamus. Even deeper lies the midbrain. This has lots of different areas, one called the peri-aqueductal grey (PAG). The PAG is an area of nerve cells, and one of their functions seems to be defensive aggression. Interestingly, one of its other activities concerns pain. Damage to the PAG prevents both defensive responses to natural aggression, and defensive aggression after stimulating the hypothalamus. So it is downstream of the latter. We begin to see that a whole string of related structures in the brain are implicated in different sorts of aggression. Is there an 'aggression-system' (rather than an aggression-centre) in the brain? Is there more than one aggression-system

There's someone very close behind me, feeling his way towards the box. It's a man — I can hear the maleness of his level breathing. A grown man — I can hear the size of him. In another moment I shall feel his hands as they reach out towards the box and encounter my back instead.
I can't move. I can't breathe. An agonising electric coldness passes through my back as it senses the approach of those hands.
And at last the darkness dissolves in a flood of moonlight.
The level breathing behind me ends in a sharp, raucous gasp.
Neither of us moves. Neither of us breathes.

Michael Frayn. (2002) *Spies.* (Faber and Faber, London.)

Every vestige of control, of sense, of thought, went out of her as the room plunged into dark at the failure of power and she found herself whimpering like an idiot or a child. Animal sounds came out of her throat. She gibbered. For a moment, it was Fear itself that had her by the arms, the legs, the throat; not fear of the man, of any single menace he might present, but Fear, absolute, abstract. If the earth had opened up in fire at her feet, if a wild beast had opened its terrible mouth to receive her, she could not have been reduced to less than she was now.

Nadine Gordimer. (1978) *Is there nowhere else we can meet?*
Selected short stories. (Penguin Books, London.)

. . . She takes up her lamp and leaves, and I am plunged in an awful darkness.
I think it is a terrible thing to do to a child; I think it terrible, even now. I lie, in an agony of misery and fear, straining my ears against the silence — wide awake, sick, hungry, cold, alone, in a dark so deep the shifting black of my own eye-lids seems the brighter. . . . Now and then the great clock shifts its gears and chimes; and I draw what comfort I can from my idea that somewhere in the house walk lunatics, and with them watchful nurses. . . . Perhaps the wicked girl that sleeps next door is herself demented, and will come and throttle me with her hard hand! Indeed, no sooner has this idea risen in me, than I begin to hear the smothered sound of movement, close by — unnaturally close, they seem to me to be: I imagine a thousand skulking figures with their faces at the curtain, a thousand searching hands.

Sarah Waters. (2002) *Fingersmith.* (Virago, London.)

(to account for the different types of aggression or their role in different contexts)? Do they overlap? Does this tell us anything interesting about the use of aggression in our own society? Or what we might regard as its misuse?

The effective use of aggression requires some of the most sophisticated processing in the human brain. This is because aggression, by its very nature, usually involves interaction with other people. This nearly always occurs within a wider social group. The complexity of social interactions and signals includes the assessment of when and how aggression might pay off, the realisation that one is being attacked (or about to be attacked), devising a suitable strategy to avoid aggression or injury, learning about the circumstances in which either aggression or submission is appropriate, and whether, in fact the strategy chosen has succeeded, recruiting help when this is needed. All these complex events require equally complex neural processing. There is only one part of the brain that has this capability, the cerebral cortex.

Curiously enough, though the cortex is essential for social learning, anticipation of the consequences of behaviour and selection of an appropriate behavioural response, removal of the cortex in rats does not affect their ability to express aggression. So the basic mechanisms do not require the cortex. What it does is an effective assessment of when to use them. Various areas of the cortex are concerned with analysing different aspects of the environment: visual, auditory, tactile and so on, and constructing perceptions from this information, all important in detecting aggression, or the events that might lead to it. However, most neuroscientists would agree that the prefrontal lobes are the part of the cortex in humans responsible for decision-making, social awareness, and forming judgements. We have already considered some of the properties of the prefrontal lobes in Chapter 9. A subset of these lobes, the part lying at its base just above your eyes (and thus called the orbital cortex), is known to be concerned with emotions. Damage to the orbital cortex can make aggression more likely. The prefrontal cortex has an inhibitory influence on the expression of aggressive behaviour. There are connections from the orbital frontal cortex to both the amygdala and the hypothalamus, and both are inhibited by stimulation of the orbital cortex. This part of the brain seems, therefore, to act as a brake on aggressive behaviour. Just what is needed in a well-regulated and peaceful society.

But now a great fear is upon us, a fear not of one but of many,
A fear like birth and death, when we see birth and death alone
In a void apart. We
Are afraid in a fear which we cannot know, which we cannot face, which
none understands,
And our hearts are torn from us, our brains unskinned like the layers of
an onion, our selves are lost lost
In a final fear which none understands.

T S Eliot. (1888–1965) *Murder in the cathedral.*

The hurrying darkness, now gathering great speed, rushed up from the
East and swallowed the sky. There was a dry splitting crack of thunder
right overhead. Searing lightning smote down from the hills. The came a
blast of savage wind, and with it, mingling with its roar, there came a high
shrill shriek. The hobbits had heard just such a cry far away in the Marish
as they fled from Hobbiton, and even there in the woods of the Shire it had
frozen their blood. Out here in the waste its terror was far greater: it
pierced them with cold blades of horror and despair, stopping heart and
breath.

J R R Tolkien. (1954) *The lord of the rings.*
(George Unwin and Allen, London.)

The vertigo of fear began in his stomach and rose in a spiral to his brain.
He did not know what he was afraid of. He was not terrified by anything,
he was just in terror. It had the aspect of movement, of something rushing
at him, or in him, like a brown wind. Some alien intelligence wanted
desperately to shriek, yet knew that if it should utter a sound, it would be
lost; and wanted blindly to clutch, yet dared not move.

Lionel Trilling. (1947) *The middle of the journey.*
(Penguin Books, Harmondsworth, UK.)

Ralph screamed, a scream of fright and anger and desperation. His legs
straightened, the screams became continuous and foaming. He shot
forward, burst the thicket, was in the open, screaming, snarling, bloody.
He swung the stake and the savages tumbled over, but there were others
coming towards him, crying out.... He swung to the right, running
desperately fast, with the heart beating on his left side and the fire racing

Humans with damage to the orbital cortex become impulsive, and act without planning or taking into account the consequences of their behaviour. They are irritable and have short tempers, responding to minor provocation. During their brief outbursts of anger, they may take impulsive action and commit an aggressive act, but are usually indifferent to the consequences. The orbital cortex is where the neural process occurs that decides the time, place and strategy of response appropriate to anger induced by others. Different sub-regions of the frontal lobes may be concerned with different sorts of aggression. For example, damage to the orbital cortex has been suggested to be involved in what is termed 'disinhibited-nonaggressive' behaviour (i.e. socially inappropriate extravagant behaviour), while the part just above it may be more implicated in the expression of physical aggression. Overall, it seems likely that the prefrontal cortex plays a major part in the social regulation of aggression, and the way that aggressive interactions are used to determine social relationships.

Now back to the scenario of our play. Everything is the same as the first, real-life one, except that you 'know' you are in a play and that the man with the gun is part of it and thus not 'real'. During the second scenario, we can imagine something like the following: the temporal cortex tells 'you' that a man with a gun has come through the door, but your prefrontal cortex reminds 'you' that you are in a play, and that this was expected, and that nothing untoward will happen. The orbital frontal cortex then calms down the amygdala. So no fear, no hormonal changes (activation of the hypothalamus), no alterations in blood pressure (the brainstem). In the first, real-life, scenario, your prefrontal cortex is telling 'you' just the opposite, so your amygdala and the rest of the limbic system go on full alert. You might wonder at the apostrophes round the word 'you'. This is to indicate some state that represents your knowledge of yourself and what is going on around you at any given time. Of course, it is what your brain does, so to say that a part of your brain tells 'you' something is a bit tautological. At this point, I am going to resist any temptation to write even a word about consciousness, since anything I could say would only add to the intellectual floundering that characterises so much of the literature on that subject.

Most violent crime is committed by young men. They also tend to drive cars faster than others, and thus have a higher accident rate. Watch *forward like a tide. The ululation rose behind him and spread along, a series of short sharp cries, the sighting call. . . . He forgot his wounds, his hunger and thirst, and became fear; hopeless fear on flying feet, rushing through the forest towards the open beach. . . . He stumbled over a root and a cry that pursued him rose even higher. . . . Then he was down, rolling over and over in the warm sand, crouching with arm up to ward off, trying to cry for mercy.*

William Golding. (1958) *Lord of the flies.*
(Faber and Faber, London.)

He stopped still. Then all of a sudden, his heart began to behave strangely. Like a rocket set off, it began to leap and expand into uneven patterns of beats which showered into his brain, and he could not think. But in scattering and falling it made no noise. It shot up with great power, almost elation, and fell gently, like acrobats into nets. It began to pound profoundly, then waited irresponsibly, hitting in some sort of inward mockery first at his ribs, then against his eyes, then under his shoulder blades, and against the roof of his mouth when he tried to say "Good afternoon, madam." But he could not hear his heart — it was as quiet as ashes falling. This was rather comforting; still, it was shocking to Bowman to feel his heart beating at all.

Eudora Welty. (1998) Death of a traveling salesman.
In: *The collected stories of Eudora Welty.* (Virago, London.)

children on a playground anywhere in the world, and you will see boys rushing around, pushing each other, playing competitively, even aggressively, whereas the girls sit more quietly in a corner, engrossed in less physical games. All those who lecture to students like to show off a little. I project onto the screen a chemical structure, unlabelled, and tell them that this molecule has had more influence on the course of human history than any other. The next slide reveals the label. It is, of course, testosterone. Nobody laughs, but I go on doing it.

Sex (gender) differences exist in aggression, so is this attributable to testosterone or social construct? Many animals have restricted breeding seasons, to ensure that the considerable investment in young occurs at the best time of year — when there is enough food. Hence, lambs in the spring. In many species, there is a noticeable increase in aggression between the males in the season of maximum sexual activity. Stags lock horns, bulls bellow, tomcats squawl in the alleys and even male mice repel other males from their haystack territories. It would be difficult to ascribe these sex differences in aggression to social construction. Fighting is all part of the process of competing for a mate, and keeping her once one has been acquired. Part, that is, of reproductive behaviour, by now a familiar theme in the study of aggression. Nevertheless, experiments show that the aggressive component of sexuality in males is triggered by testosterone. But try giving the same amount of testosterone to females. You will not get nearly as good a result, though aggression may increase somewhat. So, testosterone alone is not enough, it needs a male brain to work on.

The interesting thing is that, as with sex, aggressive male brains are made and not born. Give a newborn female rat some testosterone just after birth (rats are born in a very immature state). Wait until she grows up and give her another shot of testosterone. Now she shows much more aggression when she's with other rats than 'controls' (i.e. normal female mice). Female mice that lie in the uterus closest to males (and hence, it is supposed, receive a small amount of spill-over testosterone) are more aggressive later in life than females lying between two other females. Interestingly, they attack other females, not males.

Now we recall our children in the playground; rough play is not restricted to those who have entered puberty. So male-type aggressive play in humans (which we assume is a rehearsal for real-life aggression)

The Functions of the Amygdala

The effect of amygdalectomy is to make it difficult for reinforcing stimuli, whether positive or negative, to become established or to be recognized as such.

> L Weiskrantz. (1965) Behavioural changes associated with ablation of the amygdaloid complex in moneys. *Journal of Comparative and Physiological Psychology* **49**, pp. 381–391.

Although we used to think of the amygdaloid body [amygdala] primarily as a modulator of hypothalamic activities, it is becoming increasingly more obvious that the functions of the amygdaloid body are considerably more complicated and diversified.

> L Heimer. (1981) In: *The amygdaloid complex*. Ed. Y Ben-Ari, pp. 3–9. (Elsevier/North Holland Biomedical Press, Amsterdam.)

Infant monkeys appear quite normal immediately after amygdalectomy, but they become increasingly abnormal with time. . . . They first began to exhibit difficulties in their social interactions at about 8 months of age, after which they were consistently subordinate to control monkeys.

> C I Thompson. (1981) Long-term behavioral development of rhesus onkeys after amygdalectomy in infancy. In: *The amygdaloid complex*. Ed. Y Ben-Ari, pp. 259–270. (Elsevier/North Holland Biomedical Press, Amsterdam.)

Despite impressive strides made with a simple model system approach [to studying the amygdala], there is still little contact between the study of simple Pavlovian conditioning and the complex associative processes that characterize mammalian adaptive behavior.

> M Gallagher and P C Holland. (1992) Understanding the function of the central nucleus: is simple conditioning enough? In: *The Amygdala; neurobiological aspects of emotion, memory and mental dysfunction*. Ed. J P Aggleton, pp. 307–321. (Wiley-Liss, New York.)

. . . There is general consensus that the neurons in the amygdala are necessary for the acquisition of Pavlovian fear conditioning. This. . . brings us one step closer to understanding the basic neurobiological processes underlying this important form of behavioral plasticity. And although we have made considerable progress in understanding these mechanisms, there is still much to be done before we crack the brain's almond.

> S Maren and M S Fanselow. (1999) The amygdala and fear conditioning: has the nut been cracked? *Neuron* **16**, pp. 237–240.

can occur without current levels of testosterone being high, perhaps because of testosterone experienced in the womb. Infant female monkeys whose mothers were given large amounts of testosterone during pregnancy also show masculine-type 'rough' play without being given further hormone. There are a number of rather rare clinical conditions that entail exposure of female human foetuses in the womb to excess testosterone. One is congenital adrenal hyperplasia (CAH), in which a genetic abnormality in the adrenals results in their making large amounts of testosterone. Little girls affected in this way may play in the rough-and-tumble manner so characteristic of boys. The converse is seen sometimes in males, who can have another genetic defect that prevents them responding to testosterone (lack of functional testosterone receptors). They play like girls.

However, we still have to account for the violence of young men. Can this be testosterone? If it is, why does this socially aberrant behaviour not continue throughout adult life (is that a whisper . . . 'but it does'. . . ?). Testosterone levels fall a little with age in men, but not nearly enough to account for this age-related observation. Even older men may have blood levels 10 times that of women. There are plentiful amounts of testosterone receptors in the limbic system, including the amygdala and hypothalamus, and they do not fall much with age either.

There are rumours of 'roid rage', aggressive outburst in those who take massive doses of testosterone or related steroids for (illicit) sporting purposes. There have been scientific attempts to replicate this: subjects have been given large amounts of testosterone (though only for a few weeks). Disappointingly, perhaps, for the investigators, they showed neither increased aggression nor heightened irritability. Whether differences in testosterone between normal men are related to aggression is still uncertain. In male prison inmates, testosterone was higher in those committing violent crimes, but is this cause or effect? Positive correlates have been found in adolescent boys and adult men between testosterone and a variety of aggressive behaviours by some investigators but not others.

But there is one important fact that all these studies have to take into account: aggression itself reduces testosterone in males. Not in the aggressor, but in the recipient, particularly if that recipient is defeated. On

The Amygdala in Man

It seems to be one of the main functions of temporal lobe cortex and temporal lobe limbic structures, especially the amygdala, to provide the link between the master storehouse of information laid down in the neocortex and the fundamental motivational drive mechanisms centered upon the hypothalamus.

> P Gloor. (1972) Temporal lobe epilepsy: Its possible contribution to the understanding of the functional significance of the amygdala and of its interaction with neocortical-temporal mechanisms. In: *The neurobiology of the amygdala.* Ed. B E Eleftheriou, pp. 423–457. (Plenum Press, New York.)

After the procedure of lesions of the amygdala. . . the child is very quiet and obedient. Hair-cutting is now normally possible with no difficulty, and even injections are accepted easily and with no force. . . .A visit to the department store or toy shop, taking him to the party in a friend's house, or even a trip by train are now performed with no special difficulty.

The violent behavior and destructiveness in such child cases, though not so seriously antisocial as in the adult cases because of their age, also are much calmed.

> H Narabayashi. (1972) Stereotaxic amygdalotomy. In: *The neurobiology of the amygdala.* Ed. B E Eleftheriou, pp. 459–483. (Plenum Press, New York.)

Amygdala stimulation (in humans) can evoke intense dream-like hallucinations, visceral sensations, emotions, and other mental phenomena. . . . Since most of the evoked mental phenomena are expressions of emotional tension, a parsimonious explanation for these observations is that artificial activation of the amygdala may produce emotional tension. Conversely, amygdala lesions appear clinically to reduce emotional tension. . . . These observations imply that the amygdala helps organize the discharge of emotional tension into consciousness.

> E Halgren. (1981) The amygdala contribution to emotion and memory: current studies in humans. In: *The amygdaloid complex.* Ed. Y Ben-Ari, pp. 395–408. (Elsevier/North Holland Biomedical Press, Amsterdam.)

the contrary, being aggressive successfully may increase testosterone, even winning a competitive tennis or football match. In troops of monkeys, the top-ranking males usually have higher levels of testosterone than subordinates; when the latter rise in rank, so does their testosterone. If, therefore, we try to relate individual differences in testosterone to aggression, we have to be very sure we know whether the testosterone is 'causing' the aggression or vice versa. In men, testosterone is a very sensitive index of stress, including such social stress as a demanding job, or a crisis at home. Physical stress, too, like those experienced by army recruits trying to qualify for 'elite' corps, can drop testosterone levels quite markedly. Soldiers in battle can have levels not much higher than those expected after castration; but once they go on leave, their levels rise again to normal (see Chapter 8).

Within their social groups, monkeys and humans try to optimise their social relationships. They also try to ensure that they are both predictable and controllable. This is part of the adjustment ('coping') process that each member of a social group undergoes. Once you have learned your place, and how to deal with its demands, then things are much better. Not only for you, as a person, but for your physiology. Much of our own social structure, with its laws, customs and formalities, has exactly this function: we know what to expect. We find uncertainty deeply disturbing. And we try to deal with those who would upset this arrangement. Anarchy is intolerable. Which brings us back to those violent young men. One explanation is that they are really replicating what can be seen in young baboons: the need to rise in the hierarchy by selective aggression, the need to acquire desirable objects (mates, money — a proxy for power and possessions) by competition, the process of becoming adult males. There is a more banal one. The frontal lobes are peculiar in that they do not fully mature in humans until late adolescence or even early adulthood. Perhaps, it is simply a case of too much testosterone and too little brain. Just what you always thought.

So far, our exploration of the brain in search of the aggression-centre has been a modular one. That is, we have considered the brain, mostly the limbic system, as a series of neural boxes (the orbital cortex, the amygdala, the hypothalamus and so on) each with a defined function. Even within these areas, we have wondered whether there might be sub-modules (the nuclei) that might be responsible for different bits of aggression. There is

'Over and over again during these days (the fall of Berlin in 1945)'
(a women) diarist wrote, 'I've been noticing that not only my feelings, but
those of almost all women towards men have changed. We are sorry for
them, they seem so pathetic and lacking in strength. The weakly sex.
A kind of collective disappointment among women seems to be growing
under the surface. The male-dominant Nazi world glorifying the strong
man is tottering, and with it the myth 'man''

Antony Beevor. (2002) *Berlin. The downfall 1945.*
(Viking Books, London.)

Everywhere, all in our generation, and Pao and I with them, caught in the
whirlpool of war. Some plunging into the current, joyous, eager for the
testing, shouting of flag and country and cause, dying for symbols.
Others, as young but unillusioned, seeing clearly the wasted sacrifice of
life and the greater death in the hardening of spirits to hatred, lying and
killing. We are all swirled into the current, rushed into experiences of
terror and exaltation. There is no true adventure save within oneself. No
experience has significance until one has received it and made it a part
of oneself in thought.

Han Suyin. (1974) *Destination Chungking.*
(Penguin Books, London.)

If we were to ask, what has been the most dangerous emotion of the last
two centuries, one possible answer might be: the nostalgia for
community, the yearning, in an age of mechanization and eclecticism, for
the sort of powerful sense of group identity that will enable you to hold
hands with people and sing along, your lucid individuality submerged in
the folly of collective delirium, united in a common cause, which of
course implies a common enemy.

T Parks. (2002) *Soccer: A matter of love and hate.*
New York Review of Books **49**, pp. 38–40.

Whether they are aware of it or not, the most widely shared interest of
human beings, old or young, rich or poor, the world over, must be that no
nation should attack another with nuclear weapons. There can be no one

another way, and it is important if we want to think about drugs to control unwanted or abnormal aggression.

We know the brain is an electrochemical machine. Different classes of neurons use distinct chemicals as transmitters to communicate with other neurons, and so 'encode' neural activity. We have already seen how chemical messages from outside the brain (the hormones) are involved in aggression and fear. Now, it is time to consider whether any of the new neurochemistry can shed any light on our quest. Let us begin with the amino-acid transmitters, like glutamate and GABA. These, we recall (Chapters 2 and 3), act rather like chemical switches, either exciting or inhibiting the next set of neurons in the circuit. They are found throughout the brain, so we will not expect them to play a special part in aggression because of their chemical structure; however, they might be the means of passing on special information in neural systems particularly concerned with aggression or fear.

As it happens, both glutamate and GABA have been implicated in aggression. Mice that have a genetic variation in one of the glutamate receptors (there are three main types) show large differences in aggression — though whereabouts in the brain this occurs is still a mystery. GABA is also interesting. This is because there is a class of drugs called 'benzodiazepines'. These include such familiar names as Librium and Valium, and are used to quell anxiety. Now, we can debate for hours whether anxiety is a subset of fear (eg. a lesser variant) or a separate emotion. Some would say that fear is focussed (on something) whereas anxiety is generalised. Clinicians rather spoil this idea by talking about 'phobias' such as arachnophobia, fear of spiders, as an anxiety disorder. Anyway, animals or people treated with Valium are less anxious and fearful. Benzodiazepines like Valium act by enhancing the neurotransmitter GABA (γ-amino-butyric acid). You may be surprised that a drug with such a general action (GABA is found all over the brain) has such a specific effect. Actually, benzodiazepines have other effects as well, some more understandable. For example, they are effective in the treatment of epilepsy, just what you would expect from an 'inhibitory' action. Why they reduce anxiety is still a trifle mysterious, but they are very useful and we can say that GABA plays a part in anxiety. Mice lacking the essential enzyme that makes GABA are very anxious, and *with any claim to be considered sane, who would not opt to be rid of weapons capable of destroying all civilised life. Yet in a world ruled by suspicion and fear and steered, if at all, by showmen rather than statesmen, no one seems willing to mention the existence of 40,000 warheads.*

John Peyton. (2001) *Solly Zuckerman. A scientist out of the ordinary.* (John Murray, London.)

rather non-aggressive (they also have epileptic fits). GABA infused into the amygdala dispels anxiety; a good example of how the right chemical in the right place is critical for a behavioural state. Oddly, benzodiazepines are said to increase aggression in people occasionally, perhaps because they make them less anxious about what will happen if they behave aggressively.

But what we are looking for is a neurochemical that is specially concerned with either aggression or fear. One that 'codes' one or the other (or maybe both). Let us try serotonin.

At first sight, it is not too promising. As we know, serotonin is distributed widely (though not uniformly) throughout the brain (see Chapter 3). It is only to be expected, therefore, that serotonin is involved in a wide range of psychological functions including sleep, appetite, pain perception, sexual activity, memory and mood control. In general, it seems to inhibit behaviour. But one of its characteristic effects seems to be to regulate reactivity to environmental stimuli. If serotonin activity is reduced, there is decreased impulse control and hyper-responsivity to external stimuli. Reduced levels of serotonin are typical of spontaneously aggressive rats or those that have become aggressive after a period of isolation. Genetic differences in isolation-induced aggressive behaviour in mice may be paralleled by differences in serotonin synthesis. Reducing serotonin in normal mice tends to make them more aggressive. Giving them drugs such as SSRIs, which increase serotonin action in the brain, reduces aggression. It is beginning to look more interesting. What about humans?

There have been many studies of serotonin and aggression in humans. Some have been carried out by measuring differences in the serotonin content of platelets in the blood (these have high amounts of serotonin). They are not much use, since what we need to know is what is happening to serotonin in the brain. One way to do this is to measure a metabolite of serotonin in the fluid surrounding the brain (samples can be taken by inserting a needle into the base of the vertebral column). This metabolite is called 5-HIAA, and the assumption is that lower levels in the spinal fluid means less serotonin being released in the brain. Some studies find that lower levels of 5-HIAA are typical of people with a history of impulsive, destructive behaviours, particularly when aggression and

War

. . . The French who had preached resistance to Germany for twenty years appeared to be dragged into war by the British who had for twenty years preached conciliation. Both countries went to war for that part of the peace settlement which they had long regarded as least defensible. Hitler may have projected a great war all along; yet it seems from the record that he became involved in war through launching on 29 August a diplomatic manoeuvre which he ought to have launched on 28 August.

Such were the origins of the second World war, or rather of the war between the three Western Powers over the settlement of Versailles; a war which had been implicit since the moment when the first war ended. . . . The British people resolved to defy Hitler, though they lacked the strength to undo his work. He himself came to their aid. . . . In 1941, he attacked Soviet Russia and declared war on the United States, two World Powers who asked only to be left alone. In this way, a real world war began. We still live in its shadow.

A J P Taylor. (1961) *The origins of the second world war.*
(Hamish Hamilton, London.)

Psychologists have become increasingly interested in principles drawn from biology, but are rightly distrustful of *analogies* between the behavior of particular animal species and particular human practices: there are so many animal species, and so many human cultures, that analogies to back up any thesis are always available. The resemblances of conflicts between ant colonies and international war are entirely superficial, and even the inter-group conflicts of chimpanzees lack all the defining features of international war. . . .

The factors that increase the likelihood of aggression between individuals are not the same as those that increase the likelihood of war between states; the processes are quite dissimilar. . . . an aggressive interaction between two individuals, group aggression, and the societal phenomenon of war can be described in similar words, but they differ in many respects. . . group aggression may involve individual aggressive propensities but also issues of group dynamics irrelevant to the behavior of individuals; and war involves issues of group dynamics but must be seen also as an institution with its constituent roles. . . .

The motivations that are responsible for individual aggression play little part in total war. Hope of material gain is unimportant, at any rate any rate among the combatants. . . . But aggressive motivation is seldom an important violence are involved. These include violent offenders, subjects suffering from personality disorders characterized by aggressive traits, alcoholics with aggressive behaviour while sober, normal adults acting out self-reported hostility; and children with a history of cruelty to animals or a disruptive behaviour disorder. It is important to bear in mind that low spinal fluid concentrations of 5-HIAA are found in a sizeable proportion of the normal population, so it is not a sufficient cause (i.e. by itself it does not necessarily lead to impulsive behaviour). For example, reducing serotonin in individuals with high 'trait' aggression (that is, an aggressive personality-type) makes them more angry, aggressive, annoyed and hostile whereas this procedure had no effect on individuals with low trait aggression. Other possible reasons for low serotonin include genetic variations in the enzyme that makes it (it is called tryptophan hydroxylase).

One of the more fascinating results of research on serotonin in humans is its possible role in suicide. Suicide can be viewed as an extreme form of self-aggression, sometimes highly impulsive. Low 5-HIAA has been found in people who kill themselves, or in those with a history of suicidal attempts. Since depression is a cause for many suicides, or attempts at suicide, researchers have had to be careful to separate the illness itself from the particular symptom of suicidal ideas or action. But the combination of impulsiveness and self-aggression fits in rather well with what we know about some of the actions of serotonin.

If serotonin is a neurochemical involved in aggression, what about its receptors? Perhaps the neurons responsible for aggression (if they exist) have a special type of serotonin receptor? This would interest drug companies, who would see a window for developing drugs that counter excess aggression. Drugs called 'serenics' have been developed that stimulate a type of serotonin receptor. Animals studies have shown that they inhibit offensive aggression without any interference with social functioning, adaptive defensive behaviour or other elements of normal behaviour such as sexual or eating behaviours. In aggressive patients, serenics reduce aggressive behaviour without inducing severe adverse effects or diminishing social relationships. However, we have already noted the complex relation between fear and aggression. Serenics may potentiate fear and anxiety reactions in rodents. So, their anti-aggressive effects may be secondary to an increase in anxiety, and this may limit their clinical usefulness.

issue in international war, and when it is, as at My Lai, it is often not condoned. ... International war may cause aggression, but aggressiveness does not cause war.

> R A Hinde. (1998) The psychological bases of war.
> *American Diplomacy*, 3rd electronic ed.

It is always silly to generalize, but I think it not unlikely that the aspects of this war (second World War) which will be most reflected in the poetry of the next few years is the danger that, in order to win it, the democracies will construct an anti-fascist political religion, and so, by becoming like their enemies, lose the peace.

> W H Auden. (1942) W H Auden speaks of poetry and total war.
> In: *The complete works of W H Auden prose.*
> Ed: E Mendelson. (Princeton University Press.)

In 1978, the anthropologist Carol Ember calculated that 90 percent of hunter-gatherer societies are known to engage in warfare, and 64 percent wage war at least once every two years. ... In 1972, another anthropologist, W T Divale, investigated 99 groups of hunter-gatherers from 37 cultures, and found that 68 were at war at the time, 20 had been at war five to twenty-five years before, and all the others reported warfare in the more distant past. Based on these and other ethnographic surveys, Donald Brown includes conflict, rape, revenge, jealousy, dominance, and male coalitional violence as human universals.

> Steven Pinker. (2002) *The blank slate.* (Allen Lane, London.)

This is not a book about the sociology of war, or even the psychology of war, but if we are to ask meaningful questions about the role of the brain in the phenomenon of war, we have to consider how it might differ from inter-personal aggression.

We should not assume that conflict between social groups relies on the same brain mechanisms as conflict within them. As we have seen, within-group aggression has a purpose, competition for resources that may aid survival. Between-group conflict (war in man) also determines resources, in humans, mostly land or water, though sometimes access to sexual partners. So the 'ultimate' biological factors underlying war and inter-personal aggression seem, at first sight, somewhat similar. One difference is that the 'pay-off', in terms of enhanced resources, may not benefit all members of the group equally, though there is always the chance that an overall improvement may trickle down to even the most lowly individual. But war is not waged by individuals in the expectation of personal gain, though sometimes corporate safety (e.g. from invasion) may play a part. Inter-personal conflict depends upon a specific objective (a gain, or avoiding a loss), and the exchange of information (signals) between individuals. This is not so in war. It also depends upon the adoption of a behavioural strategy (aggression) which is also not necessarily true for war. War is conflict between social groups, and has properties which are distinct from inter-personal aggression. Groups define other groups as different from them on the basis of a variety of attributes, a uniform, a nationality, a religion, an ethnic-related feature and so on. We discuss the survival value of belonging to a group in other chapters of this book, as well as the 'bonding' process necessary for one individual to form special relationships with others. This is one fundamental requirement for war: membership of one group and distinction from another, and the characterisation of an individual as worthy of attack purely on the basis of group membership. A second is the special role of leaders. We have already discussed the role of dominance hierarchies; these not only determine behaviour, particularly the allocation of resources, within a group, but also the behaviour of one group towards another. Human history shows the central role of leaders in the cause (and prevention) of war.

Where does the limbic system fit into all this? War may induce fear in individuals, so this will be one role. But that is not what we really need

I know that I shall meet my fate
Somewhere among the clouds above;
Those that I fight I do not hate,
Those that I guard I do not love;
My country is Kiltartan Cross,
My countrymen Kiltartan's poor,
No likely end could bring them loss
Or leave them happier than before.
Nor law, nor duty bade me fight,
Nor public men, nor cheering crowds,
A lonely impulse of delight
Drove to this tumult in the clouds;
I balanced all, brought all to mind,
The years to come seemed waste of breath,
A waste of breath the years behind
In balance with this life, this death.

    W B Yeats. (1869–1935) *An Irish airman foresees his death.*

The other expression was the trench expression. It looks quite daunting if
you don't know what it is. Any one of my platoon could have posed for a
propaganda poster of the Brutal Hun, but it wasn't brutality or anything
like that. It was a sort of morose disgust, and it came from living in
trenches that had bits of human bone sticking out of the walls, in freezing
weather corpses propped up on the fire step, flooded latrines.
Whatever happens to us can't be as bad as that.

    Pat Barker. (1995) *The ghost road.* (Viking Press, London.)

The writer Konstantin Simonov. . . saw a sight he would never forget. 'In
that place, there was rather thick forest on both sides of the autobahn, half
coniferous, half deciduous, already becoming green. A cross-cutting, not
wide, led through the forest on both sides of the motorway. . . (it was)
packed with something incredible: a terrible jam of cars, trucks, tanks,
armoured vehicles, ambulances, all of them not only pushed closely against
one another, but literally jammed over one another. . . . In this mess of
metal, wood and something unidentifiable was a dreadful mash of tortured
human bodies. . . . In the surrounding forest — corpses, corpses, corpses,

to know. Does the limbic system play any strategic part in war? We know very little about how the brain encodes the ideas of group cohesion and decision-making in times of corporate threat. I am going to suggest that the social regulation of war and its use as a political and economic instrument make it very likely that some of the most complex parts of the human brain, those responsible for appraisal, decision-making, social awareness, and personal and group identity are involved. Not a job for the limbic system, but for the cerebral cortex, particularly those areas (e.g. the frontal lobes) that execute such high-level social functions. If this is true, the study of the way that the limbic system regulates inter-personal aggression will not help our understanding of the role of the brain in war very much, even though its activity during war may play a large part in an individual's behaviour. Since war is a pervasive feature of human history, with obvious survival value, it is time we learnt more about how the brain determines why we go to war and when.

mixed with, I suddenly noted, ones who were still alive. There were wounded people lying on greatcoats and blankets, sitting against trees, some in bandages, others still without any. There were so many that apparently nobody had yet managed to do anything about them.'

Antony Beevor. (2002) *Berlin. The downfall 1945.*
(Viking Books, London.)

The sun hung on the lip of the horizon, filling the sky. I don't know whether it was the angle or the drifting smoke that half obscured it, but it looked enormous. The whole scene looked like something that couldn't be happening on earth, partly the sun, partly the utter lifelessness of the land around us, pitted scarred, pockmarked with stinking craters and scrawls of barbed wire. Not even birds, not even carrion feeders. Even the crows have given up. . . . We hadn't slept for four days. Tiredness like that is another world, just like noise, the noise of a bombardment, isn't like other noise. You see people wade through it, lean into it. I honestly think if the war went on for a hundred years another language would evolve, one that is capable of describing the sound of a bombardment or the buzzing of flies on a hot August day on the Somme. There are no words. There are no words for what I felt when I saw the setting sun rise.

Pat Barker. (1995) *The ghost road.* (Viking Press, London.)

The organizers of the anti-Vietnam War movement. . . . would one day believe they had failed because the war, regardless of everything, continued for ten more years. . . . I wondered how many times a country could be disowned by a vital and intelligent sector of its youth before something broke, something deep inside its structure that could never be repaired again. The systole and diastole, the radicalization and the return of cautionary thinking, the bursts of idealism followed by equally quick swerves back to skepticism and the acceptance of things as they are — how many times before memory catches up with the latest swelling of the ideal and squashes it with cynicism before it can mature? In a word, how long is freedom? Is this the way America grows, or is this the way she slowly dies? Are these spasms of birth of or death?

Arthur Miller. (1987) *Timebends. A life.*
(Harper and Row, New York.)

The soldiers sprang to their feet and charged, and simultaneously the second machine gun opened fire. . . . In the incomprehensible hurricane of bullets, the soldiers whirled and fell for half an hour. . . . The machine guns ceased, the guerrilleros ceased, and two hundred soldiers threw aside their arms and ran back to cover as a stampede of mules and donkeys rushed through them, hurling them to the ground and trampling them. The two hundred rose to their feet and Hectoro and the men and women of the village burst upon them firing revolvers into their chests from point blank range, and hacking their limbs with machetes. Coldly Hectoro dismounted and walked among the carnage, slicing the throats of all who still lived. . . .

Only fifty men of the brigade. . . escaped back to the camp. . . . Back on the field of slaughter the victors were both jubilant and appalled. Shaken, pale and trembling, they embraced each other and then wandered dumbly among the fallen.

"They were innocents," said Misael. "Look at them, they were all boys."

"Yes," said Pedro. "Little boys with mad leaders and fear in their hearts."

Louis de Bernieres. (1990) *The war of Don Emmanuel's nether parts.* (Martin Secker and Warburg, London.)

Chapter 11

The Rhythm of Life

We've set up a camera, scanning both the trees and the open country that borders them. And there is a couple of houses in the shot as well. It is a rather special camera, one of those that compresses an hour into a minute or two. We turn it on, and leave it for a few days.

 ˙Then we sit down to view the film. As we run it, the first thing we notice, of course, is the passing of the days: great sweeps of light, then dusk, then night; not actually darkness, for amongst its other properties, our camera also has a special infrared lens that allows it to record much of what goes on in the night. We cannot help being struck by this regular surge of light, then dark, then light again: not something we notice under normal conditions, but only when the whole process is so speeded up that we begin to see the pattern and recognise its cyclic nature. We watch the sun rush up from the East, pass over our heads, and sink into the West, like a great celestial tennis ball, but one that goes over an imaginary net in only one direction. Helped by the biologist friend who is watching with us, we begin to notice more. We notice that the leaves on the trees also seem to have a pattern. They move differently as the day passes, some open during the day, close at night. Just as we are beginning to feel quite pleased with our powers of observation, our biologist gently points out that a Frenchman named de Mairan, who was not even a biologist, but an accomplished astronomer, had also noticed the same thing (without using a high-tech camera) in 1729. And as we will see, his curiosity led him to do a simple, but striking experiment, which is what distinguishes his observation from all those who had noticed similar things before, going back to the ancient Greeks.

Not only the plants. We notice great scurryings amongst the animals, also at certain times of the day. Some species appear on our screen early in the morning, then disappear for the rest of the day, perhaps to reappear in the evening; others are active for most of the day, but rest at night; yet others (particularly the small, furry, edible ones) make their appearance only at night; we do not see them during the day. Each species follows a daily, private programme of activity, locked, it seems, to the passage of the sun. But each species has its own daily agenda. Our biologist points out that not all the nocturnal activity is due to edible rodents: quite a few predators seem also to have adopted a similar rhythm, perhaps to coincide with their food supply. Now we notice that the lights in the houses in view are also following a time pattern, going on in the evening, but turning off after a few hours. We watch the occupants of the houses appear each morning, go off about their business, then reappear each evening, regular as clockwork, as we say. Except that there is no clockwork around to time all this coherent, concerted, regular activity, so far as we can see. Not a clock in sight. Yet the whole world seems to pulse with a 24-hour period of activity.

Easy, you may say, every animal (and plant) simply responds to the sun, or the dark, and species differences are easily accounted for by assuming that the way they respond differs. So if you really are a furry edible creature, you do not wander about during the dangerous daylight, but sensibly respond to the onset of darkness as a 'get-up' signal, hoping that your worst enemies are just going to bed, or at least, if they do get up to hunt you, will have greater difficulty finding you. No doubt, had we asked anybody (even the most informed biologist) in 1729 that very question, that is the sort of answer we would have gotten. Except that de Mairan decided to do something which we like to think of as very modern: test the idea by doing an experiment. He had been watching mimosa, a plant whose leaves open during the day, but close at night. De Mairan took a mimosa and put it in a dark cupboard. Let us suppose we have 10 eminent 18th century biologists standing by. Ask them what they think will happen over the next few days to de Mairan's plants in the dark cupboard. It is a good bet that they would tell you the plant's leaves would stop moving. I rather suspect you might give the same answer. It makes sense; there is no stimulus, hence no response. Wrong. The leaves continued to open and close just as if the sun had risen; that is, as if they were in the garden. Actually, if you look very

Daily Rhythms

There is virtually neither tissue nor function that does not manifest regular changes from day to night. These diverse rhythms usually maintain distinct phase relationships to each other as well as to the entraining zeitgebers. Together, they represent a high degree of temporal order.

> J Aschoff. (1979) Circadian rhythms: General features
> and endocrinological aspects. In: *Endocrine rhythms*.
> Ed. D T Krieger, pp. 1–61. (Raven Press, New York.)

The beat of biology has been clear to Man for hundreds of thousands of years. More than three hundred years before the birth of Christ, Aristotle noted the swelling of the ovaries of sea urchins at full Moon. Hippocrates observed daily fluctuations in the symptoms of some of his patients and thought that regularity was a sign of good health. Cicero mentioned that the flesh of oysters waxed and waned with the Moon, an observation later confirmed by Pliny. However, the recognition that this behaviour was driven by an internal process rather than being a direct response to sunlight, darkness and other environmental factors, did not come until many centuries later. Today biologists regard these beats and rhythms as being the most conspicuous features of natural ecosystems.

> P Coveney and R Highfield. (1990) *The arrow of time*.
> (W H Allen, London.)

The great majority of plants and animals, invertebrate and vertebrate, have evolved, as part of their innate organization, oscillating systems whose periods are a close match to one, or more, of the major physical cycles in the environment. These oscillations with circa*dian,* circa*tidal,* circa*lunar* or circa*nnual* periods are clock-like in several respects: their periodicity is remarkably stable and homeostatically conserved in the face of environmental change; and they are readily entrained by some environmental cycle (especially the light/dark cycle in the circadian case) that not only imposes its own frequency (as zeitgeber) on the internal clock-oscillator but phases it appropriately to local time.

> C S Pittendrigh. (1981) Circadian organization and the
> photoperiodic phenomena. In: *Biological clocks in seasonal*
> *reproduction.* Eds. B K and D E Follett, pp. 1–35. (Wright, Bristol.)

carefully (it took someone else to realise this) they open and close round about 24 hours.

Animals do the same. Your pet hamster will wake up and start running in the wheel you have kindly provided for him every night at about the same time. Put him into continuous darkness, and he continues to do something very similar, though now his timing will be slightly off every day. If you measure his rhythm, you will see that, perhaps, he now begins to run every 22.5 hours (instead of 24). Borrow next door's hamster, and he will also continue to run when you put him into prolonged darkness, but this one has a rhythm of, say, 24.8 hours. So animals, like plants, do not need a daily signal to tell them when to get moving (or to go to sleep). They have an internal clock, but a clock that needs the sun (or some external event) to keep it running at 24 hours to synchronise it. But each clock is slightly different. Your electric clock at home also has an internal mechanism that keeps it going; you regulate it by changing its hands and, on some models, it is synchronised with 'external' time (i.e. the sun) by a radio signal. The distinction between generating a daily rhythm and synchronising it is important.

You can show the difference by having not one or two, but a whole room of hamsters, all running on their individual wheels. The room is in dim red light (i.e. effectively dark). Each hamster begins its daily running bout at slightly different times, because their clocks are all slightly different, as we have seen. In scientific parlance, they are said to be 'free-running', that is, their activity is unconstrained by a synchronising stimulus. Eventually, there will always be at least one hamster running, while others sleep, since they will get out of phase with one another. Now turn on the lights for about 10 minutes once per day, say at 8 am your time. Within a few days, all the hamsters are now starting their running activity at about the same time, and the interval between running bouts is now 24 hours exactly. They are synchronised. If you were to turn on the light every 23 hours, then your hamsters would run every 23 hours, their 'day' would now be 23 hours, not 24. Similarly for lights turned on every 25 hours. Interestingly, there's a limit to this: try a 30 hour or a 20 hour 'day' and it doesn't work: the hamster's internal clock cannot deviate too far from 24 hours.

But you do not need to turn on the light everyday. A light stimulus every second or third day is just as good. This shows us one of the

"The sleep-compelling centre can be likened to a faithful watchman. From his post in the stem of the brain he perceives the giving way of the waking activity of the roof-brain [cortex]; wisely then he extinguishes the lights and draws the curtain for the good repose which shall restore his master"

Bremer quoted by C S Sherrington. (1940) *Man on his nature.*
(Penguin Books, London.)

Circadian timing refers to the ability of an organism deprived of external temporal cues to express physiological and behavioural rhythms with a period of approximately 24 hours. This endogenous capacity to anticipate and thereby synchronize with changes in the outside world is of fundamental adaptive value, matching internal physiology to external cycles.

M H Hastings. (2000) Circadian clockwork: Two loops are better than one. Nature Reviews. *Neuroscience* **1**, pp. 143–146.

Defining the molecular basis of circadian timing in mammals has profound implications. . . . The circadian system is among the most tractable models for providing a complete understanding of the cellular and molecular events connecting genes to behaviour. . . . Understanding the molecular clock could increase our knowledge of how gene mutations contribute to psychopathology (for example major depression and seasonal affective disorder). . . [and] lead to new strategies of pharmacological manipulations of the human clock to improve the treatment of jet lag and ailments affecting shift workers, and of clock-related sleep and psychiatric disorders.

S M Reppert and D R Weaver. (2002) Coordination of circadian timing in mammals. *Nature* **418**, pp. 935–941.

advantages of having an internal clock, rather then depending solely on an external stimulus. You do not have to receive the stimulus every day. Useful if you live in a burrow. What is more, you can anticipate the stimulus if you have an internal clock. Hamsters do this: keep them on 12 hours of light, followed by 12 hours of darkness (a sort of artificial spring day) and they start to run just before the lights go out (remember they are nocturnal). Useful if you have to be somewhere before something else has happened. Your alarm clock has gone off.

If our camera were to be set up over a small town, we would quickly see that humans, too, show marked and reliable 24 hour rhythms. A great surge of activity at around 8 am, a peak in electricity use, then the usual traffic jams. Another peak of activity around 1 pm, and again at 5–6 pm, a different period of behaviour in the early evening, and so to bed. Put a human into a bunker, or a mine shaft, cut off from all contact with the rest of the world, something that was a popular experimental approach in the 1980s. The conditions of these experiments varied a bit, but in general the subjects could sleep, wake, eat, and read whenever they felt like it. Sometimes they could put a light on or off when they wanted; but more often they were kept on dim light which did not vary. The important point was that they had no access to external cues about time, or any idea whether it was day or night outside. And what do you observe? The emergence of the human clock, just as in hamsters. The subjects showed a regular alternation of activity and sleep. If you measured the period of this rhythm, it would be around (but not exactly) 24 hours. About a day, or 'circadian' as it is called. Some people, like hamsters, have clock rhythms that were less than 24 hours, others slightly longer. But not too much. Nobody has a 36 hour rhythm. Somewhere inside the body, a clock is ticking.

Though we have focussed on awakening and sleeping, in fact the 24 hour rhythm is made up of much more than this. All animals, including humans, have a daily body programme that follows a remarkably consistent pattern. The day (or night) is full of different bodily events, all in the right sequence, and happening at the right time. In some cases, for example, the digestive processes that follow a meal, the sequence of events depend upon each other, rather than upon an external synchronising signal. In others, there is a direct link between the

But at my back I always hear
Time's winged chariot hurrying near;
And yonder all before us lie
Deserts of vast eternity.
Thy beauty shall no more be found,
Nor, in thy marble vault, shall sound
My echoing song: then worms shall try
That long-preserved virginity,
And you quaint honor turn to dust,
And into ashes all my lust:
The grave's a fine and private place,
But none, I think, do there embrace.

Andrew Marvell. (1621–1678).

That night, in the grove of trees, seemed to her sense of subjective time —
her private time — to crawl by with intolerable slowness. The refusal of
the earth to turn faster, to bring the light round to this corner of Africa, to
initiate civil time once more, seemed to her almost a personal insult.
And in the dense blackness of that interminable night, she was highly
conscious of the clock-like systems in her own body. The beat of her
heart, the inflation and deflation of her lungs. But she knows now that our
sense of private time is not formed by the pulsing heart or the breathing
lungs but by the neural impulses of our brain.
A neuron transmits a pulse at about fifty times a second, and the impulse
travels down the branching tree of the nervous system at a speed of
approximately fifty metres a second. This neural timekeeper is never at
rest for an instant; throughout our entire life the neural race never
quickens or slows. Its regularity and constancy fulfill all the requirements
for the definition of a clock.
If this is indeed how our sense of personal time originates. . . . then one
intriguing consequence of the theory is that other primates — whose
neural impulses function identically to ours — should have a similar
sensation of personal time also.

William Boyd. (1990) *Brazzaville beach.*
(Sinclair-Stevenson, London.)

synchronising signal (the sun). This means that different events must have a different lead time. If your lunch is linked to sunrise, then your body has to have some means of assessing the passage of time, so that lunch occurs at lunch-time, not earlier. Many animals can do this; for example, you can train an animal to come for food at a certain time of day. The animal has no watch, but its internal clock tells it, in some way, when the time is right. If you move that animal across several time zones (say, take it from the UK to the US), then it will appear for food at the 'right' British time on its first day, gradually adjusting its internal clock so that, after a few days, it now arrives at the right local time. This implies, of course, that animals (and humans) can measure the passage of time quite accurately without looking at an external clock, a topic we will return to later.

Behaviour, important though it is, is not the only thing that follows a daily rhythm. Practically everything else in the human body does as well. Some hormones (like cortisol) surge in the morning, but drop in the evening: others rise during sleep. Enzymes rise and fall as the day passes: some people find they cannot drink nearly as much alcohol during the day as in the evening. Their liver enzymes that break down alcohol have a marked circadian rhythm. Drugs may have more prolonged actions at different times of the day, a fact which is still not used much in medicine. Your body temperature is higher in the evening; your blood pressure and heart rate show a similar rhythm. Your brain functions a little better at certain times of the day. All will change if you fly to New York from London, and re-synchronise your body to the new external signal. And if you were to spend time in that bunker, cut off from the rest of the world, some of your rhythms would stay in synch with each other, showing they were linked in some way; others would go off on their on their own, still with a circadian pattern but a different period. After you fly back from that great week in New York, you feel dreadful for a few days. Not just because you are back to everyday life, but because your rhythms are, for a while, desynchronised both from the external signal (day) and from each other. Disturbed rhythms are bad for your sense of well-being. They may also be bad for your health, a matter of concern to those who work night shifts, or those whose job takes them across time zones regularly, for example, air hostesses.

Thomasina: When you stir your rice pudding, Septimus, the spoonful of jam spreads itself round making red trails like the picture of a meteor in my astronomical atlas. But if you stir backward, the jam will not come together again. Indeed, the pudding does not notice and continues to turn pink just as before. Do you think this is odd?

Septimus: No

Thomasina: Well, I do. You cannot stir things apart.

Septimus: No more you can, time must needs run backward, and since it will not, we must stir our way onward mixing as we go, disorder out of disorder into disorder until pink is complete, unchanging and unchangeable, and we are done with it for ever. This is known as free will or self-determination.

Tom Stoppard. (1999) *Arcadia*. (Faber and Faber, London.)

You can easily see that this daily programme, synchronised to an external signal, is hugely important for survival. Every animal needs to relate the workings of its body, and what it does, to the passing of the day. We have already seen that edible species need a rhythm that delays their becoming a meal, but there are many other reasons why internal and external events should be synchronised. It is not just individually important; since social interaction and co-operation is a vital part of successful survival, the fact that all the members of a group are doing similar things at about the same time is essential for a co-ordinated social strategy. Animals need to go to drink together, so that they can improve their corporate awareness of danger. You need to arrive at the office with the others, so that you can work together, more effectively than working alone. For much of the time, the external environment is highly predictable, so the daily rhythm of most animals (and people) is equally predictable. Nobody has managed to abolish the daily rush-hour. Our friend the biologist knows this, so he is able to find the animals he is currently watching in the forest more often than not. He knows where they might be and what they will be doing at each time of the day. Not by external clock time, but by biological time. You know this as well: though you may like to think of yourself as a free spirit, your days are mostly predictable. If they become unpredictable (something unexpected happens), then we are into demand or stress, and a different set of defence mechanisms, a subject we discuss more fully elsewhere in this book (Chapter 4). So where do we look for the master clock, the clock that sets up this rhythm for survival? In the limbic brain, of course.

Of course, you say: but where? Since the limbic system controls eating, drinking, hormones, the cardiovascular system and many other elements make up the daily programme, it seems likely that the clock, if there is just one, might also be somewhere in this part of the brain. Let us focus a bit more: the hypothalamus is the part of the limbic system that monitors the internal environment, and thus the daily surges of physiological activity. So perhaps we should look in the hypothalamus. Despite what now may seem rather obvious, it was not until 1972 Friedrich Stephan and Irv Zucker, working in the US, did the essential experiment: they found the clock.

Time present and time past
Are both perhaps present in time future,
And time future contained in time past.
If all time is eternally present
All time is unredeemable.

. . .

Time past and time future
Allow but a little consciousness.
To be conscious is not to be in time
But only in time can the moment in the rose-garden,
The moment in the arbour where the rain beat,
The moment in the draughty church at smokefall
Be remembered; involved with past and future.
Only through time time is conquered.

T S Eliot. (1944) *Burnt Norton.*
(Faber and Faber, London.)

And the rhythm of life is a powerful beat
Puts a tingle in your fingers and a tingle in your feet
Rhythm in the playroom, rhythm in the street
Yeah the rhythm of life is a powerful beat

To feel the rhythm of life,
To feel the powerful beat,
To feel the tingle in your fingers,
To feel the tingle in your life

Flip your wings and fly to daddy
Take a dive and swim to daddy
Hit the floor and crawl to daddy

Cy Colman and Dorothy Fields. (1966)
The rhythm of life. From: Sweet Charity

Time is to clock as mind is to brain. The clock or watch somehow contains the time. And yet time refuses to be bottled up like a genie stuffed in a lamp. Whether it flows as sand or turns on wheels within wheels, time escapes irretrievably, while we watch. Even when the bulbs of the

The nerves from the two eyes pass back towards the brain. Just under the hypothalamus they meet, and many of the nerve fibres cross over. This is a neural junction, called the 'optic chiasm'. In the overlying hypothalamus lie two little balls of nerve cells (one each side). So they are called the 'suprachiasmatic nuclei' (the nuclei that lie above the chiasm). Quite a mouthful, so most scientists abbreviate them to 'SCN'. Stephan and Zucker knew that some of the nerve fibres from the eyes seemed to end in the SCN. They also knew that light (i.e. sunlight) was the most important synchronising signal for circadian rhythms. Was this where light signals regulated the clock? Or was it the clock itself? They did a classical experiment, by destroying the two little nuclei, and the clock stopped.

Two things happened. The first was that the rats with damaged SCN no longer showed the normal daily pattern of activity or drinking behaviour. They did not stop either behaviour. It just became scattered throughout the day and night, rather than showing the usual regular pattern. So the internal system was no longer in synch with the external signals. This would be very bad news indeed in the real world. But there was more. If they put their SCN-damaged rats into constant dark (or dim red light, the two seem essentially the same) then these rats had no predictable, regular, period of drinking or activity. Normal rats, of course, would all be going off on their own, individual, circadian rhythm. So damaging the SCN not only prevented synchronization, it also seemed to destroy the internal clock itself. The animal had lost the ability to be rhythmic. It was, to use an over-worked term, a breakthrough.

In the intervening years, a mass of experiments has confirmed the essential truth of the original finding. The SCN is the clock (or, at least, a clock). It behaves like one: its neurons fire during the day, not at night (it itself has a rhythm). The firing pattern in reset by light, in the way you would expect. One of the most dramatic ways to show that the SCN is the clock is to transplant it from one animal to another. Recall that each individual hamster (or rat, or any other animal) has its own individual periodicity (the rate at which its clock runs), which is only revealed when it 'free-runs' in constant darkness or dim red light. Now, take a hamster with a 24.6 hours period, and remove its SCN. Then graft an SCN from another hamster, but in this case one with a period of, say, 22.2 hours. You have guessed it: the recipient adopts the running period of the donor.

hourglass shatter, when darkness withholds the shadow from the sundial, when the mainspring winds down so far that the clock hands hold still as death, time itself keeps on. . . . Timepieces don't really keep time. They just keep up with it, if they are able.

Dava Sobell. (1996) *Longitude.*
(Fourth Estate, London.)

If you look inside your old-fashioned clock, you will see a mass of wheels, cogs and a spring. This is how it measures time. But look inside a modern electronic clock, and you'll see a very different design: transistors, a chip, and a battery, perhaps. Two pieces of equipment doing the same thing, but using completely different methods. Mechanical and electrical clocks are analogous, not homologous. They have a similar function, but a different form. Both, however, have three essential properties: a means of generating a precise time interval (a swing of the pendulum, an electronic pulse), a method for adding such intervals into larger intervals which can be transmitted as information (hands, LED numerals) and the ability to be synchronised with an external standard (eg. Greenwich mean time). Our knowledge of the brain excludes the expectation that we will find either cogs or transistors in the SCN. So how does it keep time?

The SCN uses biological means to achieve similar results to mechanical or electronic clocks. It all depends on the expression of genes, one of which is called *period*. Genes themselves do not do anything. They can only have an influence on the body by being activated ('expressed'). When they are expressed, they produce (via an intermediate molecule mRNA) one or more proteins. It is the proteins that do the job. The SCN produces the *period* protein (conventionally called PERIOD) by activating the *period* gene (and other genes, but the principle is the same). The trick is to regulate the expression of *period* so that levels of the protein PERIOD rise and fall inside the cells of the SCN with an interval of about 24 hours. This gives the basic oscillation, which we would expect to vary between animals of the same species (thus generating the different 'free-running' rhythms), but be rather constant within an individual. PERIOD (and associated proteins) is generated by a system of negative and positive feedback. Negative feedback means that as the cell produces more PERIOD in light, the protein itself inhibits the expression of its own gene (*period*). This, by itself, will produce an oscillation. As PERIOD goes up, *period* is inhibited: as *period* is turned off, PERIOD will go down (it's now dark), thus liberating *period* to make more PERIOD and so on. By now, your eyes are watering somewhat; but remember that *period* is the gene, and PERIOD is the product of the gene. However, this simple negative feedback (inhibition) is not stable enough nor does it

Nothing better than moderate sleep, nothing worse than it, if it be in extremes, or unseasonably used. It is a received opinion, that a melancholy man cannot sleep overmuch; excessive sleep is good, as an only antidote, and nothing offends them more, or causeth this malady sooner, than waking; yet in some cases sleep may do more harm than good in that phlegmatick, swinish, cold, and sluggish melancholy. . . that thinks of waters, sighing most part. . . . But, as I have said, waking overmuch is both a symptom and an ordinary cause.

R Burton. *The anatomy of melancholy.*

As you grow older, sleep somehow becomes thinner, as if the fabric of unconsciousness itself is becoming stretched and febrile; you don't go down as far or for so long; as if the permanent period of rest in the rapidly approaching future is already exerting its effect, in the way that one recovers reserves of energy as soon as the end of a boring film or dinner party finally heaves into sight. Sleep is a bank account that you put capital in when you are young and draw on as you get older; and then you run out of capital and die.

John Lanchester. (2000) *Mr Phillips.* (Faber and Faber, London.)

To sleep was so important! To lie there on one's belly, to cover one's back and just sleep. When you were asleep, you didn't spend your strength nor torment your heart — and meanwhile your sentence was passing, passing. When our life crackles and sparks like a torch, we curse the necessity of spending eight hours uselessly in sleep. When we have been deprived of everything, when we have been deprived of hope, then, bless you, fourteen hours of sleep!

Alexander Solzhenitsyn. (1974) *The Gulag archipelago.*
(Fontana, London.)

Well, naturally, we finally get around to torch songs, as guys who are singing in quartet are bound to do, especially at four o'clock in the morning, a torch song. . . which guys sing when they have a big burnt-up feeling inside themselves over a battle with their dolls.

When a guy has a battle with his doll, such as his sweetheart, or even his ever-loving wife, he certainly feels burnt up inside himself, and can have the right temporal qualities by itself to generate a circadian rhythm. The SCN cell needs a second, positive loop: one in which PERIOD activates other genes (one is called *clock*) which produce another protein (CLOCK) that increases the expression of *period*. Basically, it's as if the SCN cells have two sets of wheels, one raising the level of the 'output' proteins (PERIOD etc.), the other decreasing it. The two, of course, have to work 180° out of phase; a fail-safe mechanism. The net result is a circadian oscillation in PERIOD and associated proteins. In some way, the few thousand nerve cells in the SCN are coupled, that is, they all oscillate together. If they did not, there would be no clock. So the clock is running. We do not need a battery or a spring, because the normal metabolic machinery found within any cell supplies the energy. But animals with mutations in one or more of these genes have abnormal biological clocks and so do humans. One wonders if people who naturally get up early in the morning have slightly different genes in their SCN from those who like to sleep late.

The next problem is to synchronise the clock with the external world. As we have already seen, a light pulse given at the right time can synchronise the biological clock. Many years ago, neuroanatomists showed that some of the nerve fibres from the retina ended up in the SCN (and perhaps nowhere else in the hypothalamus). They come from special cells in the retina, different from those you use for vision. If these fibres are cut, the clock is no longer synchronised. The animal 'free-runs' as if it were in the dark. But exactly how a pulse of light alters the molecular machinery (*period* etc.) is still not really understood. But at least we know where to look: how changes in the activity of the nerve fibres from the eye entering the SCN alter the oscillations going on in its cells. Neither do we really understand why the light pulse has to arrive at the right time to be effective, though this is clearly biologically important.

Now we come to the question of how the clock in the SCN communicates its information to the rest of the brain. In our world, we 'read' our clocks by looking at the hands of the clock, or the illuminated LED figures. No hands or figures in the SCN. Now, the SCN does not itself control eating or drinking or sleeping or hormones or activity or any of the others behaviours and physiological events that we know form part of the daily programme. Many of these are, of course, the responsibility of other areas *scarcely think of anything much. In fact, I know guys who are carrying the torch to walk ten miles and never know they go an inch. . . everyone knows that at four o'clock in the morning the torch is hotter than at any other time of the day.*

Damon Runyon. (1956) *Guys and dolls.*
(Penguin Books, London.)

of the hypothalamus. But these parts need access to the time information being generated by the SCN. The obvious answer is that should be a great leash of nerve fibres leaving the SCN, carrying this information to the areas that need it. The strange thing is that there isn't. When you track the nerves leaving the SCN (and there are rather good ways of doing this), there seem to be very few. One explanation might be that there is a relay centre: the SCN sends its information to a single centre, which then distributes it as required. This is a possible scenario, for the sparse nerve fibres leaving the SCN make their way toward another group of cells in the hypothalamus, the paraventricular nucleus. This nucleus, which we discussed in more detail in Chapter 4, is an important one for adaptation. It has direct connections to the centres in the brain controlling the autonomic nervous system (hence blood pressure, heart rate and so on), a role in eating behaviour, and is an important regulator of the pituitary. In particular, it controls the release of a pituitary hormone called ACTH, which in turn acts on the adrenal glands to make them secrete cortisol. Cortisol, an essential hormone, has a very marked circadian rhythm: as we have seen, your blood levels are highest around the time you get up, but fade away to very low levels twelve hours later. If you fly to New York from London, your cortisol rhythm is amongst the last to adapt; so its also its very stable. There is some evidence that, amongst its other functions, the cortisol rhythm sends out circadian information to the other tissues of the body; they know what time of the day it is by the current level of cortisol.

But there is another possible way for the SCN to signal the time of day to other parts of the brain. About 10 years ago, an experiment was done in which in the SCN was enclosed in a sort of plastic bag. Nerve fibres could not get through, but chemicals could. Such animals still had intact rhythms. So it looked as if the SCN communicated with other parts of the brain by secreting a chemical, rather like a hormone-producing gland, instead of the more conventional method of sending signals down nerve fibres. Very recently, a protein has been identified which might actually do the job (it is called prokineticin 2). So the SCN could be a little hormone-producing gland in the brain, its message being 'time of day.' Recall that the hypothalamus contains groups of nerve cells that are well-known to produce hormones that enter the blood stream (e.g. oxytocin),

Seasonal Rhythms

Evolution has taken place in an environment subject to regular and cyclic fluctuations both of short duration, such as the diurnal cycle of night and day, and of much longer periodicities, as exemplified by the changing seasons. It is not surprising therefore that the survival of a species has required it to adapt many of its physiological processes to these cyclic phenomena, and, in particular, that reproduction be synchronized so as to ensure the maximal survival chances for both parents and offspring. Natural selection will strongly favour those individuals producing offspring at the most propitious season. . . . Such a differential survival rate will rapidly define the characteristic breeding season of any particular species. . . (and) has resulted in the establishment of annual breeding seasons.

> B Lofts, B K Follett, and R K Murton. (1982) Temporal changes in the pituitary-gonadal axis. *Memoirs of the Society for Endocrinology* **18**, pp. 545–575.

Although as students of the pineal gland we have long been struck by the rhythmicity of melatonin synthesis, we have only recently begun to appreciate the functional importance of this feature. In none of the physiological effects of pineal secretion is the significance of rhythmicity so apparent as in the photoperiodic control of seasonal reproduction in mammals. Studies in both a long- and short-day breeder now indicate that a particular characteristic of this rhythm — the duration of nightly melatonin secretion — determines whether reproduction is induced or suppressed.

> E L Bittman. (1985) The role of rhythms in the response to melatonin. *Ciba Foundation Symposium* **117**, pp. 149–169.

The central problem of how to time the days and the seasons of the year is well illustrated in Ph. Galle's engraving *The Triumph of Time,* . . . Father Time, represented by Saturn, is seen as the central figure, eating his child — a reminder of the destructive nature of time. In his left hand he holds aloft a serpent, biting its tail, an illustration of the endless cycles of time. Saturn is riding in a chariot which also carries the globe, encircled by the signs of the zodiac, representing the motion of the stars in our firmament, against which man has always measured time. The chariot is drawn by two horses, one bearing the symbol of the Sun, and one the Moon.

> R V Short. (1985) Photoperiodism, melatonin and the pineal: It's only a question of time. *Ciba Foundation Symposium* **117**, pp. 1–8.

as well as special nerve-cells that regulate the pituitary by secreting peptides, and that, in a way, all nerve cells are really hormone-producers, in that they release chemicals (transmitters) that act on the next neuron in line. So if the SCN really does transmit its time message to other parts of the brain by releasing a local hormone, this would not be too novel. But the story does not end there. All the cells in the body have the same complement of genes, but certain tissues express a particular set of genes (hence the difference between, say, the liver and the kidney). Now, the curious fact is that the *period* gene may be active not only in the SCN, but also in peripheral tissues, such as liver etc. This may indicate that they have their own clocks, perhaps 'slave' clocks that are controlled by the 'master' clock in the SCN. Since there could be different time lags between the 'slave' and 'master' clocks in different tissues, you can see how this could produce the daily circadian programme.

The daily sleep cycle is the most obvious way that animals and people divide their day up. Many of those working on sleep treat it as a distinct feature of daily life. But sleep is only part of the daily programme, and it is closely bound up with other daily changes such as hormones, metabolism, and social activity. Nevertheless, the question 'why do we sleep' can be broken down to two sub-questions: why do we need to sleep? And, why do we sleep when we do?

The first is still a puzzle, despite decades of research and generations of poetic, philosophical and even religious speculation. The fact that we really cannot say with precision why most of us spends about a third of our lives in dormancy is a hint that we need to retain our modesty about how the brain works. It is widely assumed that there is some homeostatic function related to sleep. After all, if you do not sleep, you show all the signs of a 'need'. You 'need' to fall asleep, and this need takes priority over any thing else — though, of course, in extreme conditions, sleep can and must be relegated. And if you are deprived of sleep, your brain will begin to malfunction. You become miserable, you cannot think with your usual rapidity and clarity, you may become confused, and eventually you may even begin to have hallucinations. Sleep is essential. Every interrogator knows this, which is why sleep deprivation is a favourite method of breaking down the resistance of prisoners. Much effort has been put into defining exactly why the brain needs to sleep. They include ideas that the brain

Although humans consider themselves to be largely independent of the seasons, there is now a great deal of evidence for seasonal rhythms in psychological dimensions, emotional states, and physiological, neurochemical and hormonal measures.   Patients with seasonal affective disorder (SAD) show an exaggerated seasonality: this has been defined as two or more consecutive depressive episodes in autumn or winter with remission the following spring or summer. . . . Patients experience atypical symptoms such as hypersomnia and fatigue, and changes in eating patterns are a dominant part of the clinical picture.

K Krauchi and A Wirz-Justice. (1988) The four seasons: Food intake frequency in seasonal affective disorder in the course of a year. *Psychiatry Research* **25**, pp. 323–338.

may accumulate some substance (a 'sleep-inducing peptide' was popular for a while), or may need to get rid of excess memories (like deleting those files in your computer to make room for more), or solidify those memories that you need to retain (Aldous Huxley wrote a famous novel in which children had little loudspeakers under their pillows that taught them things while they slept). Anyway, the longer you stay awake, the more likely you are to sleep, though what you do depends on a second set of factors, including whether there is anything interesting or arousing going on at the time. Which is presumably why I see the occasional student nodding off in my supposedly fascinating lectures. The accumulating sleep debt is sometimes called the 'S process'.

The second question (when do we sleep?) is easier to answer. The circadian clock in the SCN sends a signal to the sleep mechanisms. This is sometimes called the 'C process'; when the two processes coincide (ie. you have a sufficient debt and it's night) you are very likely to sleep. So damage to the SCN, as we have seen, disturbs the timing of sleep but not its amount. Every parent knows that small babies do not show much of a sleep rhythm, though they sleep quite a lot. As they grow older, their sleep solidifies into the adult pattern of about 8 hours during the night. In the very old, the pattern may begin to break down again. This is thought to be due to the maturation and subsequent degeneration of the SCN.

It is long been known that the hypothalamus, that homeostatic regulator, is important for sleep. Damage it, and sleep is very disturbed. Recently, a peptide called either orexin (there are two), or, better, hypocretin, has been discovered in the hypothalamus. Initially these peptides were thought to be important for eating, and indeed they do increase food intake (Chapter 5), but their more interesting function is as a sleep regulator. Humans, mice or dogs that lack the hypocretin receptor have narcolepsy: they cannot stay awake, and fall asleep quite suddenly at any time. The nerve fibres containing hypocretin connect with a number of other neurons in the brainstem, particularly those containing noradrenaline and serotonin. It has long been know that these systems (the amines, see Chapter 3) have a widespread distribution in the brain, just what you would expect if they controlled general functions like wakefulness. So we may be beginning to unravel how the brain sleeps (or wakes) even if the 'why' is still rather elusive.

We need to recognise that the soul is really joined to the whole body, and that we cannot properly say that it exists in any part of the body to the exclusion of the others. . . nevertheless there is a certain part of the body, where it exercises its functions more completely than in all the others. . . . I think I have clearly established that the part of the body in which the soul directly exercises its functions is not the heart at all, or the whole of the brain. It is rather the innermost part of the brain, which is a certain very small gland [the pineal] situated in the middle of the brain's substance.

R Descartes. (1649) The passions of the soul. In: *The philosophical writings of Descartes*, Vol 1. Translated by J Cottingham, R Stoothoff, and D Murdoch. (Cambridge University Press, Cambridge.)

The year was old, that day. The patient year had lived through the reproaches and misuses of its slanderers, and faithfully performed its work. Spring, summer, autumn, winter. It had laboured through the destined round, and now laid down its weary head to die. Shut out from hope, high impulse, active happiness itself, but messenger of many joys to others, it made appeal in its decline to have its toiling days and patient hours remembered, and to die in peace.

Charles Dickens. *The chimes.*

The sky turns day to night with a sunset, measures the passing months by the phases of the moon, and marks each season's change with a solstice or an equinox. The rotating, revolving Earth is a cog in a clockwork universe, and people have told time by its motion since time began.

Dava Sobell. (1996) *Longitude.* (Fourth Estate, London.)

I sit beside the fire and think
Of all that I have seen,
Of meadow-flowers and butterflies
In summers that have been;
Of yellow leaves and gossamer
In autumns that there were,
With morning mist and silver sun
And wind upon my hair.

Our biologist friend, who has been quiet during all this talk of molecular clocks and hypothalamic chemicals, now points out that we have assumed that 'day' means the same throughout the year, when, as we all know, the dawn gets earlier as spring and summer advance, and dusk later, the whole process reversing during autumn and winter. For example, in Cambridge the longest day of the year (June 21st) lasts 16 hours and 46 minutes, whereas the shortest (Dec 21st) only 7 hours 43 minutes. The further you are from the equator (which has a constant 12 hours of daylight), the bigger the annual variation. But everywhere, daylength is 12 hours on two days of the year (21st of March and September). It is obvious that the SCN circadian clock has to adapt to these changes; no good a diurnal animal assuming that dawn always happens at the same time. In fact, there is good evidence that the onset of light (and, in some cases, the onset of darkness) can alter the timing of the SCN clock. But the biologist also points out that there is quite another rhythm, the yearly one. The days get longer and longer in the first half of the year, then progressively shorter and shorter during the second (in the Northern hemisphere). If you were to draw this out on piece of paper, you would see a perfect annual rhythm. Does this matter, we ask? The biologist suppresses a smile, but instead points to a field not far away: we see lambs gambolling about. It is February: the biologist asks us if we have ever seen lambs in September. We have not.

The biologist points out that, in countries appreciably distant from the Equator, the young of nearly all wild species are born in the spring. The reason is obvious: reproduction, a biologically and socially expensive and risky business (we talk more about this in Chapter 8) needs the very best conditions to ensure that the young survive. Most animals cannot afford to breed throughout the year. They have to 'choose' the best season. That is spring and early summer, when food in most parts of the world is relatively plentiful, air temperature moderate, and rainfall adequate to provide drinking water. Recall that to arrange to have young in the spring requires some forward planning. Pregnancy lasts a predictable period (in most cases, see below), which differs by species. So to ensure that the young are born at the right time, animals have to mate at the 'right' time, which will differ depending on the duration of pregnancy (for that particular species). Which presents us with another adaptive problem:

I sit beside the fire and think
Of how the world will be
When winter comes without a spring
That I shall ever see.

J R R Tolkien. (1945) *The lord of the rings.*
(George Allen and Unwin, London.)

They would answer the call of the north in the spring, but in the fall they would come back again, barking and whooping and honking in the autumn sky, to circle the landmark of the old light and drop to earth near by to be his guests again. . . . And this made Rhayader happy, because he knew that implanted somewhere in their beings was the germ knowledge of his existence and his safe haven, and that this knowledge had become part of them, and, with the coming of the grey skies and the winds from the north, would send them back unerringly to him.

Paul Gallico. (1941) *The snow goose.* (Michael Joseph, London.)

how on earth do animals know when spring will come? Or when it is here? How do different species mate at the right (different) time? The annual baby-boom in the spring clearly shows us that they must do it somehow. Luckily, they have a means: if they could measure daylength (as opposed to the time of day) they, might be able to compute the time of year.

But can they? It all began with juncos, a type of finch, in 1925. A Swiss-born biologist named William Rowan, working in Canada, exposed some juncos to electric light after dark in deepest winter. After a few weeks, they began to sing, develop their testes, and were ready to breed, weeks before the usual date. They had some way of measuring daylength, and their reproductive system had been fooled by the artificial light onto believing it was spring (when this species usually mates). Although Rowan (who was also a talented artist) is given credit (rightly) for the first experimental demonstration of what is now called photoperiodism, it is said that the Japanese, who have an ancient culture of breeding songbirds, knew all about light accelerating breeding seasons. Later, similar experiments were done on ferrets. The female ferret is a very convenient animal. She has a vulva that swells up like a small onion when she is fertile. So you can see whether she is ready to breed without any complicated tests. This happens regularly in the spring in ferrets kept under natural conditions. That is, like most other species, they have an annual, restricted, breeding season. But put a group of out-of-season ferrets into extra light (so they get about 12 or more hours of light each day) and you will have breeding ferrets in midwinter. Many other species do the same. But not all respond to increasing daylengths. Sheep, being big animals, have a rather long pregnancy. If they waited until the spring to mate, by the time they gave birth it would be autumn or even early winter. So they breed in the autumn, thus ensuring that their young are born in the spring. If you take a ewe in the summer (when she is ordinarily not fertile) and reduce the length of her day (e.g. close the blinds at 4 pm), she will come into breeding season much earlier than normal: she thinks it's autumn.

As our biologist tells us, the biological processes required to measure the time of day (the SCN) and daylength are very different. Time of day depends upon dawn; after that, the day unfolds. Of course, a longer day

How do you know that the pilgrim track
Along the belting zodiac
Swept by the sun in his seeming rounds
Is traced by now to the Fishes' bounds
And into the Ram, when weeks of cloud
Have wrapt the sky in a clammy shroud,
And never as yet a tinct of spring
Has shown in the Earth's apparelling;
    O vespering bird, how do you know,
    How do you know?
How do you know, deep underground,
Hid in your bed from sight and sound,
Without a turn in temperature,
With weather life can scarce endure,
That light has won a fraction's strength,
And day put on some moments' length,
Whereof in merest rote will come,
Weeks hence, mild airs that do not numb;
    O crocus root, how do you know,
    How do you know?

        Thomas Hardy. (1840–1928) *The year's awakening.*

Midwinter spring is its own season
Sempiternal though sodden towards sundown,
Suspended in time, between pole and tropic.
When the short day is brightest, with frost and fire,
The brief sun flames the ice, on pond and ditches,
In windless cold that is the heart's heat,
Reflecting in a watery mirror
A glare that is blindness in the early afternoon.

        T S Eliot. *Little Gidding.* (Faber and Faber, London.)

With his marine clocks, John Harrison tested the waters of space-time.
He succeeded, against all odds, in using the fourth — temporal —
dimension to link points on the three-dimensional globe. He wrestled the

means that the daily programme may be extended. But measuring the duration of the day (or the night, either would do) requires a different detector. Furthermore, recall that a 12 hour day occurs twice a year: so animals have to know whether it is the spring or the autumn equinox. The first signals days of ease and plenty (or perhaps intolerable heat); the second, maybe a savage winter and little food. So how do animals measure daylength?

We know they need their eyes, so the detector pathway starts here. Many years ago now, there was a scientific row between two groups of researchers (see Chapter 2). One group thought that the pituitary gland, which is essential for fertility, received a nerve supply from the autonomic nervous system which thus controlled it. They removed this system in some ferrets by taking out two tiny neural ganglia in the neck of ferrets. These ganglia supplied most of the head, including the pituitary, with its autonomic nerve supply. To their delight, the ferrets no longer responded to extra light by beginning their breeding season early. The other group pointed out that the operation did not prevent the ferrets' vulvae swelling up at the 'normal' time (which made a pituitary explanation difficult), but also caused the eyelids of the ferrets to droop (this is called ptosis), so the fact they did not respond to extra light might be due to less light reaching the eyes. The debate raged on for years. Who was right? Neither, as it happens. What they did not know was that the same ganglia also supplied nerve fibres to another structure in the brain called the pineal gland. If you look at the pineal under the microscope, you will see lots of autonomic nerve fibres, whereas they are hard to see (some say impossible) in the pituitary.

In humans, the pineal gland is the size of an average pea, and it lies deep in the brain, in the midline, just under a huge vein (the vein of Galen) that drains much of the brain's interior. It is attached to the nearby brain by two tiny stalks. It has been known for centuries, and at one time excited much speculation about its possible function. Most of the ideas before the 16th century supposed that the pineal was some sort of valve regulating the flow of 'humours' through the brain. Then came Descartes, who also thought the pineal regulated what he called 'animal spirits' in the brain. Animal spirits, amongst other functions, were held to be responsible for movement. He is usually misquoted as suggesting that the *world's whereabouts from the stars, and locked the secret in a pocket watch.*

Dava Sobell. (1996) *Longitude.*
(Fourth Estate, London.)

All old and vigorous languages abound in images and metaphors which, though lightly and casually used, are in truth poems in themselves, and poems of a high and striking order. Perhaps no phrase is so terribly significant as the phrase 'killing time'. It is a tremendous and poetical image, the image of a kind of cosmic parricide. There is on earth a race of revellers who do, under all their exuberance, fundamentally regard time as an enemy.

G K Chesterton. (1958) Charles II. In: *Essays and poems.*
Ed. W Sheed. (Penguin Books, Harmondsworth, UK.)

pineal was the 'seat of the soul', in fact his idea was that the pineal was the organ in which soul and brain came together (part of his views on mind-brain relations, which continue to be debated today). Descartes apparently thought that the pineal was unique to humans, so even immortals can get it wrong. One cannot help wondering how much his ideas would have changed had he known that sheep, ferrets, hamsters, rats and all the rest have pineal glands as well.

With the dawn of the experimental age, not much evidence for any function emerged for the pineal, and it was rather forgotten. Except that it proved useful to radiologists: the pineal of humans tends to calcify, which makes it visible on X-rays. The phrase 'has no known function' tended to slip into 'has no function'. Then, in the 1960s, a group of American scientists showed that the rat's pineal was metabolically very active, and furthermore, that it produced a substance called melatonin. Melatonin is so called because it can cause intense contraction of pigment cells in frogs or tadpoles: they turn pale. In such creatures, the pineal is a third, specialised, eye, but not in mammals. Then it was discovered that the mammalian pineal had a huge autonomic nerve supply, that this supply controlled the formation of melatonin, and that melatonin was formed at night. Two French scientists reported that hamsters in which the pineal had been removed did not breed at the right time of year. Then, ferrets with no pineal failed to respond to additional light, but they began breeding just as if they had been left in natural lighting. Removal of the pineal gland in seasonally-breeding mammals prevents them adjusting their season in response to light. However, and this is important, their circadian rhythms remain unaffected. If you remove the pineal and leave the animal in natural light for long enough, it gradually begins to breed at the wrong time (this is only possible for species that live for several years), though whether there is a true free-running annual cycle (analogous to the circadian one) is still uncertain. The bottom line is that the pineal enables the animals to measure daylength. How?

The answer is the melatonin molecule. Actually, they do not measure daylength, but nightlength. The pineal begins to secret melatonin as soon a darkness falls, and continues to do so for as long as the night lasts. So all the animal has to do is measure the duration of the melatonin signal and it can deduce the duration of the night (hence the day). If you inject melatonin into sheep or ferrets or hamsters, you can induce them to respond as if they were in 'long' nights (late autumn, winter) or 'short' nights (spring, summer) depending on how long each night you give melatonin. But how do they measure the duration of the melatonin pulse (it is called an 'interval timer')? Nobody knows. There must be a set of receptor nerve cells that can add up the duration of the melatonin pulse, but where or how remains a mystery. Wherever it is, it must communicate with many other parts of the limbic system, particularly with those that control the secretion of the hormones from the pituitary (gonadotrophins) that regulate fertility. Since sleep happens at night, it is not surprising that melatonin, the night-hormone produced by the pineal gland, is a hypnotic.

There is another clever wrinkle to the way the brain reads the duration of the melatonin signal, and it accounts for the equinox problem; that is, how animals distinguish between 21st March and 21st September, both with 12 hours of daylight. Remove the pineal, so the hamsters (or whatever) have no melatonin of their own. Now give one group melatonin for 16 hours (a long night: so the animals believe they are living in winter) but the other one for 8 hours (corresponding to summer). After a week or so, give them both melatonin for 12 hours (as at the equinox). The first group respond as if the nights had suddenly become shorter (ie. its spring), the second as it they were longer (it is autumn). So the system that reads the melatonin signal has a sort of memory. It can compare what is now which what has gone before. Problem solved.

So what does man use his pineal for? Not breeding: like other 'domesticated' species, humans have only a very residual breeding season, if one at all (there are rather more births in the spring and early autumn than at other times of the year). Melatonin has recently become fashionable for all sorts of supposed benefits, none of them with much scientific support. It does have a mildly sedative action, so it is useful for jetlag. But it is not the signal that controls circadian rhythms. The human pineal continues to produce melatonin at night, though perhaps the message it wants to send is no longer being received. But it might be unwise to write off melatonin in man. History holds too many examples of scientists dismissing an organ as without function, only to have their over-confident assertion proved utterly wrong.

Knowing the time of day is a different piece of information from knowing the time of year, though both are essential for successful adaptation. The SCN synchronises the daily programme, whereas the pineal coordinates reproduction and other seasonally important events, like growing a thick coat for the winter, or shedding it in time for the hot days of summer. But the two aren't completely independent. As you will have noticed, the daily surge of melatonin is itself a circadian rhythm, so like other such rhythms it is controlled by the SCN. Damage the SCN, and you disturb seasonal as well as daily rhythms, because the pineal no longer secretes melatonin in the correct daily sequence.

Our biologist specialises in mustelids, a group of animals that includes badgers, otters, ferrets, weasels, stoats, mink and skunks. He tells us that they all give birth in the early spring, but that the ways they do this is a good example of how species use different adaptive methods for a common objective. Ferrets (known as polecats in the wild) and some species of skunk (Eastern spotted) have the simplest approach: the females become fertile and sexy in late winter/early spring (controlled by daylength), mate, and deliver their young about six weeks later. Polecats that do not get pregnant at once will go on trying until late summer/early autumn, but Eastern skunks only stay fertile for about a month, so they have to be rather efficient. Mink and the striped skunk are fertile and mate rather earlier, but deliver their young at about the same time. They do this by using a trick. The fertilised embryo is held in suspended animation for a few weeks (called 'delayed implantation' or 'diapause'). The important point is that the trigger for the embryo to be implanted into the uterus, and begin development, is also controlled by light so these species have two light-control systems (one on time of mating, the other on time of implantation). Both depend on the melatonin signal from the pineal. Other mustelids (the American badger, and the Western skunk) mate in the autumn, but suspend their embryos for longer, so that they, too, are born in the spring. But it is the European badger that takes this to extremes. The female mates in late spring/early summer, but the embryo is carried in the suspended state for almost a year (at body temperature) before implanting and beginning to develop, a feat that many scientists would not mind emulating.

By now, you must be thinking that light is the only stimulus that controls circadian and seasonal rhythms. This is not so. If you put rats into dim red light, but feed them only for an hour per day, they will synchronise their daily rhythms to the feeding schedule. Changes in temperature can regulate seasonal cycles: sheep, which normally become fertile in response to the shortening days of autumn, also respond to lowered temperature, particularly if the light is held constant. Timing breeding optimally is so important that there are multiple ways of making sure it happens. Social factors can also regulate rhythms, so a group of hamsters housed together will tend to wake, run, eat and sleep at the same time, even under constant conditions. How all the factors other than light tap into the biological clock is not really known, though the SCN does have input connections from parts of the brain in addition to the eyes, which may carry this information to it.

Although we have focussed on daily (circadian) and annual (seasonal) rhythms, it is important to note that there are other sorts as well. For example, your hormones surge about every 90 mins or so; body temperature has a 28 day cycle (as, of course, does the menstrual cycle), your heart beats regularly, and so on. Animals that live on the sea-shore experience a twice-daily rhythms of the tides, one that gradually moves across solar time because it is driven by the moon. Some of these animals have an internal clock that allows them to predict the time of high or low tide.

Rhythms represent regularities in behaviour and physiology which form essential adaptive responses to a regularly changing environment. These adaptations must be flexible even though the light cycle stays the same each year, since other important elements in the environment, such as food supply or temperature, are not nearly so reliable. So it is not surprising that both circadian and annual cycles can be modulated by factors other than light. Animals living at different latitudes also need to be able to adapt: for example, breeding in foxes living in more Northern regions begins later than in the same species nearer the Equator. The limbic system makes sure that the internal and external environments stay in concert with one another. Your body dances to the music of time.

Chapter 12

The Brain Breaks Down

Adaptation has a price. Sometimes the cost is too high, and the brain fails to cope. Persistent stress, such as a job with too much pressure but too little power of decision, predisposes us to illnesses such as duodenal ulcers, diabetes, heart disease. All are the consequences of the cost of demand. Stress is translated into illness by the brain, since this is how you become aware of the demands on you, and how you formulate your response to them. But the brain itself may succumb to stress, and this is the subject of this chapter.

Nearly everyone has, at sometime in his or her life, a stress such as a bereavement, loss of a job, or the breakdown of a relationship. Painful as these are, most people get over them in time. But not everyone. In a small proportion of people, such an adverse 'life event' (as it is called) is followed by an episode of mental illness, particularly depression (major depressive disorder or MDD). The brain has failed to cope with, or adapt to, this serious stress. Depression is a major health problem throughout the world. It used to be called a 'mental breakdown'. Despite all the defences we have against misfortune, sometimes it overwhelms us. Our adaptive power has failed us. What has happened?

Imagine a time when there were no X-rays, no blood tests, no laboratory investigations of any sort. All a doctor had was a keen eye, lots of experience, and a pen (a quill, perhaps) and paper to record the answers that you, the patient, gave to his/her questions. All he (it would have been mostly 'he') could do by way of tests was to prod you for lumps, bumps or swellings, examine you carefully for any external signs (a rash, perhaps) and even taste your urine — diabetes mellitus is named for the sweet taste physicians recognised in their patient's urine. But most of all,

When to the sessions of sweet silent thought
I summon up remembrance of things past,
I sigh the lack of many a thing I sought,
And with old woes a new wail my dear time's waste;
Then can I drown an eye, unused to flow,
For precious friends hid in death's dateless night,
And weep afresh love's long-since-cancell'd woe,
And moan the expense of many a vanish'd sight.

William Shakespeare. *Sonnet XXX*

It was the black, angry despair of curse pressure; she realized this, and yet believed as she always did that there was no reason to suppose that what she saw in these moments of lucid misery was any further from ultimate truth because it took up only one week out of four. It made so much more impression on her, after all, than whatever occurred in those three relatively placid weeks. . . .

A S Byatt. (1964) *In the shadow of the sun.*

Tears, laughter, tread so hard upon the heel
Of their evoking passions, that in those
Who're most sincere they least obey the will.

Dante. *The divine comedy. II. Purgatory. Canto XXI*
Translated by D L Sayers. (Penguin Books, Harmondsworth, UK.)

Rachel hugged Carrie goodbye at the school gate and set off in the direction of the café. Newspapers, hot coffee, the sense of privacy that only public places could give. She skimmed the paper, reading only the beginnings of paragraphs, and slipped to where she really wanted to be, in a reverie. Gazing out of the window she saw movement and pattern but no detail. She experienced herself as a dangerously unstable structure, a form held together more with glue and bits of string than nuts and bolts, that any kind of stress threatened to bend and warp, bringing the whole edifice down in a disordered unrecognizable heap. Not even stress, though; merely life. Anything that happened and impinged upon her felt dangerous.

Jenny Diski. (1986) *Nothing natural.* (Minerva, London.)

the doctor relied on careful and experienced questioning to make sure he knew exactly what your symptoms were, and for how long you had had them, whether they had occurred before, and whether anyone in your family or friends had similar problems. From such an account (doctors call this the 'history'), he would arrive at a diagnosis (decide the nature of the condition or illness from which you were suffering), make a prognosis (that is, tell you what was the likely outcome) and prescribe the appropriate treatment. That was the situation 100 or more years ago. The astonishing thing is how much progress medicine made using these simple and, to the modern mind, essential but rather primitive methods. This was thanks to the sagacity, powers of observation and the persistence of the doctors and scientists of the time. The names of many of these men (there are hardly any women) are enshrined in the diseases they were the first to describe. They did this by recognising a cluster of symptoms (what patients say they have noticed about themselves), associating this with any signs the patient might have (for example, a rash, a lump, a swelling), how the disease progressed (the prognosis) and, in some cases, making careful observations at post mortem examinations. Together, these make up a syndrome, and the recognition of a syndrome is the first, difficult step to defining an illness. Parkinson's disease, Alzheimer's disease, Addison's disease, Cushing's syndrome, Huntington's disease, Hodgkins' disease, Henoch's purpura, Meniere's disease and so on are hard-earned and wholly justified memorials to the great men who first recognised these conditions or, in some cases, to whom history has awarded this accolade.

But no matter how acute the observation, however careful the collection of cases, how much inspired insight is applied to the recognition and definition of a syndrome, this method of classifying and understanding disease will always be limited. As an example, take the case of someone who is short of breath (called 'dyspnoea'). Careful questions may elicit the fact that this has been progressive and recent; that it is associated with a pain in the chest; that the person concerned smokes and is overweight. The doctor may justifiably suspect coronary artery disease. But it could be anaemia (not enough red cells to carry oxygen in the blood can give rise to dyspnoea etc.) or an abnormality in the lung. Even if it turns out to be a heart condition, there are a number of different reasons why the heart should be failing, some common, others

"Lord Darlington wasn't a bad man. He wasn't a bad man at all. And at least he had the privilege of being able to say at the end of his life that he made his own mistakes. His lordship was a courageous man. He chose a certain path in life, it proved to be a misguided one, but there, he chose it, he can say that at least. As for myself, I cannot even claim that. You see I trusted. I trusted his lordship's wisdom. All those years I served him, I trusted I was doing something worthwhile. I can't even say I made my own mistakes. Really — one has to ask oneself — what dignity is there in that?"

K Ishiguro. (1989) *The remains of the day.*
(Faber and Faber, London.)

I dropped on my knees, and took his paw in my hand. He gave the faintest wag of his tail, and tried to raise his head; but it fell back again, and he could only look at me.

For an instant, for the briefest instant, we looked at each other, and while we looked his eyes glazed.

"Coco — I've come back. Darling — I'll never leave you any more —"

I don't know why I said these things. I knew he was dead, and that no calls, no lamentations, no love could ever reach him again.

Sliding down to the stone flags beside him, I laid my head on his and wept in an agony of bitter grief. Now indeed I was alone in the world. Even my dog was gone.

Elizabeth von Arnim. (1936) *All the dogs in my life.*
(William Heinemann, London.)

We entered the hut together our bare feet caked with soil our hats already in our hands and there we saw poor da lying dead upon the kitchen table he were bulging with all the poisons of the Empire his skin grey and shining in the gloom.

I were 12 yr. and 3 wk. old that day and if my feet were callused one inch thick and my hands hard and my labourer's knees cut and scabbed and stained with dirt no soap could reach yet did I not still have a heart and were this not he who give me life now all dead and ruined? Father son of my heart are you dead from me are you dead from me my father?

Peter Carey. (2000) *True history of the Kelly gang.*
(University of Queensland Press, Brisbane.)

rather rare. To decide between these possibilities, investigation is required: that is, appropriate tests (a chest X-ray, an electrocardiogram, blood analysis etc.). These tests not only allow the doctor to make a more accurate diagnosis, they may also tell him much more about the cause of the illness than is possible by external observation alone, skilful though this may be. Suppose, in fact, that the patient turns out to have anaemia rather than heart disease. The appropriate tests will reveal whether or not this is due to insufficient iron in the body (iron-deficient anaemia), or to other possible causes of anaemia (there are quite a few, including vitamin B12 deficiency or bone marrow failure). We know low iron can be a cause of anaemia because research has shown that iron is an essential element in the molecule of haemoglobin, the oxygen-carrying protein in the blood. Scientific research has thus given medicine two critical pieces of information. The first is basic scientific knowledge that applies to everybody: for example, why and how iron is important for normal levels of haemoglobin and why this protein is required for transporting oxygen from lungs to tissues. The second is individual information: whether the patient who now sits in front of the doctor, complaining of dyspnoea, has the blood picture compatible with low iron, or whether his/her blood levels of iron are low. Further studies using even more sophisticated tests may be needed in each case to determine why iron levels are too low: is the patient losing iron (e.g. bleeding from somewhere?); is his/her intake too low; can he/she absorb it properly etc. In some cases, genetic analysis may add to the picture. Thus, the huge advances in basic physiological knowledge, accurate information from tests on how a particular physiological process is disturbed in a given disorder, and the availability of treatments designed to correct these derangements have been the basis on which modern medicine has made its extraordinary advances in the last century. But this is not so in psychiatry.

Join me in your mind's eye, and sit behind an experienced psychiatrist as he talks to a new patient. You will be impressed by his skill (it could well be a 'her'; assume either). Deftly, he extracts the information he needs about the patient's illness: its symptoms, when it started, what effect it has on the patient's life (and the lives of those around him). Should this be a case of suspected depression, the psychiatrist will ask about the patient's mood,

We have not been happy. My Lord, we have not been too happy.
We are not ignorant women, we know what we must expect and not expect.
We know of oppression and torture,
We know of extortion and violence,
Destitution, disease,
The old without fire in the winter,
The child without milk in the summer,
The labour taken away from us,
Our sins made heavier upon us.

T S Eliot. (1888–1965) *Murder in the cathedral.*

feelings and emotions; and delicately enquire about the possibility of suicidal thoughts (about 15% of people with depression commit suicide, a substantial risk). He might ask whether there are feelings of worthlessness and hopelessness, and whether these vary during the day (characteristically, they are worse in the morning). He will ask about possible disturbances in memory and the way the patient thinks about things. Depression can have marked effects on both. He does this to establish whether the features of the patients illness fits into a pattern corresponding to depression, or to another diagnosis. Is this the first time that the patient has experienced such symptoms? Many episodes of depression are recurrences of previous episodes of illness. Has the patient suffered any personal disasters, setbacks or tragedies recently? He will ask about the family history: are any of the patients relatives affected in this way? Some forms of depression are known to be more frequent in the close relatives of those who themselves suffer from this condition.

Eventually, the consultation ends. It will occur to you that two things that go with most medical examinations are missing: the psychiatrist is not very likely to examine the patient physically (this would be highly unlikely in other medical contexts); and there is no mention of blood tests, or X-rays or any other laboratory investigation. You suddenly realise that everything depends on that folder in which the psychiatrist is writing so busily. And that what he writes depends on the nature of his questions, and the content of the answers that the patient gives him (or his relatives, for they are often consulted as well). In other words, we seem to be back in the 19th century, as if 'scientific' medicine had never been invented. This, of course, is not entirely true, for some of the treatments that the psychiatrist is able to offer are very much the product of the 20th and 21st century. But the process of diagnosis is one that would be not at all strange to a psychiatrist living and working 50 or even 100 years ago, in contrast, shall we say, to the events during a cardiologist's consultation, with its high-tech radiology, blood enzyme levels and measures of lipids and so on, which might very well baffle a doctor resurrected from a previous generation.

Why is psychiatry so seemingly backward? Why, in particular, does a diagnosis like 'depression' depend solely on the history? Why are there no blood tests and X-rays that are useful to psychiatrists? Does it matter that the diagnosis of mental illness such as depression is made without the

Life Events

... Severe losses often lead to negative thoughts about oneself and one's world, which can then generalize, thus ushering in the familiar symptoms of major depression. One severe loss may be enough to do this, and several minor losses do not seem capable of adding up to an equivalent effects. . . .

The issue (causality) can be most easily illustrated by. . . cigarette smoking. Although most instances of lung cancer are associated with heavy smoking, much less than 1% of the variance is explained. . . . This is due to the fact that variance explained takes into account not only that most people with lung cancer are heavy smokers, but also that *most heavy smokers do not have lung cancer.* Since people without lung cancer greatly outnumber those with it, the fact that most people with lung cancer are heavy smokers gets swamped. . . . This has close parallels with the findings for depression: although for the majority of people developing depression a provoking agent occurs before onset, most people experiencing a provoking agent do not develop depression.

G W Brown and T O Harris. (1989) Depression. In: *Life events and illness.* Eds. G W Brown and T O Harris. (Unwin Hyman, London.)

It has often been pointed out that close scrutiny of the (life) events reported by patients suggests that they can, at best, only be partial causes. Most of the events. . . were in the range of everyday experience, rather than catastrophic. It seems probable that in most cases these events are negotiated without illness so that some other factors must contribute to the development rates for the population. It is particularly easy to lose sight of the importance of base rates. . . when the prevalence of a disease state is relatively low, single events will be of limited value in explaining it if they exist with moderate frequency in the general population. . . the general point remains that most stressful events are not followed by psychiatrically treated depression. Some are followed by other psychiatric disorder. . . or by somatic disorder, but many do not lead to any disorder at all. . . . We must assume that there are a large number of personal factors reflecting vulnerability to events. . . they include all sorts of deficits of biologic structure and functions, . . . the kind of causative chain that is indicated by this model is a multifactorial one, in which many factors converge on the final state. . . . Although this kind of multifactorial etiology may . . . be less logically satisfying that the apparently precise distinctions posited by earlier views, it is more in keeping with appurtenances of modern medicine? Is there any need to bring a different set of science-based approaches into this field of medicine, and any immediate prospect of their being available?

Psychiatrists are no less well-trained or expert than other medical specialities. They are all trained thoroughly for many years. They are taught a great deal of clinical skill. They learn a lot of medical science. They also realise, during their training, that rather little of this science is any direct use for their everyday practice of psychiatry. In particular, they may be given lots of lectures and tutorials about recent advances in the neurosciences. At some point in their training, they may well ask themselves why so little of this fascinating stuff is helping them really understand the cause and treatment of mental illnesses such as depression. The real answer is not that studying the brain is irrelevant to psychiatry — there is general acceptance that mental illnesses are the product of a brain disorder. The real answer is that neuroscience is simply not up the task, yet, of providing the information that psychiatrists need to understand, in a way that their more fortunate colleagues in other specialities do, the exact nature of the disturbance that has lead to the illness, and thus how it might be corrected. We need to ask why this is so.

Let us return, for a moment, to our patient with dyspnoea. The doctor suspects a heart condition. Now, the heart is not a mystery. Of course, there is still plenty to be learned about it, and research into the heart continues vigorously. But the fundamental principles about how the heart works are understood. It is a rather complicated pump and schoolchildren learn about it. No mystery here. We have a clear set of ideas about how the heart works, which allow doctors to pin-point disturbances in any of these components of the heart which can lead to illness. For example, heart failure — the inability of the heart to work hard enough, can be the result of damage to its cells, damage to its valves, or its disorders in blood supply and so on. Each will result in heart failure (one symptom of which is dyspnoea) but different causes require different treatments. Different tests enable the doctor to tell which is responsible. Line up six patients with dyspnoea due to heart disease, and each one may be getting a different treatment. Dyspnoea, as we have seen, is not a diagnosis but a symptom. It may not even be due to heart disease.

Now, let us go back to our patient with depression. Or, rather, to his psychiatrist. The patient has gone home, and we are left with his doctor, empirical data and our knowledge of the complexity of psychological relationships and brain mechanisms in general.

E S Paykel. (1979) Recent life events in the development of depressive disorders. In: *The psychobiology of the depressive disorders. Implications for the effects of stress.* Ed. R A Depue. (Academic Press, New York.)

It is hypothesized that major life events may act as specific precipitants (of depression) by inducing rhythm disruptions and thus take on a direct link to the biomedical features of depression. It may be that some of the specific psychosocial precipitants of depressive disorder. . . may be particularly potent in their ability to trigger these biological desynchonizations through the capacity of interpersonal relationships and social demands to act as potent synchonizing factors for biological rhythms.

C L Ehlers, E Frank, and D J Kupfer. (1988) Social zeitgebers and biological rhythms. *Archives of General Psychiatry* **45**, pp. 948–952.

It was curious. . . that the first medicine was not a herbal preparation or a surgical procedure, but simple kindness; odd, because the struggle of the pioneering mad-doctors had always been to establish that illness of the mind was organic, a physical malfunction, to be treated in the same way as an illness of the liver or the foot, the brain being such an organ, entirely compatible to the others — if more complicated. Yet, one did not treat cirrhosis or a broken metatarsal with kindness, so here was the paradox. . . . To the patient with the broken tibia, you gave a pair of crutches; to the one with an abscess, you gave a bandage, but surgery came before crutches or bandage. Kindness to the lunatic was like the support of bandage; the odd thing about psychiatry. . . was that its cart had come before its horse; its task was to discover its primary treatments, the cures of surgery or apothecary. (the novel is set in the late 19th century)

Sebastian Faulks. (2005) *Human traces.* (Vintage Books, London.)

who is very well-informed and scientifically-trained. Let us ask him some questions. Our first might be: is this patient actually suffering from depression? The psychiatrist agrees that he almost certainly is. We ask him how he comes to the conclusion. He says that psychiatrists have a set of criteria on which they base their diagnoses. As it happens, our psychiatrist is involved in a research project on depression. He says that there exists an agreed set of symptoms that define depression, and shows them to us. They are set out on a large book called the Diagnostic and Statistical Manual of Mental Disorders (DSM), and our psychiatrist tells us that this is essentially a book written by a committee. He also says that this book is now accepted as the gold standard by which diagnoses are made. No reputable scientific psychiatric journal would ever accept a research article (a paper) which did not use these criteria. This, he tells us, is very useful: it makes sure that everyone studying depression is using the same set of decision rules about diagnosing this condition, whether they work in New York, London, or anywhere else. At least, he says, we are all studying the same illness. We ask to see the section of DSM on depression.

Several things immediately stand out. The first, not surprisingly, in view of our recent experience in psychiatric out-patients, is that there is no mention of anything other than symptoms. The second is that we see a long list of symptoms, and the statement that at least five of these (there are nine altogether) must have been present for at least two weeks to qualify the patient as having depression (MDD). There are two 'key' sets of symptoms required for a diagnosis of depression — depressed mood and loss of interest or pleasure; without these, major depressive disorder is not diagnosed even if the others are present. We wonder why five are needed; is this a reflection of something real, or an attempt to apply precision where none exists? What if someone feels worthless and fatigued for weeks, and thinks about suicide, but does not have one of the two 'key' symptoms? And why two weeks? We also note that there seems to be a let-out clause: there may be other ways to account for these symptoms (e.g. recent bereavement), and the psychiatrist has to be sure that the patient's symptoms are not accounted for by a 'medical' condition — by which is meant other pre-existing abnormalities; for example, excess secretion of certain hormones, or taking illicit drugs. These can also result

Depression

The idea is that the amount of depression in a culture will be related to the size of the enterprises people pursue. In the environments we evolved in, marriages lasted only a few years, efforts to get food were successful or not in a few days, and even social competitions lasted only months or a few years. Now, by contrast, most people are engaged in efforts that require gigantic initial investments. If they don't work out, the option of leaving and starting over may not only be difficult, it may be impossible. So, people persist in efforts that seem hopeless precisely because they have no alternative. I wonder of the frequency of depression in modern life might arise from the size of the enterprises people now engage in, the large groups in which they compete for status and mates, and the difficulties of starting a major enterprise afresh.

R N Nesse. (1999) The evolution of hope and despair.
Social Research **66**, pp. 429–469.

Depression is not a single disease; the term is used loosely to describe a plethora of illnesses that have some core symptoms in common. . . .

It has been estimated that over 50% of patients suffering from chronic pain also express clinically diagnosable symptoms of depression. However, chronic pain, like depression, is not a single disease.

G Blackburn-Munro and R E Blackburn-Munro. (2001)
Chronic pain, chronic stress and depression:
coincidence or consequence? *Journal of*
Neuroendocrinology **13**, pp. 1009–1023.

For more than 2000 years there has been a tradition in Western medicine that has equated health with harmony in physical and emotional life. In this tradition, disorders have been understood as disruptions of optimal relationships between different elements, and the restoration of health has been thought to require a restoration of balance. While we now know that this paradigm is oversimplified and for some disorders inaccurate, the concepts of harmony and balance nevertheless form the basis for an increasingly sophisticated model of how the body reacts with and adapts to a changing environment — a model of how what we call stress disturbs the body's normal homeostasis, and how in response the in depressed mood. We also see that DSM lists a number of other conditions, some of whose symptoms overlap with MDD, but which have added ones that qualify then for a different diagnosis (label). We point out the similarity between dyspnoea and depression, in that both are something a patient tells you about — a real problem that interferes with their life and which they regard as 'abnormal'. How do you know, we ask the psychiatrist, that depression is not a symptom rather than a disease? And, how do you know that depression, whether a symptom or a disease entity, represents an abnormality in the brain?

If depression is a symptom, this alters our view of how it might be caused, and how we might understand the role of the brain. A symptom might well be a part of several distinct mental illnesses, just as dyspnoea can be a feature of heart, respiratory or blood disorders. Of course, even if it were a symptom, depression might still represent a common disturbance of brain function, just as breathlessness reflects a common response of the neural structures controlling respiration to a mismatch between what is needed (an adequate amount of oxygen) and what the cardiovascular system can deliver. Nevertheless, if depression is a symptom there would certainly be less rationale for recognising MDD as a distinct illness, and we should begin asking a set of different questions about the origin and cause of mental illness such as 'depression.' At present, most psychiatrists would give depression a central position in the classification of mood disorders, and this has a huge influence on the way we think about it. There is a 'chicken-and-egg' situation: if depression is a discrete illness, then there will be an equally discrete cause; but to find that cause we have to assume the illness. Our psychiatrist thinks it is highly likely that MDD is a distinct illness, but is modest and intelligent enough to recognise that this opinion is based on clinical experience, overlain with a strong dose of professional compliance.

Can we measure depression, and bring a little scientific rigour into what has seemed, so far, as a very qualitative argument? We are now joined by a clinical psychologist, who specialises in measuring mental function. This includes mood states. The psychologist explains that mood can be measured in various ways. All, however, depend on the patient answering or responding to questions. In other words, we are back to the symptoms. The questionnaires used by the clinical psychologist are body mobilizes a group of highly specific mechanisms to defend and maintain this balance.

D Michelson, J Licinio, and P W Gold. (1995) Mediation of the stress response by the hypothalamo-pituitary-adrenal axis. In: *Neurobiological and clinical consequences of stress. From normal adaptation to PTSD.* Eds. M J Friedman, D S Charney, and A Y Deutch, pp. 225–238. (Lippincot-Raven, Philadelphia.)

Unlike other species, we display an extraordinary range of apparently aberrant mental processes and resultant behaviours — at one extreme, we call this mental illness, and at the other, creative genius.

Kelly Morris. (2002) Does art work in mental health? *Lancet* **360**, pp. 1104.

A common medical school joke defines a psychiatrist as a nice Jewish boy who can't stand the sight of blood. . . . In dealing with depression, psychiatrists. . . do experience their full share of medical responsibility for decisions that will help determine if the patient will live or die. . . the threat to life is in the patients own hands — the threat of suicide.

Depression is probably the most common of the major mental illnesses. . . . Thus, it is not surprising that Nathan Kline, a well-known American psychiatric authority on depression concluded that "more human suffering has resulted from depression than from any other single disease, medical as well as psychiatric, affecting mankind."

S H Snyder. (1976) *The troubled mind.* (McGraw-Hill Book Company, New York.)

It is customary to define psychiatry as a medical speciality concerned with the study, diagnosis and treatment of mental illnesses. This is a worthless and misleading definition. Mental illness is a myth. Psychiatrists area not concerned with mental illnesses and their treatments. In actual practice, they deal with personal, social, and ethical problems in living.

T S Szasz. (1972) *The myth of mental illness.* (Paladin, St Albans.)

Psychiatry is a medical discipline long on disorders and short on explanations. . . . Psychiatrists tend to split up into two camps, based on purported explanation — hence biological, dynamic, behavioural, and even the eclectic — and go to war with one another. . . .

so constructed that they reflect the common symptoms associated with depression (fatigue, loss of pleasure, suicidal thoughts, difficulty in getting to sleep etc.). Some focus more heavily on physical symptoms (tiredness etc.), others on psychological ones (feelings of guilt etc.). All these can be part of MDD. You might say that the way these questionnaires are constructed reflect our prejudice about what depression is, but the psychologist defends his questionnaire by saying that it measures what patients really complain about (it has clinical validity), that when he (or another psychologist) uses it several times on the same person he gets the same result (it is reliable) and that when he adds up the total score this gives a good indication of who is, in fact, ill and how ill they are (it is sensitive and specific). Finally, he points out that as patients get better, their questionnaire scores reflect this, and may predict whether or not they relapse — as we have seen, depression has an unfortunate habit of recurring.

You can measure breathlessness by getting a patient to walk along a moving belt at a given speed, and seeing either how long he can go on, or the maximum speed of the belt that he finds tolerable. Both depression questionnaires and exercise machines thus allow clinicians to assess how incapacitated their patients are, and whether they are responding to treatment. All very useful, but not at all helpful in our quest for the cause of the illness underlying the symptom. For the patient with dyspnoea, the exercise machine is only the start of a considerable clinical investigation. For the depressed patient, apart perhaps from some additional psychiatric questioning, it's as far as it gets. On an exercise machine, the doctor can measure the level of oxygen in the blood as the patient walks faster or changes in the ECG, thus gaining access to an independent (and physiologically relevant) index of cardiovascular function. The psychiatrist cannot measure anything apart from adding up the score on the mood questionnaire.

So how do we know that mood itself is a property of the brain? Does this mean that depression (a disturbance of mood) is the result of brain malfunction? Taking us to lunch, we pass a friend and colleague of the clinical psychologist, a neuroscientist who is collaborating with him on a research project, and whose expertise lies in the relation of brain to behaviour. Sensing, perhaps, that he is facing a sceptical audience, the

Psychiatry is a medical discipline. It is capable of medical triumphs and serious medical mistakes. We don't know the secrets of human nature. We cannot build a New Jerusalem. We can describe how our explanations for mental disorders are devised and develop, and where they are strong and where they are limited. We can clarify the presumptions about what we know and how we know it. With more research, steadily, we can construct a clinical discipline that, while delivering less to fashion, will bring more to patients and their families.

> P B McHugh. (1995) Witches, multiple personalities, and other psychiatric artefacts. *Nature Medicine* **1**, pp. 110–114.

Unipolar major depression is one of the most serious mental health disorders whose adverse outcomes include chronic mental and physical ill health, social difficulties, and successful suicide. The disorder occurs across the lifespan, but the nature, characteristics, and outcomes of the condition may vary with age. It is unclear if children, adolescents, adults, and the elderly who present with depressive illness are necessarily suffering from the same disorder with common aetiologies or will respond to the same treatments.

> I M Goodyer. (2003) Preface to: *Unipolar depression, a lifespan perspective*. Ed. I M Goodyer. (Oxford University Press, Oxford.)

psychologist invites him to join us. Our psychiatrist, a man with literary tendencies like many others in his speciality, reminds us that mood and temperament were once confidently ascribed to bodily 'humours'. After all, it was none other than Galen, influenced by Hippocratic ideas, who proposed that an excess of black bile was responsible for melancholia (depressed mood). This was a conceptual leap, since it ascribed an observable mental state of an individual (his mood) to an underlying physiological state (too much black bile). This implied not only that a major attribute of someone's personality might be regulated by a bodily function, but also that something might be done about it; if only one could change the amount of black bile. Galenic physicians did so by advice on diet and exercise, but also by bleeding their patients. This stimulates the psychologist who, like many of his profession, finds firing verbal darts at medics irresistible, to point out that the latter treatment, though at best harmless and certainly not effective, held sway for centuries and was universally accepted by the medical profession as a basic therapy. How many others, he says, used with equal certitude today, may fall into the same category? The discussion, now becoming animated, is helped along by the newly-arrived neuroscientist pointing out that Galen's drawing of the brain was completely inaccurate, yet was also accepted for centuries. All Galen, or anybody else, had to do, was to look inside the head of a corpse to see how wrong it was. Nobody did, or thought to do so. Or perhaps, the psychologist adds, they did but were afraid to go against the prevailing view. After all, he points out, established opinions in the medical profession are still hard to displace, even in the 21st century.

We are into a discussion of evidence-based medicine. This, we are told, is the real difference between ancient 'primitive' science, based on thought; conjecture; prejudice and suggestion, and the 'new' medicine. As with many other advances in medicine, this came from outside it. The great scientists of the 15th century and after were the ones who laid down the rules upon which today we lean. Galileo, Newton and many others convinced the rest of the world — though so slowly, and with what difficulty — that the old ideas were figments of the human imagination, whereas today, the psychiatrist confidently states, we need evidence, not opinions. The neuroscientist will ask: really? what about having a good idea? Or different interpretations of a given piece of evidence? After all,

Emotion

Darwin thought that emotional expression was primitive and of little adaptive significance for modern Englishmen. Even in the case of animals, he greatly emphasised one function of emotions, communication, and gave relatively little attention to other possible benefits. Thus, the father of evolutionary theory started off research on emotions by minimizing their adaptive significance for humans and neglecting the full range of benefits they offer for animals. . . .

While debate continues about whether there are or are not basic emotions, there seem to be good reasons for thinking that certain emotions are fundamental capacities of the organism. Furthermore, there is substantial agreement on what these emotions are: Happiness, sadness, anger and fear — with love, surprise and disgust also often mentioned.

R N Nesse. (1999) The evolution of hope and despair.
Social Research **66**, pp. 429–469.

Emotions are a basic component of human experience, but their exact nature has been elusive and difficult to specify. This is due to a number of causes, including the fact that so many systems of the body are involved in emotion. A second problem has been the tendency to separate emotion from cognition or rational thought processes.

A S Baum. (1994) In: *The encyclopaedia of psychology*. 2nd Ed.
Ed. R J Corsini. (John Wiley and Sons, New York.)

Philosophers have neglected the topic of the emotions, or else assimilated the emotions to either belief or desire. I shall establish the uniqueness of emotion, and the related notion of an "attitude". In any analysis attention must be paid to the phenomenology of emotion, to the function of emotions in our lives, and to the circumstances in which particular emotions arise. Emotions, I claim, are singularly related to satisfied or frustrated desire.

Richard Wollheim. (1991) *On the emotions.*

Emotion, as a human experience, is a commonly recognized psychological state, and many ordinary words describe different kinds of emotions — anger, fear, happiness, sorrow etc. . . . Experimental study of the emotions since the beginning of the 20th century has yielded many isolated facts, but it has not been possible to develop a single self-consistent theory covering all aspects of emotional experience and behaviour.

Encyclopaedia Britannica. (1970) (William Benton, Chicago.)

science thrives on dispute. Pick up any copy of any scientific journal, and it is not long before you will find scientists disagreeing with each other. Evidence-based science has not, it seems, removed uncertainty, or room for argument, or replaced the need for great ideas with the routine business of collecting more data. We still need our Harveys, Hunters and Kraepelins — original minds who not only can interpret and collate the mass of information but who can see what is needed next.

Attempts to understand how depression is associated with brain function are a good example of the way that two major strands of information about any illness try to come together. On the one hand there is knowledge about the neural basis of emotion. This is derived mostly from experimental studies on the brain. On the other, there is understanding depression as a clinical phenomenon, related to maladaptation. This comes from observations on patients, and resulting experience of the variety and outcome of depression. Firstly, of course, we have to accept that the first strand is relevant to the second. Is depression a disorder of emotion? Clinicians do not often talk about 'emotion' but of 'mood'. Depression, most psychiatrists agree, is a disorder of mood; that is, it is the presence of an abnormal, inappropriate, incapacitating mood state. Experimental psychologists hardly ever study 'mood' but something they call 'emotion'. Clinical psychologists, in the other hand, measure mood state, or assert that they do. Are they all talking about the same thing?

Emotion is a central state that one individual experiences: there is no way that anyone else can experience your emotion, though they can infer you are in an emotional state by either looking at you (you look angry, fearful, happy and so on) or by asking you how you feel. Or you tell them that you feel angry or whatever, and that your heart is beating wildly; that is, you access your own feelings and physiology and then give this state a label. The label depends on the language you speak, its vocabulary, and the way that humans classify their emotional states. So there are physical components of emotion as well as psychological ones. Emotion is something we all think we know about, like 'consciousness', but it is one of those words that, as soon as you try to define them, seems to slip from your grasp. Before we consult our psychologist, let us see what philosophers have had to say.

Emotion is a topic that, more than any other, has bedevilled students of mental life. The peculiar characteristics of emotional behaviour and experience have been repeated stumbling blocks in the attempt to see human nature as rational, intelligent or even sublime.

R L Gregory (ed). (1987) *The Oxford companion to the mind.*
(Oxford University Press, Oxford.)

Much in animal behavior substantiates the notion that strong emotions evolved chiefly in mammals and to a lesser extent in birds. The attachment of domestic animals to humans is, I think, beyond question. The apparently sorrowful behavior of many mammalian mothers when their young are removed is well-known. One wonders just how far such emotions go. Do horses on occasion have glimmerings of patriotic fervor? Do dogs feel for humans something akin to religious ecstasy? What other string of subtle emotions are felt by animals that do not communicate with us?

Carl Sagan. (1977) *The dragons of Eden.*
(Hodder and Stoughton, London.)

Philosophers have also been intrigued by emotion. The classical intellectual question 'what do you mean by...' is much derided, but wholly essential. Define the question and you are halfway to the answer is a good academic principle. The philosopher Susan James, in her book, '*Passion and action: The emotions in seventeenth century philosophy*' shows how this question of definition preoccupied even Aristotle. She includes emotions in 'passions' as do many other philosophers. Passions, she writes, are generally thought to be thoughts or states of the soul. Our psychologist, and even our psychiatrist, might have problems with the last word in that sentence, but let us dodge, for the moment, whether substituting 'brain' for 'soul' would be helpful or even equivalent. James makes the point that classifying passions implies a more-or-less articulated conception of what they are and how they operate. Aristotle, she tells us, made a list. This included anger and mildness, love and hatred, fear and confidence, shame and esteem, kindness and unkindness, pity and indignation, envy and emulation. Several things are noteworthy about this list. Firstly, it is made up of pairs of words that represent opposites. This makes us wonder if there are intervening points: that is, are we dealing with a 'binary' state (one or the other) or a continuous scale (a current emotional state can be on some imaginary line connecting the two extremes). Which one we choose will influence our view of how emotion is constructed, and how it may become pathological. Secondly, notice that Aristotle has given a list of pairs. This seems to imply that there are several distinct categories of emotion. If this is true, then each pair (or emotional 'dimension') may have separate representations in the brain. They may also be able to occur simultaneously and independently (that is, the presence of one emotion does not imply, or even necessarily influence, that of another). This will also influence how we think about disordered brain states. However, if we accept Aristotle's list (note that 'sadness' doesn't appear, but that 'fear' does), we cannot accept that one can have maximum 'love' together with maximum 'hate' simultaneously, since they are on the same dimension. These two ideas — that one can categorise emotions on a dimension (or scale) and that there are separable dimensions, each representing a distinct emotion, have dominated thinking in this area ever since. Of course, there have been many variants in the years since Aristotle. Practically, every philosopher of note has, at

Alexus: Jealousy is like
A polished glass held to the lips when life's in doubt:
If there be breath, 'twill catch the damp, and show it.

Cleopatra: I grant you, jealousy's a proof of love
But 'tis a weak and unavailing medicine;
It puts out the disease, and makes no show,
But it has no power to cure.

John Dryden. (1677) *All for love.*

Jealousy is the most dreadfully involuntary of all the sins. It is at once one
of the ugliest and one of the most pardonable. Zeus, who smiles at lovers'
oaths, must also condone their pangs and the venom which these pangs
engender. Some Frenchman said that jealousy was born with love but
does not always die with love. . . . Jealousy is a cancer, it can kill that
which it feeds on, though it is usually a horribly slow killer.

Iris Murdoch. (1973) *The black prince.*
(Chatto and Windus, London.)

He suspected she had replaced him with another lover. He interpreted her
every gesture to others as a code of promise. She gripped the front of
Roundell's jacket once in a lobby and shook it, laughing at him as he
muttered something, and he followed the innocent government aide for
two days to see if there was more between them.

Michael Ondaatje. *The English patient.*
(Bloomsbury Publishing Co., London.)

The stormy sadness of her thoughts oppressed her. Had she tried to think
them all out aloud, one by one, she would not have had sufficient words
or time enough till dawn. But out here, in the street, these comfortless
reflections flew at her in clusters, and she could deal with them together,
in the short while it took her to walk a few times from the monastery gate
to the corner of the square and back.

Boris Pasternak. (1958) *Doctor Zhivago,*
Translated by Max Hayward and Manya Harari.
(Wm Collins and Co. Ltd., London.)

some point, wrestled with emotion. Prominent amongst them was Descartes, who separated reason from emotion, and elaborated a complex account of passions, together with a series of (entirely conjectural) physiological events in the heart, nerves and, famously, the pineal gland. Descartes also had his list of 'primary' passions, which did include sadness (the others were wonder, joy, love, hatred and desire). Just as we see colours as a compound of three primary ones (blue, green, red) so Descartes thought that all emotions were a blend of his six primaries. If we accept this general idea, it has different implications for the way we might imagine emotions are coded in the brain. Even in the 17th century, it is striking that without any empirical evidence, Descartes and others were able to associate emotions with the brain. He also recognised that changes in emotional and bodily states go together. The relation between perception, thoughts (cognition), memory and emotion which so fascinated Descartes also continues to be a subject of interest, nowadays not only for philosophers but also for psychologists.

It is time to see what psychology has to offer. Let us begin by looking at several undergraduate textbooks of psychology. These are mostly written by academic psychologists, who are naturally interested in bringing order and clarity to their subject. Turn to the chapter on 'emotion' and you may not be too impressed. You will find that psychology struggles to define emotion, like everybody else. This is both comforting (it makes the rest of us seem less stupid) and dispiriting (since they are the professionals). Experimental psychologists tend to see emotions in terms of the way they try to measure it. Since this usually involves either rewards or punishment (pleasure or pain) they often define emotions as 'affective' states produced by these events. Such a definition is hardly helpful. It leaves unanswered the problem of how one defines an 'affective' state as opposed to anything else. It also blurs the boundaries between 'emotion', 'motivation' and even 'cognition'. In any case, much of the experimental work on emotion is actually on 'fear' or 'anxiety' or, rather, conditions that are presumed to result in accentuating such emotions in the animals subjected to them. There are those who do study 'reward', though this often does not include the emotional state that accompanies it. Although understanding the neurology of fear is hugely important, focussing on one category of emotion omits any possible analysis of an equally important

His left hand patted around the air searching for something: a shot of whiskey, his pipe, a whip, a shotgun, the Democratic platform, his heart — Vera Louise never knew what. He looked hurt, deeply, deeply hurt for a few seconds. Then his rage seeped into the room, clouding the crystal and softening the starched tablecloth. . . . Sweat poured from his temples and collected under his chin; soaked his armpits and the back of his shirt as his rage swamped and flooded the room.

> Toni Morrison. (1992) *Jazz.* (Chatto and Windus, London.)

Jealousy gripped him. He did his best to distract himself with work. He blamed himself, and attempted to control what he realized was a form of madness that threatened to render him ridiculous; but he was unable to prevent it. He ascertained that Pemberton (whom he had seen walking with his wife) was a married man, but that did not prevent the jealousy flaring up again and again, like a running fire that resists all attempts to stifle it. Anyone who has ever been jealous recognizes the horrible truth of his account.

> Claire Tomalin. (2003) *Samuel Pepys. The unequalled self.*
> (Penguin Books, London.)

question: how are different emotions encoded in the brain? Are they all represented in the same place, but by different combination of neural activity? Or are there separable neural systems devoted to distinct emotional states? Most textbooks, if they grapple with a definition at all, produce some variant of a diagram that depicts emotion on two (sometimes more) scales. These scales are 'orthogonal'; that is, they suggest that there are two dimensions of emotions at right angles (and thus independent) of each other. Each scale goes from one extreme to the other. For example, there may be a scale from 'ecstasy' to' terror'. In between these two extremes are a number of intervening points, and each may be labelled in some way (e.g. elation, pleasure, apprehension, fear). The orthogonal scale might go from 'rage' through 'sadness' to 'relief'. The labels vary according to the particular interest of whoever writes the textbook; there seems no agreement on categories or labels. Furthermore, are the intervening labels simply arbitrary gradations between the two extremes, or definable states in their own right? Nevertheless, we can see here a familiar pattern. Emotion has a dimension (that is, there are categories of emotional states) and a value (that is, we can position an individual's current emotion at some point within a dimension). This is not logic-chopping. We need a clear idea of what psychological process we are dealing with if we are to understand the role of the brain in emotion (what is there to explain?) and its relation to mental illness (is depression a disorder of a particular emotion?). Recall that Papez ascribed emotion as the defining function of the limbic system (Chapter 1). Even Charles Darwin, in his book, '*Expression of the emotions in man and animals*' never seems to define what an emotion is, though he lists quite a few.

What about emotion and mood? As we have seen, experimental psychology talks of emotion, clinical psychology of mood. Are they the same? Moods are variously defined as emotions that persist (but for how long?) or continue when the 'stimulus' — that is, the provoking event that induced the emotional response — is no longer present. That seems to undervalue memory or the capacity to appraise the significance of whatever it was that caused the emotion in the first place. Other psychologists prefer the idea that moods represent a (temporary) shift in outlook, such that any external event is more likely to be appraised in a particular emotional light — that is, result in a given emotional reaction or reacted

Emotion and the Brain

We should not elevate the neurological over the behavioural or cognitive, or foster this idea among the general public. We should strive to develop and understand a new model in which a human being moves from one psychophysical state to another, describable on different levels by different specialists. Causation flows between these states and not between the levels of description.

> J Herlihy and J Gandy. (2002) Causation and explanation.
> *The Psychologist* **15**, pp. 248–251.

The tendency which I want to resist is to speak of 'emotions' and 'motives' as if they are classificatory terms for lumping together states of mind such as fear, anger, jealousy, and the like. Psychologists often set down what they consider man's instincts or basic drives to be. They then go on to catalogue his basic motives and emotions and are somewhat embarrassed to find that states of mind like fear and jealousy occur in both lists. So they try to make motives derivatives from emotion, or emotion an aspect of. . . motivated behavior. . . . All such treatments, in my view, misconceive both how the concepts of 'emotion' and the concept of 'motive' work. For these terms are not classificatory ones; they are rather terms which are used to relate states of mind such as fear, anger, and jealousy to distinctive frames of reference, those of activity and passivity.

> R S Peters. (1965) Emotion, passivity and the place of Freud's
> theory in psychology. In: *Scientific psychology: principles and*
> *approaches*. Eds. B B Wolman and E Nagel. (Basic Books.)

The natural empathizer can perceive fine shifts of mood, all the intermediate shades of an emotion in another person that might otherwise go unnoticed. Take hostility, for example. Some people only notice a few shades of hostility. . . in contrast, a good empathizer might recognize fifty shades of hostility. . . . Empathy can be compared to colour vision in this way. Some people notice just a few shades of blue, whilst others notice a hundred. My colleagues. . . and I recently completed an emotion taxonomy. . . and discovered that there are 412 discrete. . . human emotions.

> S Baron-Cohen. (2003) *The essential difference.*
> (Allen Lane, London.)

The identification of an entire neural system that can be cogently conceptualized as a representation of the physiological condition of the body to in a way that depends on the prevailing emotion. Philosophers such as Ryle refer to 'dispositions': features than incline someone to experience a particular emotion in a given situation. It is easy to see that the boundary between 'mood' (an emotional state) and 'cognition' (the way we think about something) is not sharp, and neither should it be, since both will affect each other. The clinical psychologist will tell us that he has measures for mood. For example, a test called the Profile of Mood States (POMS) asks the subject a number of questions about how they have felt over the past few days or weeks (depending on the exact purpose of the questionnaire) and then delivers a score of six mood states (tension-anxiety, depression-dejection, anger-hostility, vigour, fatigue, confusion-bewilderment). Despite the fact that mood is supposed, by some, to be persistent emotion, you can see that not all the terms used for mood are the same as those for a list of emotions.

Let us go with the idea that a mood is a persistent emotional state. If depression is an illness, this implies that it is maladaptive. That is, being depressed represents a state that is not only unpleasant, maybe even 'painful', but one that impairs normal function, just like any other illness. Indeed, as we have seen, the DSM criteria for MDD make this one condition for the diagnosis to be made. It is obvious that being sad — even very sad — is not necessarily maladaptive or out of the normal. Someone who has just lost a great deal of money, or someone they love, or his/her job would be expected to be sad. Note that all these events involve loss of some sort. Being in this state might very well have an adverse influence on their everyday life, so impairment of function by mood itself is not depression. However, imagine someone who is in such a state of sadness, but one that is completely disproportionate to any possible recent loss. Let us also assume not only that they are sad, but very sad: that is, on any scale of mood, they would score at the top end for the dimension 'sadness'. Is this being depressed?

The question is an important one. If depression is a condition of extreme, but normal, 'sadness' but in an 'abnormal' (that is, inappropriate) situation, then our search for its cause will focus on why an extreme emotional state is triggered in the wrong circumstances. Since how we react has to be 'adaptive', that is, fit in with our requirements to cope successfully with whatever demands life puts on us, to be overwhelmed has several fundamental implications. . . . These findings signify the cortical representation of feelings from the body as a likely basis for human awareness of the physical self as a feeling entity. This association provides a fundamental framework for the involvement of these feelings with emotion, mood, motivation and consciousness. . . .

A key feature that distinguishes pain, temperature and other bodily feelings from touch is their inherent association with emotion. . . . These feelings all have not only a sensory but also an affective, motivational aspect.

A D Craig. (2002) How do you feel? Interoception:
The sense of the physiological condition of the body.
Nature reviews: Neuroscience **3**, pp. 655–666.

Natural selection doesn't give a fig for our happiness or sadness; brain mechanisms express these responses in whatever ways promote the long-term success of our genes.

R N Nesse. (1999) The evolution of hope and despair.
Social Research **66**, pp. 429–469.

There never has been any doubt that, under certain circumstances, emotion disrupts reasoning. The evidence is abundant and constitutes the source for the sound advice with which we have been brought up. Keep a cool head, hold emotions at bay! Do not let your passions interfere with your judgement. As a result, we usually conceive of emotion as a supernumerary mental faculty, an unsolicited, nature-ordained accompaniment to our rational thinking. If emotion is pleasurable, we enjoy it as a luxury; if it is painful, we suffer it as an unwelcome intrusion. In either case, the sage will advise us, we should experience emotion and feeling in only judicious amounts. We should be reasonable.

A R Damasio. (1995) *Descartes' error.*
(Picador, London.)

What neural mechanism underlies the capacity to understand the emotions of others? Does this mechanism involve the brain areas normally involved in *experiencing* the same emotion? We performed an fMRI study in which participants inhaled odorants producing a strong feeling of disgust. The same participants observed video clips showing the emotional facial expression of disgust. Observing such faces and feeling disgust activated the same sites in the anterior insula and to a lesser extent in the anterior cingulate cortex.

with the 'wrong' mood would be maladaptive, and impair normal function. At this point, our psychiatrist will tell us that depression has more than one dimension, as the DSM criteria make clear; it's not simply sadness. But let us stick, for the moment, to this simple argument. Assuming the 'wrong emotion' approach will send us off on a search in the brain for the way it matches an emotional response to the 'right' circumstances. Depression, then, is a failure of this system: the patient, has the wrong (or maladaptive) emotional reaction to an event in his/her life. This approach has its attractions. After all, we know that depression may follow an adverse 'life event' (one that usually includes the loss of something we value) a friend, a lover, a job, and so on. But not everyone who experiences such a life event becomes depressed. Furthermore, the questionnaires that psychiatrists and clinical psychologists use to measure depression are continuous: that is, anyone, whether depressed or not, will be able to score something on the test. As the score rises, the likelihood of a diagnosis of depression becomes greater, since the questions are related to the symptoms of depression. Research psychiatrists commonly use a cut-off point (a minimum score) to decide whether someone is currently depressed or not, and to assess recovery. All this suggests that the boundary between depression and normal emotion is blurred, though depression may represent depths of emotion not often (or perhaps ever) experienced by 'normal' people. If we accept this, then our enquiry for a neural 'cause' of depression will make us ask about how we relate a 'stimulus' (a set of external events) to an emotional 'response' and how this might go wrong.

But there is another possibility. Depression is common and strikes one regardless of one's class, gender, intellectual ability and education. This does not mean, by the way, that these factors do not influence the chance of its occurring. But it can happen to anybody. Including some very articulate writers, who have told the rest of us what it is like to be depressed. Listen to what they say down the ages (see the box). An academic; a novelist; a scientist (though one with considerable literary abilities), a psychologist; a renowned poet; a travel writer, all sufferers from depression, and all agreeing that what they experienced was outside the normal. Our neuroscientist, who has learned the art of scepticism as part of his training, points out that the days of introspective psychology

Thus, as observing hand actions activates the observer's motor representation of that action, observing an emotion activates the neural representation of that emotion. This finding provides a unifying mechanism for understanding the behavior of others.

B Wicker, C Keysers, J Plailly, J-P Royet, V Gallese and G Rizzolatti. (2003) Both of us disgusted in *my* insula: The common neural basis of seeing and feeling disgust. *Neuron* **40**, pp. 655–664.

went out with William James. Why should we believe what people say about their own emotional state, particularly when they have been so evidently ill?

The clinical psychologist, who prides himself on an objective approach to his subject, nevertheless, reminds us that both the diagnosis of MDD and the scales used by researchers such as he, all depend on patients self-reports; so why start disbelieving them now? Depression, according to these witnesses, represents an emotional state outside the norm. Is it a neural state which should never occur in a healthy person, but, by its very existence marks an individual as having a mental illness? If we accept this, then our search for the roots of this illness in the brain is rather different: we are looking for something in the brain that occurs only in a pathological (abnormal) state. Pathologists can distinguish cancer cells from normal ones. Will there come a day when we can recognise a 'depressed' brain by something that is observable within it? An abnormal chemical? A strange set of neurons? It suddenly becomes clear that whether we think of an affective disorder like depression as an extreme variant of the normal (though, perhaps, occurring under inappropriate circumstances) or as an abnormal state becomes critically important for the way we think about the illness itself, for how we investigate its cause in the brain, and the kind of treatments for which we search.

We should not forget that other mental illnesses may also be associated with intolerable stress. An event that threatens life itself and spells extreme danger may be followed by a disorder graphically and accurately called 'post-traumatic stress disorder' usually abbreviated to PTSD. Earthquakes, war, fires, rape and car accidents may result in PTSD, a condition that has some unusual and characteristic features. To you and me, the sound of a helicopter passing over head may simply be a minor irritant. But there are those who were in Vietnam during the 1960s–70s in whom this innocuous sound may provoke a very different, and altogether more damaging reaction. Suddenly, they are back in that forest clearing, the sound of the helicopter deafeningly close, their comrades lying mutilated round them, expecting any moment to feel bullets tearing through them too. Unspeakable terror grips them now, as it did then. Their heart pounds, their pulse races. Even though it is twenty years or more since this happened. Even though they avoid hearing helicopters if they can, they are not free. Depressed,

My pain's past cure, another Hell,
I may not in this torment dwell,
Now desperate I hate my life,
Lend me a halter or a knife.
 All my griefs to this are jolly
 Naught so damn'd as Melancholy
 Robert Burton. (1641) *The anatomy of melancholy.*

In ways that are totally remote from normal experience, the grey drizzle
of horror induced by depression takes on the quality of physical pain. . . .
For those who have dwelt in depression's dark wood, their return from the
abyss is not unlike the ascent of the poet. . . trudging upwards out of hell's
black depths into. . . the shining world.
 William Styron. (1992) *Darkness visible: a memoir of madness.*
 (Vintage books, New York.)

Sadness is to depression what normal growth is to cancer.
 Lewis Wolpert. (1999) *Malignant sadness.*
 (Faber and Faber, London.)

Which way I fly is hell; myself as Hell;
And in the lowest deep a lower deep
Still threat'ning to devour me open wide,
To which the Hell I suffer seems a heaven.
 John Milton. (1608–1674) *Paradise lost.*

When he was in a phase of depression, I had known him insomniac for
four or five nights together. He would lie open-eyed through the minutes
of the night, and then another, having to face his own thoughts. Until, his
control broken, he would come to my room and wake me up: should we
drive over to George Passant and make a night of it? Or to our friends in
London? Or should we go for a walk all night? The melancholy, the
melancholy shot through with sinister gaiety, had been creeping upon him
during the past few weeks. He could not throw it off, any more than a
disease. When it seized him, he felt that it would never let him go.
 C P Snow. (1951) *The masters.* (Penguin Books, London.)

anxious, finding it difficult to relate even to those near them, let alone colleagues at work, they drift into semi-isolation. There are even those who carry with them to this day such scars from the second world war, 60 years or more ago. PTSD is a kind of malignant memory, uneradicable, and, it has to be said, very difficult to treat. Anyone with PTSD has his/her own 'trigger' that induces such 'flashbacks' as these episodes are called, one that is ineluctably associated with the traumatic event. But, just as not everyone who has a severe loss gets depressed, so not everyone exposed to the horrors of personal peril in war, or a life-threatening earthquake, gets PTSD. Some, it seems, are more vulnerable than others.

Medicine is not only about putting things right that have gone wrong (treatment) but also about prevention. We immunise those at risk of getting tuberculosis. What do we know about individual differences in vulnerability to depression? We know that only some people exposed to 'loss' (life events) get depressed, just as, during a flu epidemic, some will get ill, whilst others will not. Are there recognisable features in individuals that predispose them to becoming depressed? If there were, this might not only allow us to recognise such people, and perhaps offer some preventive treatment, it might also suggest additional 'causes' of depression. But first we must draw a clear distinction between 'risk' and 'cause'.

A war breaks out, and a group of journalists go to the front-line. All are provided with bullet-protective vests, but for some reason not all these vests are the same. Some are more effective than others. Some, indeed, are virtually useless. As the war proceeds, more and more journalists are wounded, but some are not. At its end, we can try to analyse whether receiving a wound is at all predictable. We look at where the journalists have been: those spending a lot of time in the fiercest battles clearly had the greatest chance of being wounded. Amongst this group, those with the better-quality vests had, obviously, the least chance of injury. But even though wearing the 'useless' vests increased the risk of a wound, a few of these journalists in the most dangerous places remained undamaged. Conversely, though the best quality vests provided much better protection, a few of those wearing these received wounds (even in the safer areas, though this was rare). There are two factors (at least) representing 'risk': exposure to danger and the quality of the protective vest. So, there is both a predictable element in risk and one apparently due to 'chance' (scientists

I could not stand the pain any longer, could not abide the bone-weary and tiresome person I had become.
Kay Redfield Jamison. (1996) *An unquiet mind.*
(Alfred A Knopf, New York.)

Depression is such a cruel punishment. There are no fevers, no rashes, no blood tests to send people scurrying in concern. Just a slow erosion of the self, as insidious as any cancer. And, like a cancer, it is essentially a solitary experience. A room in hell with only your name on the door.
Martha Manning. (1995) *Undercurrents.* (Harper, San Francisco.)

When I was younger, so much younger than today,
I never needed anybody's help in any way.
But now these days are gone, I'm not so self assured,
Now I find I've changed my mind and opened up the doors.

Help me if you can, I'm feeling down
And I do appreciate you being round.
Help me, get my feet back on the ground,
Won't you please, please help me.
The Beatles. *Help!*

There is a certain clarity where nothing interest, engages or motivates you. The clarity is not a window on the world — which is all black anyway — but solely on the insurmountable task of moving into a less tortured mental space.
Kate Baillie. (2002) The black window. *Planet* **151**, pp. 69–73.

call this 'stochastic'). But neither is the 'cause' of the wound. The cause is the damage inflicted by a bullet. The consequence is variable, and depends on which tissue has been damaged and the extent of this damage.

What do we know about the risk for depression? It has been known for quite some time that certain sorts of people seem to have an increased chance of getting depressed after the severe stress of an unwelcome life event. Not everyone agrees about what these factors are, but in general they fall into three categories: the person's social environment (their quality of life and the support of friends and partners), their psychological makeup (for example, their tendency to be rather anxious), and whether they have relatives that have been or are depressed. The latter might be either an 'environmental' feature (being part of family that has depressed people in it) or a 'genetic' one (being in a family that has a gene or genes for the risk for depression). It is quite difficult to decide which. And a major risk for depression is a previous episode of being depressed. So here we have a good example of differences in susceptibility to stress (a life event, say) which can, in part, be accounted for by features that distinguish one person from another. Like any other illness, there are several contributing factors, some unrelated, some not. But being able to define and even to measure these risks does not tell us how they alter the brain to make it vulnerable to depression.

But there are some other clues. The first is that women are about twice as liable to get depressed as men. There have been many attempted explanations for this, but it is striking that this sex difference appears only at puberty. Pre-pubertal children also get depressed (this used to be denied) but the sex ratio is almost one. During and after puberty, it changes. So, perhaps the rapid increase in sex hormones at and after puberty has something to do with risk? I am sorry to say that the trail goes rather cold at this point, though we should remember that many women experience a cyclic change in mood during the week or so before they menstruate (pre-menstrual tension or syndrome) which suggests that these hormones can affect mood. It also suggests that we should look inside the body as well as outside it for risk factors.

An unwelcome stress, particularly one that is unexpected or outside the control of the individual concerned, raises cortisol levels (Chapter 4). There is a condition called Cushing's syndrome (named after the American

PTSD

On the morning of March 7, 1957, an oil tanker collided with a freighter in the Delaware River. Intense explosions in the tanker killed eight men instantly, including all the officers, but the rest of the crew survived in spite of being surrounded by fire on the ship and in the water. In the short term, psychological symptoms such as nervousness, tension, or anxiety were common in the survivors. . . of the 34 men, 4 showed severe psychiatric disorder. When the men were seen a few years later, the amount of psychological deterioration that had taken place was impressive. At least 26 of the 353 men had received some form of medical help for complaints of a psychiatric nature. . . .

> G W Brown. (1989) Life events and measurement. In: *Life events and illness*. Eds. G W Brown and T O Harris. (Unwin Hyman, London.)

. . . It is clear from scientific observations that PTSD and its symptoms are present across cultures, with the only differences being the culturally specific expression of symptoms and the indigenous ways in which sufferers deal with them. Studies have shown that cross-cultural similarities and consistencies greatly outweigh cultural and ethnic differences.

> T Elbert and M Schauer. (2002) Burnt into memory.
> *Nature* **419**, p. 883.

Perhaps there are no more vivid memories than those which are stored in the brains of soldiers who have experienced excruciatingly horrible combat situations. Witness the account. . . of a 50-year-old Viet Nam veteran who cannot hear a clap of thunder, see an Oriental woman, or touch a bamboo placemat without re-experiencing the sight of his decapitated friend. Even though this occurred in a faraway place more than 28 years ago, the memory is still vivid in every detail and continues to produce the same state of hyperarousal and fear as it did on that fateful day.

> W A Falls and M Davies. (1995) Behavioral and physiological analysis of fear inhibition. In: *Neurobiological and clinical consequences of stress: from normal adaptation to PTSD*. Eds. M J Friedman, D S Charney, and A Y Deutch, pp. 177–202. (Lippincot-Raven, Philadelphia.)

"I can't get the memories out of my mind! The images come flooding back in vivid detail, triggered by the most inconsequential things, like a door slamming or the smell of stir-fried pork. Last night I went to bed, was having neurosurgeon who described it). It is caused by very high and abnormal levels of cortisol, usually as a result of a tumour of the adrenal or pituitary glands. It is a dangerous condition, and has to be treated. Such people have a number of characteristic signs: they are often rather fat, have peculiar stripes on the bodies, and high blood pressure. Some have a form of diabetes. And nearly all of them are depressed. Not surprising, you might think: they are ill, and they do not look or feel too good. Not so; as soon as you remove the tumour, their depression lifts. It is a characteristic of the condition. What is more, if you give people prolonged courses of cortisol-like hormone (corticoids: sometimes done for arthritis and other conditions), they may get depressed as well. It is looks as if cortisol itself can either induce depression or increase the risk for it. But there is more.

Recall that there is a daily rhythm of cortisol (Chapters 4 and 11). Each morning, cortisol surges into your blood, but as the evening approaches, levels go right down. Everyone has a different rhythm: my cortisol may rise slightly higher than yours each day, and yours may vary from day to day. So some people have characteristically somewhat higher 'high tides' than others. Now, here's the striking fact: women and adolescents with higher morning levels have a greater risk of becoming depressed after an unwelcome life event. The daily higher levels of cortisol seems to sensitise their brains to react to adversity by depression. Cortisol seemingly pushes them nearer the brink, but the life event pushes them over the cliff. Recall a similar situation for cortisol and brain damage (Chapter 4). And, we may think, depression is a form of brain dysfunction — reversible damage. What we do not yet know is what happens to cortisol after the life event itself and whether this also plays a part.

Now let us try and put together two facts about the body and depression: women get it more often, and higher cortisol levels in the morning are a risk factor. We can measure cortisol levels in the saliva, and these give us quite a good indication of those in the blood (and the brain). Female salivary levels of cortisol in the morning are about 20 percent higher than males — but not before puberty. Might this be one reason why women are more prone to depression than men — they are somewhat nearer the 'edge'? It is possible, though we cannot be sure yet. Why does puberty increase cortisol levels? It is known that oestrogen can increase cortisol (this happens during pregnancy).

a good sleep for a change. Then in the early morning . . . there was a bolt of crackling thunder. I awoke instantly, frozen in fear. I am right back in Vietnam, . . . I' m sure I'll get hit in the next volley and convinced I will die. My hands are freezing, yet sweat pours from my entire body. I feel each hair on the back of my neck standing on end. I can't catch my breath and my heart is pounding. I smell a damp sulfur smell. Suddenly I see what's left of my buddy Troy, his head on a bamboo platter, sent back to our camp by the Viet Cong. . . . The next bolt of lightning and clap of thunder makes me jump so much that I fall to the floor. . . ."

D S Charney, A Y Deutch, J H Krystal, S M Southwick, and M Davis. (1993) Psychobiologic mechanisms of posttraumatic stress disorder. *Archives of General Psychiatry* **50**, pp. 294–304.

Studies of concentration camp victims indicated that profound and protracted stress may have chronic or permanent effects no matter what the predisposition of the prestress personality. . . . As just one example, 99 percent of the 226 Norwegian survivors of a Nazi concentration camp in World War II had some psychiatric disturbances when intensively surveyed years after their return to normal life. . . 87 percent had cognitive disturbances such as poor memory and inability to concentrate, 85 percent had persistent nervousness and irritability, 60 percent had sleep disturbances, and 52 percent had nightmares.

M J Horowitz. (1986) *Stress response syndromes.* 2nd ed. (Jason Aronson Inc, New Jersey.)

In animals, exposure to severe stress can damage the hippocampus. Recent human studies show smaller hippocampal volume in individuals with . . . posttraumatic stress disorder (PTSD). Does this represent the neurotoxic effect of trauma, or is smaller hippocampal volume a pre-existing condition that renders the brain more vulnerable (to PTSD)? In monozygotic twins, discordant for trauma exposure, we found evidence that smaller hippocampi indeed constitute a risk factor for the development of stress-related psychopathology. . . .

M W Gilbertson *et al.* (2002) Smaller hippocampal volume predicts pathologic vulnerability to psychological trauma. *Nature Neuroscience* **5**, pp. 1242–1247.

This does not explain why some women have higher cortisol than others. One obvious reason is that those with higher levels have more stressful lives. But this does not seem to be the case. We simply do not know, but there are some intriguing possibilities. The first is a genetic one. There may be individual differences in genes (polymorphisms — we discuss them in Chapter 13) that result in differences in the shape of the daily cortisol rhythm. But which genes? There are some that are candidates, but whether they are really responsible is still to be found out. A second possibility is that things happen at a very early stage in life that have long-standing effects on cortisol. This is known to occur in animals. Separate a tiny new-born rat pup or an infant monkey from its mother for a few hours, and when it grows up its cortisol system reacts more vigorously to stress. This idea — that the brain is peculiarly susceptible to adversity early in life — may apply to many other characteristics (Chapter 13). For example, we know that early parental neglect can have longstanding results on later behaviour. Recently, it has been found that children whose mothers suffered from post-natal depression (this impairs maternal behaviour) have higher morning cortisol when they are about 13–14 years old. So, similar 'programming' of cortisol by early adversity may occur in rats and humans.

But there may be other factors we know about that make the brain more or less vulnerable to the stress of a life event. We have already considered the role of serotonin (5HT) in stress (Chapter 3). Recall that low serotonin increases the response of the brain to many events outside the body, such as something painful, or food, or a sexual stimulus. Many cases of depression are treated by drugs (e.g. Prozac) that increase serotonin. Does this mean that low serotonin 'causes' depression? Many psychiatrists believe so. This is because of the effect of the drug (people get better faster), the fact that depressed people seem to show deficient serotonin responses, and you can reawaken a depressive mood in some people who have been depressed but who are now recovered by lowering their brain serotonin (you give them a drink low in tryptophan: explained in Chapter 3). I interpret these results differently. To me, it seems more likely that serotonin influences the impact of an adverse life event: you need your serotonin when you are in trouble. If this is true, then individual differences in serotonin might also contribute to the risk of

. . . The path in front of the veranda was made of large round water-worn pebbles, from some sea beach. They were not loose, but stuck down tight in moss and sand, and were black and shiny, as if they had been polished. I adored those pebbles. I mean literally, adored; worshipped. This passion made me feel quite sick sometimes. And it was adoration that I felt for the foxgloves at Downe (Darwin's house), for the stiff red clay out of the Sandwalk clay-pit; and for the beautiful white paint on the nursery floor. This kind of feeling hits you in the stomach, and in the ends of your fingers, and is probably the most important thing in life. Long after I have forgotten all my human loves, I shall still remember the smell of a gooseberry leaf, or the feel of the wet grass on my bare feet; or the pebbles in the path. In the long run, it is this feeling that makes life worth living, this which is the driving force behind the artist's need to create.

Gwen Raverat. (1952) *Period piece.* (Faber and Faber, London.)

No man believes that many-textured knowledge and skill — as a just idea of the solar system, or the power of painting flesh, or of reading written harmonies — can come late and of a sudden; yet many will not stick at believing that happiness can come at any day and hour solely by a new disposition of events. . . .

George Eliot. (1966) *Felix Holt.*

She was walking on before him so lightly and so erect that he longed to run after her noiselessly, catch her by the shoulders and say something foolish and affectionate into her ear. She seemed to him so frail that he longed to defend her against something and then to be alone with her. Moments of their secret life together burst like stars upon his memory. A heliotrope envelope was lying beside his breakfast-cup and he was caressing it with his hand. Birds were twittering in the ivy and the sunny web of the curtain was shimmering along the floor: he could not eat for happiness.

James Joyce. (1914) *Dubliners.*
(Penguin Modern Classics, Harmondsworth, UK.)

To like something is to succumb, in a small but contentful way, to death. But dislike hardens the perimeter between the self and the world, and depression. Cortisol can alter serotonin, which might be one way. Another is that not all the enzymes and proteins that control what serotonin does in your brain are the same in all people. We discuss this further in the next chapter.

But, I hear you ask, what causes depression? Where and what is the 'bullet'? All sorts of ways have been tried of examining the brains of people who have died whilst depressed (often by suicide). Despite all sorts of claims, there isn't yet any accepted stigma in the brain characterising depression. There is certainly evidence that people with depression may have altered serotonin systems, but this is a long way from the simple assertion that too little causes this illness. Reducing serotonin (see Chapter 3) does not reliably result in depressed mood unless the person has already been depressed (itself a fascinating fact which still needs explaining). So why do SSRIs (drugs that increase serotonin) aid recovery? Perhaps for a similar reason that putting a plaster over a cut aids healing. Insufficient serotonin, in my view, is a risk factor for reacting to stress by becoming depressed, and increasing it helps the recovery process — recall that most untreated depressives get better, though they may relapse. And drugs that act on other substances in the brain also increase the rate of recovery. Absence of a plaster does not cause the cut!

Inevitably, given their potent effects on behaviour, peptides have been implicated. Corticotropin-releasing factor (CRF), a peptide we mentioned in Chapter 4, and which plays a central part of the brain's response to stress, is one. There are reports of high CRF in the fluid surrounding the brain in some depressives. Is this a cause of depression? There are problems: not all agree that depressives have high CRF; and even if they did, it might have more to do with the anxiety and the high cortisol that is typical of some cases of depression. Giving CRF to animals does not make them depressed, it makes them anxious (see Chapter 4).

Recently, scanning the living brains of depressed people has shown a small over-active area at the front part of the limbic cortex. It is quite close to the orbitofrontal cortex (see Chapters 5 and 10) — the region at the base of the front of the brain that has so much to do with emotional responses. But what this means — is it the 'cause' of depression or a consequence — and what the over-activity signifies, are still mysteries. Another plausible site is the amygdala. As we mentioned in Chapters 4 *brings a clarity to the object isolated in its light. Any dislike is in some measure a triumph of definition, distinction, and discrimination — a triumph of life.*

John Lanchester. (1996) *The debt to pleasure.*
(Henry Holt and Company, New York.)

Happiness is out there, back there, in association with those sights and sounds, and to retrieve it is to retrieve them also, to bring them crowding into the dark bedroom at three in the morning: mocking. Perfect happiness, past happiness, pluperfect.
Unhappiness. . . . is a very different matter. Unhappiness is now, not then at all. Unhappiness in like being in love: it occupies every moment of the day. It will not be put aside and like love it isolates; grief is never contagious.
Loss clamped her every morning as she woke; it sat its grinding weight on her and rode her, like the old man of the sea. It roared in her ears when people talked to her so that frequently she did not hear what they said. In interrupted her when she spoke, so that she faltered in mid-sentence, lost track. A little less, now; remissions came and went. The days stalked by, taking her with them.

Penelope Lively. (1983) *Perfect happiness.*
(William Heinemann, London.)

Everyone suddenly burst out singing;
And I was filled with such delight
As prisoned birds must find in freedom,
Winging wildly across the white
Orchards and dark-green fields; on-on-and out of sight

Siegfried Sassoon. (1886–1967) *Everyone sang.*

"I have been contemplating on emotion."
"Emotion," said Dr Ramis.
"Yes," said Stephen. "Emotion, and the expression of emotion. (In your book) you treat of emotion as it is shown by the cat, for example, the bull, the spider — I, too, have remarked the singular intermittent brilliance in the eyes of lycosida: have you ever detected a glow in those of the mantis?"

and 10, there is plenty of evidence suggesting that the amygdala has a central role in emotional responses, particularly (but perhaps not exclusively) those that are learned. Some evidence from imaging studies on depressives' brains also points to the amygdala. So, to end this chapter, here are a few speculations. Depression is caused by a reversible chemical event in the brain, probably part of the limbic system: the amygdala and limbic cortex are prime candidates (as already noted, they have plentiful connections with each other). Depression is not a variation of 'normality' so do not expect more or less of a 'normal' chemical. Certain rather serious illnesses are treated by giving patients peptides called 'cytokines': these are the chemicals mostly associated with the immune system, though they have many other functions. One of their most troublesome side effects is that the patients become depressed. Certain infections (such as influenza) activate cytokines and can be followed by depression. Some cytokines can also activate the pituitary to cause the adrenal to secrete more cortisol. There has been a suggestion (without very much evidence so far) that cytokines in the brain (where they are normally absent or present in very small amounts) might be responsible for some cases of depression. Cytokines are activated by stress as well as infections. In which case, it is an example of the price paid for an adaptive response being too high — and thus maladaptive. My money is on that being at least partly true.

Finally, back to cortisol. People with depression can also have high cortisol (though only in about half the cases), but this occurs in the evening rather than in the morning. This high cortisol may alter the way they view themselves and the world, and so prolong recovery. There is increasing interest in using drugs that block some of the actions of cortisol to treat certain sorts of depression (e.g. those that do not respond to the more usual anti-depressants). Very recently, DHEA, a second adrenal hormone, has been found to be reduced in some cases of depression. This is interesting because DHEA can also block some of the actions of cortisol on the brain. A combination of high cortisol and low DHEA seems to predict slow recovery from an episode of depression. Whether this finding can be translated into new therapy remains to be seen.

Depression wrecks lives. It also increases the risk of some other illnesses, including heart disease. Its prevalence shows how the inability

"Never, my dear colleague: though Busbequius speaks of it," replied Dr Ramis with great complacency.

"But it seems to me that emotion and its expression are almost the same thing. Let us take your cat: now suppose we shave her tail, so that it cannot shall I say perscopate or bristle; suppose we attach a board to her back, so that it cannot arch; suppose we then exhibit a displeasing sight — a sportive dog, for instance. Now, she cannot express her emotions fully: Quaere: will she feel them fully? She will feel them, to be sure, since we have suppressed only the grossest manifestations; but will she feel them fully?"

Patrick O'Brian. (1970) *Master and commander.*

(Harper Collins, London.)

of the brain to cope with stress can have a major impact on human affairs. It is beginning to seem that the black bile of yesteryear is being replaced by more modern chemicals. But let us not pretend: we have a long way to go before we can feel confident about really understanding the causes and course of this most devastating stress-related maladaptive illness.

Emotion and Reason

The neural basis of affect we can suppose need not entail much neural superstructure. It might use chemical reinforcement. This lets us stress the roof-organ (cortex) of the forebrain as especially cognitive, with below it the old kernel-organ of the forebrain especially related to 'affect'; and we remember that every cognition has, potentially at least, an emotive value. . . .

C S Sherrington. (1940) *Man on his nature.*
(Penguin Books, London.)

Intellect and emotion are inseparably bound up in expressive and receptive musical experience, but although a good deal is known about the neuroanatomical and neurophysiological substrate of emotion we do not know why music moves us as it does. Proust (1913) wrote of "keys of tenderness, of passion, of courage, of serenity" which awaken in us the emotion corresponding to the theme; music is then the image of these emotions, but that thought is only a partial answer to our problem. In the absence of any expectation of an immediate solution we turn to the poets, and in this case to Addison, "Music the greatest good that mortals know and all of heaven we have below."

R A Henson. (1977) The language of music. In: *Music and the brain.* Eds. M Critchley and R A Henson, pp. 233–254.
(Heinemann Medical Books, London.)

The Oxford dictionary defines affect as "feeling, emotion, desire especially as leading to action." Within these definitions are the germs of several ideas. . . . First, although affect is a felt experience and thus dependent on the nature of sensory input, it leads to behaviour. Second, behavior labelled as emotional manifests itself through response patterns. Third, emotional behavior is to be distinguished from reasoning. This distinction suggests that there may be different processes and different brain systems involved in the expression of emotion and reason.

S D Iversen and P J Fray. (1982) Brain catecholamines in relation to affect. In: *The neural basis of behavior.*
(Spectrum Publications, New York.)

I think we can reasonably say that the concept of emotion as disorganized response. . . is held fairly commonly amongst psychologists. . . . In this respect, we find that almost all of the discussion of emotions is in terms of such emotions as fear, anger, excitement, and their variants such as startle, anxiety, and rage. In other words, most of the attention is given to those emotional processes that seem to fit, at least half-plausibly, the idea of emotions as disorganized or disorganizing reactions. Some passing mention is usually made of other emotions such as delight, joy, affection, and love; but the space devoted to these is negligible in comparison. . . in speaking about the relation of learning to emotion, almost all. . . talk in terms of the problem of 'control' of emotion . . . . Emotion, in other words, is something to outgrow!

R W Leeper. (1948) A motivational theory of emotion
to replace "emotion as a disorganized response".
Psychological Review **55**, pp. 5–21.

Our lives. . . are a constant dance between. . . surges of ancient emotions and their impulsive behaviours on the one hand, and the slower cognitions and admonishments of the evolutionarily later cerebral cortex on the other.

Ian Robertson. (1999) *Mind sculpture*.
(Bantam Books, London.)

To begin, let us grant, on the basis of much evidence, that a general pattern of sympathetic discharge is characteristic of emotional states. Given such a state of arousal, it is suggested that one labels, interprets, and identifies this state in terms of the characteristics of the precipitating situation and one's apperceptive mass. This suggests, then, that an emotional state may be considered a function of a state of physiological arousal and a cognition appropriate to this state of arousal. The cognition, in a sense, exerts a steering function. Cognition arising from the immediate situation as interpreted by past experience provide the framework within which one understands and labels one's feelings. It is the cognition that determines whether the state of physiological arousal will be labeled 'anger', 'joy', or whatever.

S Schachter. (1975) Cognition and peripheralist — centralist controversies
in motivation and emotion. In: *Handbook of psychobiology*.
Eds. M Gazzaniga and C Blakemore, pp. 529–562.
(Academic Press, New York.)

There is a long tradition of understanding emotion and cognition as distinct from each other. This tradition extends back at least to Plato. . . . An increasingly influential modern version of this theory is based on data from the neurosciences and depicts emotion and cognition as occurring in different parts of the brain. Cognition is theorised to be mediated principally in the neocortex and hippocampus, emotion principally in the amygdala, hypothalamus and visceral nervous system of the lower brain stem. Such views. . . (argue) for the existence of independent, separate systems for emotion and cognition.

We argue that (these statements) share three shortcomings. They tend to differentiate emotion from cognition by linking emotion with sensation, but there are difficulties both in associating emotion with sensation and in dissociating the sensory from the cognitive. They tend to overestimate the autonomy of different areas of the brain and thereby overstate the extent to which different aspects of mental processes can be differentiated anatomically of functionally. Finally, they have difficulty accounting for the various cognitive aspects of the emotions.

W G Parrott and J Schulkin. (1993) Neuropsychology
and the cognitive nature of the emotions.
Cognition and Emotion **7**, pp. 43–59.

Emotional expression. . . is a pivotal processing component because music has the power to elicit strong emotional responses. It takes as input emotional-specific musical features, such as mode (eg. major or minor) and tempo (e.g. fast or slow) as computed by the melodic and temporal pathways, respectively. What is currently unclear is to what extent this emotion expression analysis component is specific to music as opposed to being involved in more general kinds of emotional processing.

I Peretz and M Coltheart. (2003) Modularity of music processing.
Nature Neuroscience **6**, pp. 688–691.

Having thus considered all the functions belonging solely to the body, it is easy to recognize that there is nothing in us which we must attribute to our soul except our thoughts. These are of two principal kinds, some being actions of the soul and others its passions. Those I call its actions are all volitions, for we experience them as preceding directly from our soul and seeming to depend on it alone. On the other hand, the various perceptions or modes of knowledge present in us may be called its passions, in a general sense, for it is often not our soul which makes them such as they are, and the soul always receives them from the things that are represented by them. . . .

The perceptions we refer only to the soul are those whose effects we feel as being in the soul itself, and for which we do not normally know any proximate cause to which we can refer them. Such are the feelings of joy, anger and the like, which are caroused in us sometimes by the objects which stimulate our nerves and sometimes also by other causes.

R Descartes. (1649) The passions of the soul. In: *The philosophical writings of Descartes*, Vol 1. Translated by J Cottingham, R Stoothoff, D Murdoch. (Cambridge University Press, Cambridge.)

But an advantage infinitely superior to all physical goods, and one of which we undeniably partake owing to the harmony of the human race, is that of attaining, through communication of ideas and the progress of reason, the intellectual regions, of acquiring the sublime notions of order, wisdom, and moral goodness, of nourishing our sentiments on the fruits of our knowledge, of raising ourselves though the grandeur of our souls above the weakness of our nature, and of equalling, in certain respects through the art of reasoning, the celestial intelligences; until finally, by combating and vanquishing our passions, we gain the power to dominate man and imitate Divinity itself.

Jean-Jacques Rousseau. (1861) *A letter from Jean-Jacques Rousseau.* Translated by Arthur Goldhammer, *New York Review of Books* **50**, pp. 31–32.

Shouts rise again from the water
surface and flecks of cloud skim over
to storm-light, going up in the stem.
 Falling loose with a grateful hold
 of the sounds towards purple, the white bees
swarm out from the open voice gap. Such "treasure":
  the cells of the child line run back
  through hope to the cause of it; the hour
is crazed by fracture. Who can see what he loves,
  again or before, as the injury shears
   past the curve of recall, the field
  double-valued at the divine point.
 . . .

  And constantly the
 child line dips into sleep, the
more than countably infinite hierarchy of
 higher degree causality conditions
setting the reverse signs of memory and dream.
 "Totally confused most of the time" — is
  the spending of gain
  or damage mended
  and ended, aged, the
  shouts in the rain: in
  to the way out.
  J H Prynne. (1999) Again in the black cloud. In: *Poems.*
   Bloodaxe books. (Newcastle upon Tyne, UK.)

"Well, it all depends on what you mean by psychology, dear doctor. If you mean Oedipus and dogma, unseen and unprovable mechanisms, a church of true believers in the great universal truth that will have no other, then you are wrong. . . .

 If, however, you mean that the biological illness of the psychotic mind finds shape and character in the individual life of the patient and is moulded by it, as water flooding a plain will be diverted by the topography of the valley, then you speak true."
[the novel is set in the late 19th century]
 Sebastian Faulks. (2005) *Human traces.* (Vintage Books, London.)

Shame and disgrace cause most violent passions, and bitter pangs.
Generous minds are often moved with shame to despair for some publick
disgrace. . . . The most generous spirits are most subject to it. Aristotle,
because he could not understand the motion of Euripus, for grief and
shame drowned himself. Homer was swallowed up with this passion of
shame, because he could not unfold the fisherman's riddle. Sophocles
killed himself, for that a tragedy of his was hissed off the stage, Lucretia
stabbed herself, and so did Cleopatra, when she saw that she was reserved
for a triumph, to avoid the infamy. . . . A grave and learned Minister. . .
was one day as he walked in the fields for his recreation, suddenly taken
with a lask or looseness, and thereupon compelled to retire to the next
ditch; but being surprised. . . by some Gentlewomen of his Parish. . . was
so abashed, that he never did shew his head in publick, or come into the
Pulpit, but pined away with Melancholy.

> R Burton. *The anatomy of melancholy.*

In the introduction to his selection from Tennyson's poems W H Auden
writes: "There was little about melancholia that he didn't know; there was
little else that he did." . . . Tennyson's melancholia had its roots in his
sense of isolation in an alien universe. His sensibility was out of all
proportion greater than his love; his awareness of life unwarmed by any
feeling that he belonged to it or it to him.

> Hugh Kingsmill. (1949) The progress of a biographer. In: *The best of*
> *Hugh Kingsmill.* Ed. Michael Holdroyd. (Victor Gollancz, London.)

"Marvin!" he exclaimed. "What are you doing?"
"Don't feel you have to take any notice of me, please," came a muffled drone.
"But how are you, metalman?" said Ford.
"Very depressed."
"What's up?"
"I don't know," said Marvin, "I've never been there."
"Why," said Ford squatting down beside him and shivering, "are you
lying face down in the dust?"
"It's a very effective way of being wretched," said Marvin. "Don't
pretend you want to talk to me, I know you hate me."
"No I don't."

"Yes you do, everybody does. It's part of the shape of the Universe. I only have to talk to somebody and they begin to hate me. If you just ignore me I expect I shall probably go away."

D Adams. (1979) *The hitch hikers guide to the galaxy.*
(Pan Books, London.)

Tom was experiencing for the first time in his life (and no doubt he was lucky to have escaped it so long) that blackening and poisoning of the imagination which is one of the worst, as well as one of the commonest, forms of human misery. His world had become uncanny, full of terrible crimes and ordeals, and punishments. He felt frightened and guilty, anticipating some catastrophe which was entirely his own fault, yet also brought about by vile enemies whom he detested. It was no good appealing to reason and common sense, telling himself it was all just a dotty episode which he could put behind him and soon laugh about.

Iris Murdoch. (1984) *The philosopher's pupil.*
(Penguin Books, London.)

His narcotics were powerless to aid him, for when after a prodigious dose he sank into a grey slumber, it was filled with shapes that haunted him when he awoke, and waved enormous sickly-smelling wings above his head, and filled his room with the hot breath of rotting plumes. His habitual melancholy was changing day by day into something more sinister. There were moments when he would desecrate the crumbling and mournful mask of his face with a smile more horrible than the darkest lineament of pain.

Mervyn Peake. (1946) *Titus Groan.*
(Eyre and Spottiswoode, London.)

Poor Molly. It began with a tingling in her arm as she raised it outside the Dorchester grill to stop a cab; a sensation that never went away. Within weeks she was fumbling for the names of things. Parliament, chemistry, propeller she could forgive herself, but less so bed, cream, mirror. It was after the temporary disappearance of acanthus and bresaiola that she sought medical advice, expecting reassurance. Instead, she was sent for tests and, in a sense, never returned. . . . Molly,

restaurant critic, gorgeous wit and photographer, the daring gardener
who had been loved by the Foreign Secretary and could still turn a perfect
cartwheel at the age of forty-six. The speed of her descent into madness
and pain became a matter of common gossip; the loss of control of bodily
function and with it a sense of humour, and then the tailing off into
vagueness interspersed with episodes of ineffectual violence and muffled
shrieking.

Ian McEwan. *Amsterdam*. (Jonathan Cape, London.)

And may at last my weary age
Find out the peaceful hermitage,
The hairy gown and mossy cell
Where I may sit and rightly spell
Of every star that heaven doth show,
And every herb that sips the dew:
Till old experience do attain
To something like prophetic strain.

These pleasures, Melancholy, give,
And I with thee will choose to live.

John Milton. *From: Il Penseroso*

Dearest
I feel certain I am going mad again. I feel we can't go through another of
those terrible times. And I shan't recover this time. I begin to hear voices
and I can't concentrate. So I am doing what seems the best thing to do.
You have given me the greatest possible happiness. You have been in
every way all that anyone could be. I don't think two people could have
been happier until this terrible disease came. I can't fight any longer. . . .
Everything has gone from me but the certainty of your goodness. . . .
I can't go on spoiling your life any longer.
I don't think two people could have been happier than we have been.

Quentin Bell. (1976) Suicide letter from Virginia Woolf.
In: *Virginia Woolf*. (Triad/Paladin, St Albans.)

Hippocratic medicine explained health and disease in terms of 'humours',
basic juices of fluids. . . . These crucial vitality-sustaining juices were blood,

choler (or yellow bile), phlegm, and melancholy. . . . Humoral balance also explained the temperaments, or what would, in later centuries, be called personality and psychological dispositions. . . .   There was boundless explanatory potential in such rich holistic interlinkages of physiology, psychology and bearing, not least because correspondences were suggested between inner constitutional states ('temper') and outer physical manifestations ('complexion').   Analogy-based explanatory systems of this kind were not just plausible but indispensable so long as science had little direct access to what went on beneath the skin or in the head.

. . . The Paris of Flaubert, Baudelaire, Verlaine, and Rimbaud, held that true art — as opposed to the good taste favoured by the bourgeoisie — sprang from the morbid and pathological: sickness and suffering fired and liberated the spirit, perhaps with the aid of hashish, opium, and absinthe, and works of genius were hammered out on the anvil of pain.

. . . When Van Gogh painted himself, who can say whether he was painting madness? — all that is clear is that he was painting misery.

Roy Porter. (2002) *Madness, a brief history.*

(Oxford University Press, Oxford.)

Hormones and Depression

Collectively, all these studies suggest that glucocorticoids can damage hippocampal neurons over the life time. Such neurotoxicity, while surprising, is not without precedent. An extensive literature demonstrates that stress and/or glucocorticoids can be neurodegenerative in other situations; they can disrupt normal aspects of development, including damaging developing neurons. Furthermore, glucocorticoids impair the capacity of nervous tissue to recover from injury.

R M Sapolsky. (1992) Stress, *The aging brain, and the mechanisms of neuron death.* (MIT Press, Cambridge Massachusetts.)

Classically, depression has been thought of as melancholia, and its mood alterations have been associated with melancholic signs and symptoms such as loss of appetite and weight, loss of libido, and the inability to sleep. Internally, melancholic depression is marked by intensely painful arousal and an obsessional preoccupation with personal inadequacy and the inevitability of loss. . . . These signs and symptoms. . . strongly suggest the possibility that the pathophysiology of melancholic depression is related to a central excess of CRH (corticotropin-releasing hormone).

D Michelson, J Licinio, and P W Gold. (1995) Mediation of the stress response by the hypothalamo-pituitary-adrenal axis. In: *Neurobiological and clinical consequences of stress: From normal adaptation to PTSD,* Eds. M J Friedman, D S Charney, and A Y Deutch, pp. 225–238. (Lippincot-Raven, Philadelphia.)

If corticosteroids (cortisol) play. . . a crucial role in remembering stressors, one might wonder what will happen in endogenously depressed patients in which steroid levels are chronically elevated. The increased steroids will probably intensify all kinds of negative experiences which will then be remembered. It might well be that the remembering of all these negative events plays an important role in the development and maintenance of the depression. . . . These studies show that for endogenously depressed patients stressful events are experienced as more unpleasant which might indicate that they are intensified by increased corticosteroid levels.

B W M M Peeters and C L E Broekkamp. (1994) Involvement of corticosteroids in the processing of stressful life events. A possible implication for the development of depression. *Journal of steroid Biochemistry and Molecular Biology* **49**, pp. 417–427.

IL-1beta (a cytokine) serum concentrations were significantly elevated in (postviral depressed patients and major depression) compared to controls. The serum concentrations of IL-1beta were higher in the postviral group than in the major depression group; this difference was not significant. These data confirm previous suggestions of elevated IL-1beta levels in major depression and postviral depression. IL-1beta is known to induce depressive symptoms as well as sickness behaviour and may contribute to the hypothalamic pituitary adrenal axis hyperactivity found in mood disorders.

> B M Owen, D Eccleston, I N Ferrier, and A H Young. (2001) Raised levels of plasma interleukin-1beta in major and postviral depression. *Acta Psychiatrica Scandinavia* **103**, pp. 161–162.

Although there can be little doubt that the primary etiologic factor in major depression originates centrally, its manifestation and persistence may be dependent, at least in part, upon the resulting steroid milieu reaching the brain.

> B E P Murphy. (1991) Steroids and depression. *Journal of Steroid Biochemistry and Molecular Biology* **38**, pp. 537–559.

Our findings indicate that severe psychiatric reactions occur in approximately 5% of steroid-treated patients, and that a large proportion of these patients have affective and/or psychotic symptoms. Psychiatric disturbances usually occur early in the course of steroid therapy. Female sex, lupus erythematosus and high does of prednisone may be risk factors for the development of a steroid-induced psychiatric syndrome.

> D A Lewis, R E Smith. (1983) Steroid-induced psychiatric syndromes. *Journal of Affective Disorders* **5**, pp. 319–332.

According to the influential WHO World Health Report 2001, about 450 million people have mental and neurological disorders. This amounts to 12.3% of the global burden of disease, and will rise to 15% by 2020. . . . The brain and mind unction as a unity, but neurologists and psychiatrists do not. . . . There is a need for greater professional and public awareness of the role of the brain in mental illness and the mind in brain illness, based on modern knowledge of the brain and mental function arising from the neurosciences and the psychological and social sciences. Such an understanding. . . would greatly facilitate a breakdown of the barriers of misunderstanding and stigma surrounding these common diseases, which already amount to about a quarter of the global burden of disease.

> E H Reynolds. (2003) Brain and mind: A challenge for WHO. *Lancet* **361**, pp. 1924–1925.

Chapter 13

Individuality

So we are nearing the end of our enquiry into the brain's role in survival. We have seen how there are general systems in the brain defending us against too little energy, not enough water, damaging temperatures, hostile neighbours, as well as those ensuring that we are well looked after. We have also seen how our brain helps us to look after ourselves, when we are young, ill, or under threat from others. The brain also ensures that we procreate so that others survive, for some time, after us. But individuals differ in how well they cope, so that not everyone in a flu epidemic gets infected, only a few that are infected die, not all those with a severe loss in their lives gets depressed, some resist the midday burning sun better than others, only some (though how many) of those deprived of food and water and shelter in St Petersburg in that terrible winter of 1942 died. The dice roll, and we carry into the game of survival the gamble of what each of possesses in terms of defence or our ability to adapt. What do we know about this?

Individuality means different things. You think of yourself as an individual: that means you are different from anybody else in the world. Your biological make-up is different — there is unlikely to be anyone identical to you anywhere, unless you happen to have an identical twin, and even he/she will have differences. You look out into the world from the 'person' lying somewhere just behind your eyes: everyone else looks at you. Your experience is different from anybody else's; even though the fabric of your life may be made up of familiar threads, the exact way they are woven makes a pattern different from others. Even if someone else had, extraordinarily, experienced everything you have experienced, the results would still be different, since the 'you' to which all this has

Individuality

From the new development of genetics even more far-reaching consequences ensue. For the evolution of man and society arises from what individual men and women do, and from the purposes they have in doing it; in other words, from their character, which in the long run is conditioned by genetic processes. What we have now come to understand is that these genetic processes are entirely at the mercy of the system of breeding. . . .

The coming of the great man is not predictable. In his origin, there are two sources of uncertainty, one genetic, the other environmental. The genetic source is that the creative individual is always a unique recombination arising from outbreeding. . . . The environmental source of uncertainty lies almost entirely in the organic world outside mankind. . .

. . . We have now learnt that intelligence is of many kinds. It has to be measured not on one scale but many. And its diversity, if lost, cannot easily be recovered. We have therefore to preserve these diverse habitats, along with their diverse inhabitants, from damage which civilization has so far so wantonly wrought upon them.

C D Darlington. (1969) *The evolution of man and society.*
(Allen and Unwin, London.)

We already know the laws that govern the behaviour of matter under all but the most extreme conditions. In particular, we know the basic laws that underlie all of chemistry and biology. Yet we have certainly not reduced these subjects to the status of solved problems; we have, as yet, little success in predicting human behaviour from mathematical equations.

Stephen Hawking. (1988) *A brief history of time.*
(Bantam Press, London.)

The self is not born out of the realm of consciousness, only the noticing of it is (i.e., self-awareness). According to this view, the self can exist without awareness of its own existence. Even in we as self-aware individuals, self-awareness is not continuously present. In the middle of a difficult challenge, such as swimming away from a shark, you will try to get to shore and be quite aware of what is happening, but you will probably not be thinking to yourself, "Here I am swimming away from a shark." You will think about it only when you get to shore and safety.

R R Llinas. (2001) *I of the vortex.* (MIT Press, Cambridge, Massachusetts.)

happened is different from anybody else. Whether you are a socialite or a recluse, shy or outgoing, other people make up a large part of your pattern of life. Whilst we all think of ourselves as individuals, making our own decisions, in fact much of what we all do is influenced, determined or directed by the other people, their priorities as well as our own needs.

If all this sounds familiar, of course it is. Each individual is just that because of a particular genetic mix, and the influence this has on physical and mental abilities. But genes are only a starting point: the environment shapes the genetic mould, in ways that are sometimes influenced by the genes themselves, sometimes not. Robert Yerkes, a famous primatologist, wrote that a chimpanzee, kept alone, was not a chimpanzee at all; he meant that not only the physical environment, but also the social one, was necessary to realise what a complex creature like a chimpanzee (and surely man) was really designed for. We carry our individuality though our lives, calling upon different aspects of its survival equipment at different times, and under different circumstances. The survival of an infant needs different equipment from that of a young adult; a harsh physical environment may call upon equipment that is otherwise little used; social adversity requires still other resources. All men may be born equal, but they are certainly not born identical. Where do we start to try and make some sense of this utterly complex picture?

Let's start with our genes. You may have been surprised about how little we have discussed genes in detail. After all, this is the age of molecular biology, that most astonishing science, and the unravelling of the human genome, that most astonishing accomplishment. A gene is a segment of DNA and it codes for a corresponding segment of RNA. RNA, in turn, codes for a protein, which itself may be modified by other proteins (enzymes). It is the proteins that actually do the work in cells: they determine how we function. We all carry the same set of genes; or, rather, a similar set of genes. Your genes for, say, making the proteins that make serotonin are similar to mine, but may not be the identical. Here is the first source of individuality.

Genes are made of long strings of four chemicals, called 'bases'. The bases are: A (adenine); T (thymine); C (cytosine); G (guanine). The code consists of any three bases (eg. ATT or CGA). Each gene is a long string of triplets. Each triplet codes for a similar triplet of RNA (there is one

Popper argues that this model (falsification as the essential mark of scientific discourse) applies also to Darwin's theory of evolution. The species encounters a problem of adaptation as a result of change in the environment; it needs to evolve genetically or become extinct. Mutations spontaneously occur, which in Popper's view function as possible solutions; most are fatal to the organism in question, which is then eliminated. But a new mutation may prove resistant to elimination, and hence come to characterize the species — until a new problem of adaptation comes along. A mutation is like a new conjecture that invites refutation; natural selection consists in the elimination of bad conjectures.

Colin McGinn. (2002) Looking for a black swan. *New York Review of Books* **49**, pp. 46–50.

Nature, that fram'd us of four elements
Warring within our breasts for regiment,
Doth teach us all to have aspiring minds:
Our souls, whose faculties can comprehend
The wondrous architecture of the world,
And measure every wandering plant's course,
Still climbing after knowledge infinite,
And always moving as the restless spheres,
Wills us to ware ourselves and never rest,
Until we reach the ripest fruit of all,
That perfect bliss and sole felicity,
The sweet fruition of an earthly crown.

Christopher Marlowe. (1564–1593) *From: Tamburlaine the great.*

"Here's what I think, Mr Wind-up Bird," said May Kasahara. "Everybody's born with some different thing at the core of their existence. And that thing, whatever it is, becomes like a heat source that runs each person from the inside. I have one too, of course. Like everybody else. But sometimes it gets out of hand. It swells or shrinks inside me, and it shakes me up. What I'd really like to do is find a way to communicate that feeling to another person. But I can't seem to do it. They just don't get it. . . ."

Haruki Murakami. (2003) *The wind-up bird chronicle.*
Translated by Jay Rubin. (Vintage, London.)

base different in RNA). Each RNA triplet codes for a single amino acid. Proteins are made of long strings of aminoacids (up to several hundred) coded by the long strings of bases in the gene. Peptides are made by chopping up the amino acid strings that make proteins into shorter ones (say 20–50 or so). The chopping is itself done by other proteins, the enzymes, also made by different genes. So it all starts with a gene which we can think of as a long necklace, made up of four differently coloured beads. The order of the beads matters, as you can see. The cell knows when one 'necklace' (gene) starts and finishes, and each of our 46 chromosomes is a huge stretch of thousands of necklaces (genes) strung together. It reads off the code from each gene to make a protein.

During the formation of eggs in the mother and sperm in the father, the genes are shuffled, so that each of us gets a unique selection of half the genes from our father and the other half from our mother. Which is why, if you have six sons (or daughters), they are all different. This is the basis of individuality, and also of selection, since the mix of genes each inherits may play a major role in their ability to survive.

How do genes differ between people? The beads (bases) on a gene can vary between individuals. Perhaps this is not surprising. It is extraordinary enough for such a complex system to be replicated during the process of forming eggs and sperm. No wonder some genes contains errors: they are called mutations. One base can be replaced by another. A triplet changes. It may not matter. If ATT changes to ATC, then the gene still makes the same aminoacid (isoleucine) in the usual position in the protein — there is often more than one code for each amino acid. But suppose it changes to ATG, then the amino acid changes, to a different one — methionine. So the chain of amino acids making up the protein alters, ever so little. This might not matter much. On the other hand, it might.

This is because the shape of a protein matters. Proteins fold in complicated ways, and this can affect how well they do their job. Although great progress is being made, the exact way that the sequence of amino acids alters protein folding, and how this can change function, is still not fully understood. A single alteration of a base is called a polymorphism because the gene can exist in several forms (two, if there is a single polymorphism, but more if there are many). Each gene has hundreds and hundreds of known polymorphisms. There are about 30000–40000 genes

We are now in a position to compare the gradual increase through evolutionary time of both the amount of information contained in the genetic material and the amount of information contained in the brain of organisms. The two curves cross at a time corresponding to a few hundred million years ago and at an information content corresponding to a few billion bits. Somewhere in the steaming jungles of the Carboniferous Period there emerged an organism that for the first time in the history of the world had more information in its brain than in its genes.

Carl Sagan. (1977) *The dragons of Eden.*
(Hodder and Stoughton, London.)

Why, all delights are vain; but that most vain,
Which with pain purchased doth inherit pain:
As, painfully to pore upon a book
To see the light of truth; while truth the while
Doth falsely blind the eyesight of his look:
Light seeing light doth light of light beguile:
So, ere you find where light in darkness lies,
Your light grows dark by losing of your eyes.

William Shakespeare. *From: Love's labour's lost.*

In all past ages in the history of mankind, most of those who peered into the future will probably have thought that the current, familiar, state of things would continue much as it was. Man stood at the centre of his world; he regarded himself as being, not evolving. But many people have not yet properly absorbed the fact that the revolution triggered by Darwin's theory has utterly destroyed this anthropocentrism. Once the theory of evolution had become established... then logically it was scarcely possible to avoid the argument that man was more likely to have created God in his own image, as Bernard Shaw had so tellingly phrased it, than the other way round. Man saw himself as a unique creature among millions of other sorts of living and extinct beings . . : he had to justify his own existence, stand on his own two feet, or confess his inadequacy.

H Wendt. (1972) *From ape to Adam: The first million years of man.*
(Thames and Hudson, London.)

in the human genome (the number keeps going down). Genes do not act singly, but together. There are 23 pairs of chromosomes in the human genome. One or more polymorphisms may occur on both pairs of genes (each pair of chromosomes has the same genes in general) or on only one. There may be as many as 3 million alternative triplets in the human genome. Each combination will alter one or more proteins in several ways. Try and work out the possible combinations: you cannot, they are astronomical, though perhaps not infinite. These single base polymorphisms (they are called SNPs, pronounced as 'snips') are only one sort of mutation. Sometimes whole lengths of DNA are omitted or replicated. More individual variation, sometimes very obvious (as in 'single gene' diseases such as Huntington's disease or cystic fibrosis), more often mostly unnoticeable. That does not mean they do not matter.

Let me give you a recent example. Chapter 2 is mostly about serotonin, but let us recall one or two known facts about it. The brain's serotonin system is activated by stress. This may help the brain resist the stress or adapt to it. Released serotonin is sucked back into the nerves that contain it by a special protein (an uptake protein) which limits its action. The gene that makes this protein has a polymorphism (in this case one that involves a 'repeated' sequence). So a person can have either two 'short' forms (fewer repeats), two 'long' ones, or one of each. You cannot tell by looking at them. But should such a person be exposed to a 'life event' (a bad stress), then something extraordinary emerges. Those with two 'short' genes (and hence a slightly altered duration of action of serotonin) are more likely to become depressed (see Chapter 12). Those with two 'long' forms are less likely, those with one of each are in between. Here is a clear example of the interaction between the environment and the genes. Life events do not happen to everybody (the environment varies). When they do, how well someone adapts depends on their genetic makeup (a known polymorphism). If they never have a life event, perhaps this polymorphism never matters. Of course, reactions to life events or any other stress are more complex then this, but the point is made. It is a start of the journey to understanding how individuality (both of experience and genetic makeup) can determine who lives, or how they live. Variations in some proteins may also matter. Brain-derived growth factor (BDNF) is known to play a major role in the way the brain grows during development. We

Genes

The concept of the cell has evolved a long way from its original characterization as a simple unit of living matter: The cell has become an organism in which the controlled and integrated actions of genes produce specific sets of proteins that build characteristic structures and carry out characteristic enzymatic activities.

> J Darnell, H Lodish, and D Baltimore. (1986)
> *Molecular cell biology.* (Scientific American Books.)

What weird engines of self-preservation would the millennia bring forth? Four thousand million years on, what was to be the fate of the ancient replicators? They did not die out, for they are past masters of the survival arts. But do not look for them floating loose in the sea; they gave up that cavalier freedom long ago. Now they swarm in huge colonies, safe inside gigantic lumbering robots, sealed off from the outside world, communicating with it by tortuous indirect routes, manipulating it by remote control. They are in you and me; they created us, body and mind. They have come a long way, those replicators. Now they go by the name of genes, and we are their survival machines.

> R Dawkins. (1976) *The selfish gene.*
> (Oxford University Press, Oxford.)

There is every reason to believe that the DNA of, say, a human being codes for such features as nose shape, music talent, quickness of reflexes, and so on. Could one, in principle, learn to read off such pieces of information directly from a strand of DNA, without going through the actual physical process of *epigenesis* — the physical pulling-out of phenotype from genotype? Presumably, yes, since — in theory — one could have an incredibly powerful computer program simulating the entire process, including every cell, every protein, every tiny feature involved in the replication of DNA, of cells, to the bitter end. The output of such a *pseudo-epigenesis* program would be a high-level description of the phenotype.

> D R Hofstadter. (1979) *Godel, Escher, Bach: An eternal golden braid.*
> (Penguin Books, Harmondsworth, UK.)

In times past, when writing materials were in short supply a scribe would often reuse a manuscript rather than obtain a new parchment. The manuscript would be turned through 90°, and overwritten. These overwritten manuscripts bearing the imprint of more than one text are known as palimpsests. The now know it is also important in the adult brain. There is a 'SNP' in BDNF which adds to the risk of abnormal behaviour in children who have been abused. Note the way this sentence is written: the BDNF polymorphism the experience of abuse separately increase the chances of this happening; together that risk is increased further.

This science is only just beginning. There may be many instances of polymorphisms influencing all sorts of responses, for instance to drugs. But we do not yet understand whether polymorphisms control things like: why some people get fat (though there is a genetic variation in the leptin receptor which results in enormous obesity: see Chapter 5), why others response to stress by having heart attacks, why some may be aggressive, or prefer a certain sort of mate, or withstand severe cold better than others. But we can see the way forward, into this immense jungle of genetic complexity.

There are some tempting sign-posts. Recall all the peptides, amines and steroids that together make up much of the chemical language of the limbic system. Polymorphisms are rife in the genes that make these molecules and, possibly more importantly, the receptors that detect them and are responsible for how they function in the brain. We have seen how the peptide NPY is a major regulator of food intake (Chapter 5). Polymorphisms occur in both the gene making NPY and its receptors. They have been associated with differences in blood lipids, and there is a recent study showing that one variant may protect against obesity. There are also polymorphisms in the receptor molecule for cortisol, the stress hormone (Chapter 4). Do these play a part in individual differences in the way we respond to stress? A good deal of attention is now focussed on polymorphisms in the genes of the angiotensin system (Chapter 6) as a possible risk factor for high blood pressure. But do they also play a part is the ability to resist salt or water deprivation? Are there polymorphisms in the oxytocin receptor (Chapter 9) that could account for variations in people's ability to 'bond' (fall in love) with others? There are reports that a particular polymorphism in the oxytocin receptor is more common in autistic people, who characteristically have problems in 'empathising' with others and thus have difficulties forming social bonds.

Until quite recently, it was assumed that all genes obeyed Mendelian rules. At their simplest, these state that genes exist in two forms: 'dominant' genetic record is a complex palimpsest. Variation among modern individuals is shaped by cumulative past processes. Extracting information on any one past period or event requires careful interpretation to isolate it from previous and subsequent processes. In addition, natural selection is ever present, potentially influencing any variation that affects phenotypic fitness.

> M A Jobling, M E Hurles and C Tyler-Smith. (2004) Origins, peoples and disease. *Human evolutionary genetics.* (Garland Science, New York.)

Complex organisms cannot be construed the sum of their genes, nor do genes alone build particular items of anatomy or behavior — as they operate through complex interactions with other genes and their products, and with environmental factors both within and outside the developing organism. We fall into deep error, not just harmless oversimplification, when we speak of genes "for" particular items of anatomy or behavior. . . .

To cite an example of this fallacy, in 1996 scientists reported the discovery of a gene for novelty-seeking behavior — generally regarded as a good thing. In 1997 another study detected a linkage between the same gene and a propensity for heroin addiction. Did the 'good' gene for enhanced exploration become the 'bad' gene for addictive tendencies? The biochemistry may be constant, but the context and background matter.

> Stephen Jay Gould. (2002) *I have landed.*
> (Jonathan Cape, London.)

and 'recessive'. If you got a 'dominant' copy from your father, and a 'recessive' one from your mother, then you would be likely to 'express' your father's gene. If the reverse, then your mother's. If you got two dominant copies, your genetic makeup might be the same as if you had only one; however, in some cases, you would express more of the genes than if you got only one dominant copy. Someone with two copies of the same gene (either dominant or recessive) is called 'homozygous'. Blood groups are a classic example of Mendelian inheritance, though in fact there are two dominant genes (A and B) and one recessive one (O). If you inherit A from one parent and B from the other (recall that you get only half the genes from each parent), you are heterozygous, and have blood group AB. If you have either two As (homozygous) or one A and an O (heterozygous) you are group A. You can only be group O if you have two O genes. But it is becoming clear that this Mendelian system cannot account for all the known effects of gene mixtures.

A couple of decades ago, the story took an amazing and unexpected turn. It had always been assumed that a gene's action depended only on its structure, irrespective of the parent from which it came. So, for blood groups, it does not matter whether you inherit an A from your mother or your father. But there are a small number of genes (less than 100 in man) for which this is not so. Some only are operative if they come from your mother, others only from your father. They are called 'imprinted' genes and their existence turned classical genetics on its head. Imprinted genes, though few in number, may have a very significant role in survival. For example, one of them (it is called *peg1*) is only active if inherited from the father. It is effect is to increase the growth and survival of the foetus. This is intriguing: it seems as if the male transmits a gene that helps ensure that his offspring (who carry his genes) will survive. It is in his interest to do so. But it gets even more intriguing. For *peg1* is expressed in the limbic system of the female (not the cortex), and females lacking it make very poor mothers. So inheriting a paternal *peg1* not only increases prenatal and postnatal growth of the baby, but also ensures that the father's second generation has a good mother. Another contribution to his gene's long-term survival. Oxytocin, which we saw played a role in maternal behaviour (Chapter 9), is reduced in females lacking paternally-imprinted *peg1*.

The Individual and Society

Social organisations consist of a number, often a large number, of individuals interacting in a regular manner. . . . What research on social interaction has done is to show how the model of man needs to be revised to take account of his social nature. We have seen that for the survival of the group, satisfaction of biological needs and the continuation of the species, cooperation in groups is necessary in animals and men; that there are innate tendencies to respond to others, which in man in particular require experiences in the family for their completion. . . . it seem likely that there is an innate moral sense, evolved to keep aggression under control; we have seem that sympathy appears in young children, and that taking account of the of the point of view of the other is an essential ingredient in interaction. . . . This basic equipment, partly innate, partly acquired from the culture, leads to the formation of interpersonal bonds, small social groups and social structures.

M Argyle. (1969) *Social interaction.*
(Tavistock Publications, London.)

. . . The proportion of all the ill health and death in the United States that stems from simple genetic disorders that are potentially curable by a 'genetic fix' (of which we do not yet have a single successful example) is very small, as compared with what can be done by less damaging workplaces, less pollution, and better nutrition. Magna Carta was all very well for the barons, but it didn't do much for the peasantry.

Richard Lewontin. (2002) The politics of science.
New York Review of Books **49**, pp. 28–31.

Anthropologists refer to man's extremely complex learned behaviour as 'culture'. Culture embraces all the political, ideological, and technological aspects of society and is transmitted from generation to generation by teaching and learning rather than by genetic inheritance. There are certainly basic, genetically controlled human behavioural patterns, but those which differ from population to population appear to be due mainly to social differences in learned behaviour. . . . The quality which has been constantly selected throughout human evolution is educability.

D Pilbeam. (1970) *The evolution of man.*
(Thames and Hudson, London.)

A consistent theme of this book is to try to reconcile the existence of an enormous cerebral cortex in humans and all its attendant functions (thought, planning, decision-making, social awareness and so on) with the activity of the more 'primitive' limbic system ('primitive' in the sense that it exists in much the same form in other mammals). It is possible to construct cells containing only maternally imprinted genes, and mix them with 'normal' embryonic cells. Astonishingly, the maternal cells end up in the neocortex, not the limbic system. What this means is still being discussed: one suggestion is that it has something to with the extension of maternal behaviour in primates well outside the hormonally-controlled postnatal period more typical of other mammals (such as rodents) thus ensuring continued care during the slow development that characterises primate infants (including humans). It is the cortex that is responsive to social needs, it is argued, and the presence of maternal genes in the decision-making cortex focuses the mothers attention on her child. But what do they do in males? The reason for the existence of imprinted genes is still the subject of rather baffled debates. However, it seems that imprinted genes are particularly concerned with growth and homeostatis.

Do not let all this, fascinating as it may be, lull you into thinking that genes are the only formative influence on the brain we bring to the survival battle. The brain passes through a period during which it is particularly sensitive to either environmental or biochemical events. Individual differences in the way these occur can have long-lasting — some would say permanent — effects. This 'critical' period occurs during early life. For example, separate a baby rat from its mother for an hour or so for a few days; when it becomes an adult, it will show exaggerated stress responses compared to its sibling that has experienced a more tranquil maternal environment (see Chapters 4 and 12). Prenatal 'stress' may also have long-term effects: treat rat embryos with a hormone similar to cortisol (the stress hormone) and they show reduced growth, but also insulin resistance and abnormal levels of stress hormones as adults. There may be a link between these 'experiential' or environmental influences on later behaviour and adaptability, and those of certain genes. One of the ways that an imprinted gene from, say, the father is 'silenced' (turned off) is by a process called methylation. Interestingly, there is some

Individual Differences

Gender differences in cognition is a relatively new and increasingly 'hot' topic. For decades, neuroscientists treated humanity as a homogeneous mass, ignoring the self-evident truth apparent to every man and woman in the street: that males and females are different. But we are finding out increasingly that one ignores gender differences in cognition at one's peril. . . . Very little has been said about gender differences in general cognitive styles. In particular, next to nothing has been said. . . about gender differences in the general approach to decision making, about what we call here *adaptive* decision making.

> E Goldberg. (2001) *The executive brain: Frontal lobes and
> the civilised mind.* (Oxford University Press, Oxford.)

Ordinary people with common sense have long recognized the importance of different stages during the development of an organisms, at any rate long before physiologists began profaning the secrets of the [brain] with their electrodes. Chief among them have been those interested in education, and who have known that there are certain periods in the life of an individual when the brain is maximally receptive to certain kinds of training and that a similar training outside these periods is comparatively ineffectual. . . . Western society has inherited an aphorism, commonly, but wrongly, attributed to the Society of Jesus. 'Give us a child until the age of seven and you can have him for life'. . . . If there is cynicism in this aphorism, there is also a profound physiological truth. . . . No wonder that Sigmund Freud considered that, psychologically, the child is the father of the man.

> S Zeki. (1993) *A vision of the brain.*
> (Blackwell Scientific Publications, Oxford.)

Personal uniqueness itself says something useful: molecular biology has made individuals of us all. Genetics disproves Plato's myth of the absolute, that there exists one ideal form of human being from which there are rare deviations such as those who have an inborn disease.

> S Jones. (1993) *The language of the genes.*
> (Harper Collins, London.)

. . . When famine is associated with a decline in food production. . . we have to go beyond the output statistics to explain why it is that some parts of the population get wiped out, while the rest do just fine. Famines survive by divide-and-rule. For example, a group of peasants may suffer entitlement evidence that early life experience in baby rats (the quality of maternal care) can alter the methylation of some genes; for example, the receptor for their adrenal corticoid hormone (corticosterone). So both genetic and 'epigenetic' factors (as these are called) can have similar effects, and both will be long-lasting.

Baby rats are born very immature compared to some other species (e.g. guinea pigs). A baby female rat, injected with a small dose of testosterone five days after birth, shows no apparent ill-effects. Wait until she has grown up, and you will see some striking alterations. She fails to show the regular ovarian cycles typical of normal females (4–5 days, see Chapter 8) and, even if given normal amounts of ovarian hormones (oestrogen and progesterone) is reluctant to mate. But give her some testosterone, and pair her with another, normal, female, and she tries to mate like a male. Exposing the brain of a little female to a brief pulse of testosterone at a crucial stage (it does not work if you wait until she is 20 days old) has resulted in permanent and biologically important changes in brain function. She has been masculinised.

Take away the testes of a male baby rat at 5 days or earlier, and the opposite occurs. He grows up with a brain that seems to be 'feminine': his pituitary can 'cycle' like a female's, he is reluctant to mate with a sexy female, but inject him with oestrogen etc. and he shows the typical sexual posture of a female. He has been 'feminised'. So, testosterone present in the brain during the 'critical' period masculinises it, but absence of testosterone results in the default condition of 'feminine'. Testosterone has two actions: during early life, it 'programmes' the brain towards 'masculinity;' later, this latent trait needs more testosterone for it to be apparent. One steroid hormone, two very different (but related) actions solely dependent on the timing of exposure of the brain to testosterone. Exposure to testosterone during early life can differ between individuals and thus contribute to individual patterns of sexuality. Note that the action of testosterone during development is independent of the genes that determine 'maleness' or 'femaleness'. What the genes do is to ensure that testosterone is present (male) or not present (female) during the critical period. What about oestrogen, the typical hormone of the ovaries? It has the same effect as testosterone (recall that testosterone can be converted to oestrogen in Chapter 8). So the 'female' genes (two X chromosomes) losses when food output in their territory declines, perhaps due to a local drought, even when there is no general dearth of food in the country. The victims would not have the means to buy food from elsewhere, since they would not have anything much to sell to earn an income, given their own production loss. Others with more secure earnings in other occupations or in other locations may be able to get by well enough by purchasing food from elsewhere. . . . Famines are highly divisive phenomena.

. . . Famines and other crises thrive on the basis of severe and often suddenly increased inequality. This is illustrated by the fact that famines can occur even without a large — or any — diminution of total food supply. . . .

Amartya Sen. (1999) *Development as freedom.*

(Oxford University Press, Oxford.)

ensure that the ovaries produce nothing during the critical period. A 'Y' chromosome (male) causes the infantile testes to secrete testosterone (but possibly in variable amounts).

In species with longer pregnancies, and thus more mature newly-borns (e.g. sheep, monkeys, guinea pigs), the critical brain period occurs well before birth. What about humans? As you can imagine, the results on rats and other rodent species have excited a good deal of interest. How far do gender differences in humans depend on something as simple as a timed pulse of testosterone? And do individual differences in sexuality also relate to the same early biochemical experience? It seems to be true (at least in part) for monkeys, though the amount of experimental evidence is much less than for easily obtained rodents. You cannot give pregnant women extra testosterone, but there are some natural experiments. One is the result of a genetic defect that prevents a 'male' responding to his own testosterone. Such individuals grow up to be female in appearance and outlook. Another is a second genetic defect that results in the adrenal gland producing abnormally large amounts of testosterone in girls (see Chapter 8). These babies not only look masculinised, but they tend to play more like boys during childhood; they do not show markedly increased incidences of transsexuality but they do tend more towards homosexuality (lesbianism); again, note the individual variation. There have been suggestions that 'lack' of testosterone during early life in boys might predispose towards either transsexuality or homosexuality, but the evidence is lacking. Incidentally, excess foetal testosterone has been proposed to encourage the development of autism, a condition much more common in boys than girls. It is certainly possible that sex hormones during the critical period may alter the brain in ways that are only indirectly concerned with sexuality, including aggressiveness, and the nature of confiding relationships or emotional reactions to others.

As we have seen, early adversity (a mother with post-natal depression) can result in apparently long-lasting alterations in cortical levels in adolescents (Chapter 12). We are all familiar with evidence that a neglected childhood seems to predispose to later antisocial behaviour, difficulties with relationships and even psychiatric illness. Human infants are born very helpless and immature. Whilst hormonal critical periods in humans seem to occur prenatally, the behavioural ones may be delayed

It was at this time that Etienne began to understand the ideas that had been vaguely buzzing round in his head. Until then all he had had was an instinct to rebel, in the midst of the inarticulate discontent of his comrades. All sorts of questions had occurred to him: why poverty for some and wealth for others? Why should the former be ground under the hell of the latter, without any hope of ever taking their place? The first step forward had been the realization of his own ignorance. . . knowing nothing he dared not talk about the things most on his mind, such as the fact that all men are equal, and equity demands a fair share for all of the things of this world.

Emile Zola. (1885) *Germinal*. Translated by L W Tancock.

(Penguin Books, Harmondsworth, UK.)

In the past men were handsome and great (now they are children and dwarfs), but this is merely one of the many facts that demonstrate the disaster of an aging world. The young no longer want to study anything, learning is in decline, the whole world walks on its head, blind men lead others equally blind and cause them to plunge into the abyss, birds leave their nests before they can fly, the jackass plays the lyre, oxen dance. Mary no longer loves the contemplative life and Martha no longer loves the active life, Leah is sterile, Rachel has a carnal eye, Cato visits brothels, Lucretius becomes a woman.

Umberto Eco. (1984) *The name of the rose*.

(Picador, London.)

His work survived as he claimed it would. We inherit his struggle to achieve supreme fictions in art, to associate art with social change, to bring together individual and social impulse, to save what is eccentric and singular from being sanitized and standardized, to replace a morality of severity by one of sympathy. He belongs to our world more than to Victoria's. Now, beyond the reach of scandal, his best writings validated by time, he comes before us still, a towering figure, laughing and weeping, with parables and paradoxes, so generous, so amusing, and so right.

Richard Ellmann. (1987) *Oscar Wilde*.

(Hamish Hamilton, London.)

until after birth. Different parts of the human brain may 'mature' at different times. There may be more than one critical period, some to hormones or other chemical signals, others to more complex behavioural events in the social environment.

Though we are sadly lacking in detail, we can begin to discern the outlines of the process of developing individuality. I mean here, not individual differences in abilities, or ways of thinking — though these are very relevant to survival — but differences in the survival mechanisms themselves. Somewhere in the brain, probably the limbic system, lie subtle distinctions that bias our ability to adapt and to cope with life's exigencies. Unlike those intrepid war correspondents in Chapter 12, we have not one, but a whole wardrobe of bullet-resistant jackets — each 'jacket' represents an ability to resist a demand, each 'bullet' a different stress. Some jackets may be better than others. Some may change over time. Their strength lies in a combination of genes (shuffled during egg and sperm formation, carrying various polymorphisms), exposure of the brain to certain chemical signals at critical, sensitive, periods, and the quality or nature of experiences early in life (even before birth, some would say). It is easy to see how these three sets interact. Genes may alter the way the brain responds to chemical signals, as well as triggering those signals in the first place. Outside events may trigger chemical events in the brain (transmitter release) or hormone secretion. Adverse experiences in early life may have greater or lesser long-term consequences depending on genes, or previous hormonal exposure or both. This is the basis of individuality. Though I limit this discussion to the 'limbic' brain, it would be foolish to ignore the role of the great cerebral cortex, itself responsible for perception, decision-making and the ability to weigh up a situation, and many other things besides. Similar influences, or even different ones, may be going on during the development of the cortex: together they represent the human survival system. Together, they steer you through the river of life, keeping you clear of the rocks for the most part; if they fail, then surely you will sink.

There is a rather striking example of the importance of individual differences in the limbic brain and the cortex. Show 20 people a ham sandwich and a typewriter (to use a famous example) and all will agree on which is which, and what is what. That is the cortex: it needs to be accurate

Six hundred years ago, a man was what he was born to be. Satan and the Church, representing God, did battle over him. He, by reason of his choice, partially decided the outcome. But whether, after life, he went to hell or to heaven, his place among other men was given. It could not be contested. But, since, the stage has been reset and human beings only walk on it, and, under this revision, we have, instead, history to answer to. We were important enough then for our souls to be fought over. Now each of us is responsible for his own salvation, which is in his greatness. And that, that greatness, is the rock our hearts are abraded on.

Saul Bellow. (1963) *Dangling man.*
(Penguin Books, London.)

I am the descendant of a race whose imaginative and easily excitable temperament has at all times rendered them remarkable; and, in my infancy, I gave evidence of having fully inherited the family character. As I advanced in years it was more strongly developed; becoming, for many reasons, a cause of serious disquietude to my friends, and of positive injury to myself. I grew self-willed, addicted to the wildest caprices, and a prey to ungovernable passions. Weak-minded, and beset with constitutional infirmities akin to my own, my parents could do but little to check the evil propensities which distinguished me.

Edgar Allan Poe. (1956) William Wilson. In: *Selected tales*
Ed. John Curtis. (Penguin, Harmondsworth, UK.)

He began to wonder whether we could ever make psychology so absolute a science that each little spring of science would be revealed to us. As it was, we always misunderstood ourselves, and rarely understood others. Experience was of no ethical value. It was merely a name men gave to their mistakes.

Oscar Wilde. The picture of Dorian Gray.
In: *Stories.* (Collins, London.)

about analysing the environment or you will not survive for long. Do it ten times and you will get the same answer. But then ask the 20 about how they feel about the ham sandwich. Those that have just eaten find it rather unappealing, whereas those that missed lunch might find it very attractive. A few hours later, these responses might be reversed. A vegetarian, or an orthodox Jew, or someone with a food allergy to ham, might never want the ham sandwich. Nobody, of course, tries to eat the typewriter. In contrast the analytical cortex, the functional activity of the limbic system is highly variable, either in the long or shorter term, depending on wants, preferences and social customs. The latter, of course, are themselves highly variable across time and region, and represent another major influence on individual differences — this time between groups, though social structure is all about differences in individual roles. Although I have emphasised the essential flexibility of the limbic system, I do not mean to imply that all the cortex is so rigid: decision-making, for example (a function of the frontal lobes, see Chapter 12) is not always so predictable, though in fact most people make the expected decisions most of the time. The point is that an inherent adaptability is an essential part of the flexible limbic brain, whereas it would be a huge disadvantage in the analytical part of the sensory cortex.

We are at the start of really defining individuality. Curiously, nearly all biological and medical research has been on groups: how a particular sort of animal or person at a particular time in its life or under particular circumstances, adapts or fails to adapt, recovers or dies. Of course, this is not always the case: the science of genetics, for example, is concerned with individual differences as well as group characteristics. But only now, when we can read small differences in the genetic makeup of individuals, are we beginning to try to understand how these differences will influence current or future survival. We need to bring equivalent precision to our understanding of all the other events, social and circumstantial, that shape individual lives, before we can begin to understand what we already know to be true: that individuality is the stuff of selection, survival and success. Is this biological determinism? Not at all, just as our fairly precise knowledge of the risks of car accidents is still unable to predict with certainty that John Smith will have one on April 8th. God may or may not play dice, but there is still something called chance.

Genetic Change

The study of polygenic inheritance and of the effects of selection upon graded, measurable characters is still in its beginnings. . . . The people who study it are confronted by strange and at present inexplicable phenomena. . . . It is not true that we now know how to control our own evolution — if by 'control' is meant directing it towards some predetermined goal. We are not entitled by our present knowledge to put a genetical construction upon the inheritance of differences in temperament or character; all we do know about the matter is what we have leant from the evolution of tameness or docility in domesticated animals: that some such characters are under some kind of genetical control.

P B Medawar. (1960) *The future of man.* (Methuen and Co., London.)

. . . When we contrast the physical with the social laws under which man finds himself here below, we must grant that Physiology and Social Sciences are in collision. Man is both a physical and a social being; yet he cannot at once pursue to the full his physical and his social end, his physical duties (if I may so speak) and his social duties, but is forced to sacrifice in part one or the other. If we were wild enough to fancy that there were two creators, one of whom was the author of our animal frames, the other of society, then indeed we might understand how it comes to pass that labour of mind and body, the useful arts, the duties of a statesman, government, and the like, which are required by the social system, are so destructive of health, enjoyment, and life.

J H Newman. (1952) *The idea of a liberal education.*
Ed. H Tristram. (Harrap, London.)

[There is the view that] organ- and organism-level matters will eventually succumb to [a] reductionist approach: understand the genome and everything else will follow. . . . [It is] important to note that this issue is still hotly debated amongst evolutionary biologists. It is not accepted by all of them by any means that microevolution will eventually explain macroevolution. . . . Stephen J Gould even goes so far as to say that future evolutionary theory 'will restore to biology a concept of organism'. . . . Readers will find powerful critiques of Gould's position in Richard Dawkin's *The blind watchmaker* and Edward Wilson's *The diversity of life*. . . . Highly developed organisms themselves, and the organs and systems of which they are composed, must impose very severe restrictions indeed on what can now be successful as a variation. . . . Perhaps it would be better therefore to picture genes as severely restricted prisoners rather than free-roving 'selfish' entities: Prisoners of the

I hope I have persuaded you that much the most important part of this individuality lies in the brain. Longer legs and sharper claws may be useful, even essential, so I am not going to dismiss individual differences in these sorts of attributes. But it is in the brain that our real individuality lies, both as a most extraordinary species and as individually unique members of that species. We have shaped our environment to a degree quite unlike that of even the most inventive animal species, largely to provide us with the staples of life. That, I have suggested, has not too much to do with the limbic system, but with the enormous flowering of the cortical brain. But deep within that brain, busy as it has been throughout mammalian evolution (and beyond), is your faithful servant, your limbic system, a collection of still half-mysterious nerve cells, talking to each other in a dimly-understood chemical language. It is as busy in you as in your primeval ancestors, and it is doing the same thing: keeping you alive. Your ingenious cortex has made its job that much easier.

I began this book with Charles Darwin, the most influential biologist of all time. This is what he wrote about survival:

"All that we can do, is to keep steadily in mind that each organic being is striving to increase at a geometrical ratio; that each at some period of its life, during some season of the year, during each generation or at intervals, has to struggle for life, and to suffer great destruction. When we reflect on this struggle, we may console ourselves with the full belief, that the war of nature is not incessant, that no fear is felt, that death is generally prompt, and that the vigorous, the healthy, and the happy survive and multiply."

That says it all; don't you think?

successful physiological systems carrying them. . . . Far therefore from molecular biology 'explaining' physiology, physiology (in the sense of an understanding of the logic of life) will be totally necessary for an understanding of what all the molecular biology means.

> D Noble and C A R Boyd. (1993) The challenge of integrative physiology. In: *The logic of life.* Ed. D Noble and C A R Boyd. (Oxford University Press, Oxford.)

Wouldn't it be nice if an organism could react to an environmental challenge with a slew of new mutations, and not wasteful, random, ones, but mutations for traits that would allow it to cope? Of course it would be nice, and that's the problem — chemistry has no sense of niceness. The DNA inside the testes and ovaries cannot peer outside and considerately mutate to make fur when it's cold and fins when it's wet and claws when there are trees around, or put a lens in front of the retina as opposed to between the toes or inside the pancreas.

> S Pinker. (1997) *How the mind works.* (Allen Lane, London.)

Even if [an] alteration in social structure of a group is due to a behavioural change in a single key individual, we cannot be sure that this member was not predisposed to the act by a distinctive capability or temperament conferred by a particular set of genes. And then how can the relative contributions of the genetic component be estimated? . . . . Uncertainty extends even to the famous cultural innovations of the Japanese macaques of Koshima Island. At the age of 18 months, a female monkey 'genius' Imo invented potato washing in the sea, a skill which then spread through the Koshima group. At the age of four years she invented the flotation method of separating wheat grains from sand. . . . Did Imo's achievements result from a rare genetic endowment, likely to occur in only some of the macaque troops picked at random? Or was she well within the range of variation of most of the local population, so that any troop first encountering the sea and certain foods under the same conditions. . . might have responded with the inventions? If the former, the drift could be said to be primarily genetic drift; if the latter, it was primarily tradition drift.

> E O Wilson. (1975) *Sociobiology. The new synthesis.* (Belknap Press, Cambridge, Massachusetts.)

Estragon: All the dead voices
Vladimir: They make noises like wings
E: Like leaves
V: Like sand
E: Like leaves
V: They all speak together
E: Each one to itself
V: Rather they whisper
E: They rustle
V: They murmur
E: They rustle
V: What do they say?
E: They talk about their lives
V: To have lived is not enough for them
E: They have to talk about it
V: To be dead is not enough for them
E: It is not sufficient
V: They make a noise like feathers
E: Like leaves
V: Like ashes
E: Like leaves
V: Say something!
E: I'm trying
V: Say anything at all!
E: What do we do now?
V: Wait for Godot

Samuel Beckett. (1956) *Waiting for Godot.*
(Faber and Faber, London.)

Not all the roots of American life are uprooted, but almost all, and the spirit if the supermarket, that homogenous extension of stainless surfaces and psychoanalyzed people, packaged commodities, and ranch homes, interchangeable, geographically unrecognizable, that essence of the new postwar SuperAmerica is found nowhere so perfectly as in Los Angeles' ubiquitous acres. One gets the impression that people come to Los Angeles in order to divorce themselves from the past, here to live or try to live in the rootless pleasure world of an adult child.

> Norman Mailer. (1999) *The time of our time.*
> (The Modern Library, New York.)

Those who visit India. . . have not been told often enough or in a popularly comprehensible way that the experience of the east is simply not accessible to the western mind, except after almost total re-education. Yet the common fallacy that sitting for extended periods of time in the lotus position gets you halfway past the wheel of existence is not only not being denied, but is currently being actively propagated by many ashrams currently in vogue. The gurus have ignored a primary difference between themselves and their disciples.

The Eastern master when asked, "What is the Answer?" has traditionally replied "Who is Asking?" In that lies a central difference between Eastern and Western thought. The East is not concerned with intellectual aggrandizement, so much so that Jung testily called the Eastern mind childish, a mind that didn't ask even ask questions, but simply perceived them. In a tradition where the question asks itself and the answer replies itself and all that remains is to establish the identity of the asker, clearly the Occidental is going to experience serious difficulty in eliciting any information at all, be it spiritual, physical or just the fastest way to get to the next town.

> Gita Mehta. (1993) *Karma cola* (Penguin Books, New Delhi.)

Such are the visions. The solitary traveller is soon beyond the wood; and there, coming to the door with shaded eyes, possibly to look for his return, with hands raised, with white apron blowing, is an elderly woman who seems (so powerful is this infirmity) to seek, over the desert, a lost son; to search for a rider destroyed; to be the figure of the mother whose sons have been killed in the battles of the world. So, as the solitary traveller advances down the village street where the women stand knitting and the men dig in the garden, the evening seems ominous; the figures still; as if some august fate, known to them, awaited without fear, were about to sweep them into complete annihilation.

> Virginia Woolf. (1958) *Mrs Dalloway.* (Hogarth Press, London.)

Author Index

Subject Index